Probiotics and Prebiotics in Pediatrics

Probiotics and Prebiotics in Pediatrics

Special Issue Editors

Francesco Savino
Yvan Vandenplas

MDPI • Basel • Beijing • Wuhan • Barcelona • Belgrade

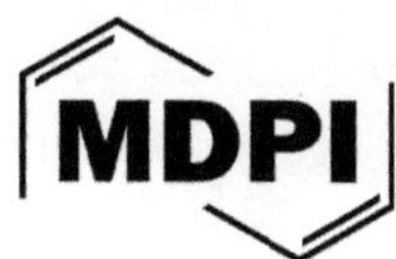

Special Issue Editors
Francesco Savino
Universitaria Città della Salute e della Scienza di Torino
Italy

Yvan Vandenplas
Vrije Universiteit Brussel
Belgium

Editorial Office
MDPI
St. Alban-Anlage 66
4052 Basel, Switzerland

This is a reprint of articles from the Special Issue published online in the open access journal *Nutrients* (ISSN 2072-6643) from 2018 to 2019 (available at: https://www.mdpi.com/journal/nutrients/special_issues/probiotics_and_prebiotics_in_pediatrics)

For citation purposes, cite each article independently as indicated on the article page online and as indicated below:

LastName, A.A.; LastName, B.B.; LastName, C.C. Article Title. *Journal Name* **Year**, *Article Number*, Page Range.

ISBN 978-3-03897-950-0 (Pbk)
ISBN 978-3-03897-951-7 (PDF)

© 2019 by the authors. Articles in this book are Open Access and distributed under the Creative Commons Attribution (CC BY) license, which allows users to download, copy and build upon published articles, as long as the author and publisher are properly credited, which ensures maximum dissemination and a wider impact of our publications.
The book as a whole is distributed by MDPI under the terms and conditions of the Creative Commons license CC BY-NC-ND.

Contents

About the Special Issue Editors

Francesco Savino is the Chief Pediatrician of Unit S.S.D. Sub-intensive care of early infancy at the Children's Hospital "Regina Margherita" of Città della salute e della Scienza of Torino. He is also a professor of the School for Pediatricians of the University of Torino. His research interests include minor digestive problems in infancy: colic, gastroesophageal reflux, and metabolism of early childhood—in particular hormones such as leptin, IGF-1, ghrelin, and adiponectin of breast-fed and formula-fed infants. He also directs a project on gut microbiota in colicky infants which focuses on treating breastfed colicky infants with probiotics. Dr. Savino also leads or participates in several other studies for investigating hormones in breast milk. He has participated in clinical trials involving gut microflora, probiotics, and new formulas for treating infantile colic, and is an active teacher of medical students and mentor to research trainees. Dr. Savino organized a scientific International Meeting on Advances on Infantile Colic.Dr. Savino recently published two Cochrane reviews as corresponding Author: "Pain relieving agents for infantile colic" 2016-CD009999, and "Dietary treatment for infantile colic" 2108. CD011029He is an author of more than 133 scientific reports.

Yvan Vandenplas studied medicine and trained in pediatrics (1981–1986) at the Vrije Universiteit Brussels. He became Head of the Unit for Pediatric Gastroenterology and Nutrition in 1987, and is Head of the KidZ Health Castle at the University Hospital Brussels (UZ Brussel) and the Chair of Pediatrics since 1994. Yvan's main interests are gastro-esophageal reflux (diagnostic procedures, treatment), eosinophilic esophagitis, infant nutrition, probiotics and prebiotics, cow's milk protein allergy, functional gastrointestinal disorders, and Helicobacter pylori. He has published many original research and review papers on topics such as infant nutrition, gastro-esophageal reflux, and functional gastrointestinal disorders. He is now one of the Associate Editors of the *Journal of Paediatric Gastroenterology and Nutrition*. He is also the Chair of the ESPGHAN Special Interest Group on "Gut Microbiota & Modifications". Yvan has more than 450 publications listed in Medline, and over 1000 oral presentations at different international meetings.

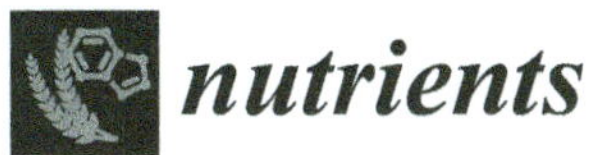
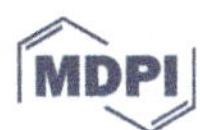

Editorial

Probiotics and Prebiotics in Pediatrics: What Is New?

Yvan Vandenplas [1,*] and Francesco Savino [2]

1 KidZ Health Castle, UZ Brussel, Vrije Universiteit Brussel, 1090 Brussels, Belgium
2 Department of Pediatrics, Ospedale Infantile Regina Margherita, Azienda Ospedaliera, Universitaria Città della Salute e della Scienza di Torino, Piazza Polonia, 94, 10126 Turin, Italy; francesco.savino@unito.it
* Correspondence: yvan.vandenplas@uzbrussel.be

Received: 11 February 2019; Accepted: 15 February 2019; Published: 19 February 2019

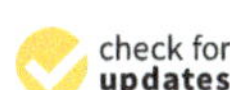

Probiotics and prebiotics are a hot topic in pediatric research. Human milk oligosaccharides have been recognized to enhance the development of a bifidogenic microbiome in infants. In this issue, many different clinical conditions are discussed in which probiotics and prebiotics can interfere with the microbiome. This editorial for a special issue of *Nutrients* contains 17 papers, a mixture of reviews and original research, reflecting the broad and evolving interest and researches in this topic, such as diarrhea, atopic diseases, infantile colic, celiac, necrotizing enterocolitis, constipation. However, in the pediatric age, manipulation of that microbiome still leads to inconclusive results as studies provide often contradictory data. The inconclusive data may be explained by the fact that dysbiosis is likely to be only one of several interfering factors causing these different conditions. In conclusion, the manuscripts in this issue raise a lot of aspects and questions and offer challenges for future research.

The evolution of knowledge on this topic in recent years has allowed us to conclude that there is currently sufficient enough evidence to conclude that the role of the gastro-intestinal microbiome during the first month of life is crucial for a balanced development of the immune system. The interest in the human microbiome and its interplay with the host has exploded and provided new insights on its role in conferring host protection and regulating host physiology, including the correct development of immunity [1,2]. *Bifidobacterium breve* is the dominant species in the gut of breast-fed infants and it has also been isolated from human milk. It has antimicrobial activity against human pathogens, it does not possess transmissible antibiotic resistance traits, it is not cytotoxic and it has immuno-stimulating abilities [3]. Probiotic supplementation during pregnancy and in the neonatal period might reduce some maternal and neonatal adverse outcomes [4]. The current evidence on the efficacy of probiotics for the management of pediatric functional abdominal pain disorders, such as functional constipation, irritable bowel syndrome, functional abdominal pain is rather disappointing as no single strain, the combination of strains or synbiotics can be recommended for the management of these conditions [5].

Allergic individuals have a different microbiome than non-allergic. The "microbiota hypothesis" ties the increase in allergy rates observed in highly developed countries over the last decades to disturbances in the gut microbiota [6]. Diaz et al showed that infants with non-IgE mediated allergy have a different microbiome compared to healthy infants, while being on an elimination diet [7]. Moreover, the protein source (formula of vegetable origin, casein or whey hydrolysate) result in a different composition of the microbiome [7]. The clinical relevance of these findings needs to be further investigated. Lactobacillus (L.) administration might also be of interest in children with chronic immune disorders, such as asthma [8]. Results of a prospective, double blind, randomized Chinese study with four groups (*L. paracasei*, *L. fermentum*, their combination and placebo) showed lower asthma severity and better Childhood Asthma Control Test scores [8]. The group treated with both probiotics improved most, as increased peak expiratory flow rates and decreased IgE levels were shown [8]. Thus, lactobacillus administration, at least the strains tested, can contribute the clinical improvement in children with asthma [8]. A meta-analysis showed that *L. rhamnosus GG* was ineffective in the reduction of atopic dermatitis [9].

Infantile colic is a common condition, occurring in about 20 % of all infants, of unknown pathogenesis that causes frustration and anxiousness in families, which then seek effective management [10]. Dysbiosis and chronic inflammation are likely to be part of the pathophysiologic mechanisms of infantile colic [11]. A study from Ukraine showed that a combination of *L. rhamnosus* 19070-2 and *L. reuteri* and a small amount of a prebiotic, fructo-oligosaccharide (FOS), resulted in a significant decrease of crying time compared to the natural evolution in the placebo group [12]. These data confirm previous literature, mainly using *L. reuteri* alone, showing that lactobacilli decrease infantile colic in exclusively breastfed infants [13]. A probiotic mixture was also shown to reduce crying time in exclusively breastfed infants compared to placebo, although no differences between the groups were found regarding anthropometric data, bowel movements, stool consistency or microbiota composition [14]. Unfortunately, data on the outcome of probiotic administration in formula fed infants presenting with infantile colic are still missing. *L. reuteri* DSM 17938 may be considered for the management of breastfed colic infants, while data on other probiotic strains, probiotic mixtures or synbiotics are limited in infantile colic [5].

The ESPGHAN working group on probiotics and prebiotics recommended considering the addition of some probiotic strains to oral rehydration therapy in the management of infants with acute gastroenteritis [15]. The additional benefit of *L. reuteri* DSM 17938 and zinc was evaluated compared to oral rehydration alone in a study, including 51 children with acute gastroenteritis [16]. Although there was a trend that the probiotic and zinc supplemented group did better, the outcome was not statistically significant better [16]. Two other large trials, with *L. rhamnosus GG* reported also a negative outcome [17,18]. *Bacillus clausii* was tested in six randomized controlled trials, including 1298 [19]. Data arising from the pooled analysis showed that *Bacillus clausii* significantly reduced the duration of diarrhea with a mean difference of -9.12 hours only compared with control. Stool frequency was not significantly different after *Bacillus clausii* administration compared with the control group [19]. A randomized trial in India with *Bacillus clausii* compared to placebo reported a statistically significant difference in duration of diarrhea of only six hours, with a difference of one defecation per day at day 4 [20]. These findings question the importance of the selection of patients, and the strain selection of the probiotic. Shortening of the duration of diarrhea might have been shown to be statistically reduced, but may lack clinical significance of benefit [19].

The use of probiotics among very low-birth-weight infants is constantly increasing, as probiotics are believed to reduce the incidence of severe diseases, such as necrotizing enterocolitis (NEC) and late-onset sepsis and to improve feeding tolerance [21]. According to feeding type, the beneficial effect of probiotics was confirmed only in exclusively human milk-fed preterm infants [22]. Fifty-one randomized controlled trials were included in a review by the ESPGHAN working group on pre- and probiotics, involving 11,231 preterm infants [23]. Most strains or combinations of strains were only studied in one or a few trails [23]. Only 3 of 25 studied probiotic treatment combinations showed a significant reduction in mortality rates [23]. Seven treatments reduced NEC incidence, two reduced late-onset sepsis, and three reduced time until full enteral feeding [23]. Among human milk fed infants, only probiotic mixtures, and not single-strain products, were effective in reducing late onset sepsis [22]. Human milk oligosaccharides (HMO) have a strong prebiotic effect, and stimulate the development of a bifidogenic microbiome in breastfed infants.

HMOs may support immune function development and provide protection against infectious diseases directly through the interaction of the gut epithelial cells or indirectly through the modulation of the gut microbiota, including the stimulation of the bifidobacteria [24,25]. The limited clinical data suggest that the addition of HMOs to infant formula seems to be safe and well tolerated, inducing a normal growth and suggesting a trend towards health benefits [24]. Gut immaturity in preterm infants leads to difficulties in tolerating enteral feeding and bacterial colonization and high sensitivity to NEC, particularly when breast milk is insufficient [26]. The HMOs diversity and the levels of

Lacto-N-difucohexaose I were found to be lower in samples from mothers of infants that developed NEC, as compared to non-NEC cases at all sampling time points [27]. Lacto-N-difucohexaose I is only produced by secretor and Lewis positive mothers. This is significant, but inconsistent with associations between 3′-sialyllactose and 6′-sialyllactose, and culture-proven sepsis; and consists of weak correlations between several HMOs and growth rate [27]. However, the benefit of HMO supplementation in preterm infants is debated [26]. These findings highlight once more that a priority research topic is the understanding why about 20% of the mothers are "non-secretors", since all data suggest that infants of secretor mothers have a better health outcome than there of non-secretors.

Constipation is still a frequent functional gastro-intestinal disorder in infants, occurring in about 10 % [10]. In a Brazilian, randomized, placebo-controlled, double blind trial, fructo-oligosaccharides (FOS) or placebo was given at a dosage of 6, 9 or 12 g daily based on the infants' weight groups of 6.0–8.9 kg, 9.0–11.9 kg or over 12.0 kg, respectively [28]. Therapeutic success occurred in 83.3% of the FOS group infants and in as much as 55.6% of the control group [28]. The placebo effect in this trial was very high, suggesting again that reassurance is the cornerstone of the management of functional disorders in infants. But, compared with the control group, the FOS group exhibited a higher frequency of softer stools and fewer episodes of straining and/or difficulty passing stools [28]. Further, after one month, the Bifidobacterium sp. count was higher in the FOS group [28].

Celiac disease is a chronic autoimmune enteropathy triggered by dietary gluten exposure in genetically predisposed individuals [2]. Despite ascertaining that gluten is the trigger in celiac disease, evidence has indicated that also intestinal microbiota is somehow involved in the pathogenesis, progression, and clinical presentation of the disease [2]. Patients with celiac disease have an increased abundance of *Bacteroides* spp. and a decrease in *Bifidobacterium* spp. [2]. A six-week multispecies probiotic treatment improved the severity of irritable bowel syndrom-type symptoms, in celiac patients on a strict glutenfree diet and was associated with a modification of gut microbiota, characterized by an increase of bifidobacteria [28]. The role of prebiotics in the nutritional management of chronic conditions, such as celiac disease in patients on a glutenfree diet is a different area of interest. Iron deficiency anemia occurs in up to almost half of the patients diagnosed with celiac disease. A randomised trial with an oligofructose enriched inulin administered during three months to celiac patients failed to show a clear benefit of a bifidogenic microbiome on nutritional (ferritin, hemoglobin) and inflammatory (C-reactive protein) parameters, although a decrease in hepcidin was shown [29]. Hepcidin is a key regulator of the entry of iron into the circulation and considered to be an interesting and useful marker.

Different aspects of pro- and prebiotics in pediatrics are presented and discussed in this special issue. The overall conclusion suggests that although there is a physiologic and patho-physiological ground regarding the impact of a balanced microbiome on different health aspects in infants and children, clinical outcomes are often contradictory. Future research and trials must reveal relevant outcomes about which there is a consensus regarding. It should be mandatory to report the specific strains of probiotics. Studies should be done with commercial products. Therefore, further research on the impact of manipulation with probiotic and prebiotic of the gastrointestinal microbiome in pediatrics is still needed.

Conflicts of Interest: The author declares no conflict of interest.

References

1. Dominguez-Bello, M.G.; Godoy-Vitorino, F.; Knight, R.; Blaser, M.J. Role of the microbiome in human development. *Gut* **2019**, in press. [CrossRef] [PubMed]
2. Cristofori, F.; Indrio, F.; Miniello, V.L.; De Angelis, M.; Francavilla, R. Probiotics in celiac disease. *Nutrients* **2018**, *10*, 1824. [CrossRef] [PubMed]
3. Cionci, N.B.; Baffoni, L.; Gaggìa, F.; Di Gioia, D. Therapeutic microbiology: The Role of Bifidobacterium breve as food supplement for the prevention/treatment of paediatric diseases. *Nutrients* **2018**, *10*, 1723. [CrossRef] [PubMed]

4. Baldassarre, M.E.; Palladino, V.; Amoruso, A.; Pindinelli, S.; Mastromarino, P.; Fanelli, M.; Di Mauro, A.; Laforgia, N. Rationale of probiotic supplementation during pregnancy and neonatal period. *Nutrients* **2018**, *10*, 1693. [CrossRef] [PubMed]
5. Pärtty, A.; Rautava, S.; Kalliomäki, M. Probiotics on pediatric functional gastrointestinal disorders. *Nutrients* **2018**, *10*, 1836. [CrossRef] [PubMed]
6. Cukrowska, B. Microbial and nutritional programming—The importance of the microbiome and early exposure to potential food allergens in the development of allergies. *Nutrients* **2018**, *10*, 1541. [CrossRef] [PubMed]
7. Díaz, M.; Guadamuro, L.; Espinosa-Martos, I.; Mancabelli, L.; Jiménez, S.; Molinos-Norniella, C.; Pérez-Solis, D.; Milani, C.; Rodríguez, J.M.; Ventura, M.; et al. Microbiota and derived parameters in fecal samples of infants with non-IgE cow's milk protein allergy under a restricted diet. *Nutrients* **2018**, *10*, 1481. [CrossRef]
8. Huang, C.F.; Chie, W.C.; Wang, I.J. Efficacy of Lactobacillus administration in school-age children with asthma: A randomized, placebo-controlled trial. *Nutrients* **2018**, *10*, 1678. [CrossRef]
9. Szajewska, H.; Horvath, A. Lactobacillus rhamnosus GG in the primary prevention of eczema in children: A systematic review and meta-analysis. *Nutrients* **2018**, *10*, 1319. [CrossRef]
10. Vandenplas, Y.; Abkari, A.; Bellaiche, M.; Benninga, M.; Chouraqui, J.P.; Çokura, F.; Harb, T.; Hegar, B.; Lifschitz, C.; Ludwig, T.; et al. Prevalence and health outcomes of functional gastrointestinal symptoms in infants from birth to 12 months of age. *J. Pediatr. Gastroenterol. Nutr.* **2015**, *61*, 531–537. [CrossRef]
11. Savino, F.; Tarasco, V. New treatments for infant colic. *Curr. Opin. Pediatr.* **2010**, *22*, 791–797. [CrossRef] [PubMed]
12. Gerasimov, S.; Gantzel, J.; Dementieva, N.; Schevchenko, O.; Tsitsura, O.; Guta, N.; Bobyk, V.; Kaprus, V. Role of Lactobacillus rhamnosus (FloraActive™) 19070-2 and Lactobacillus reuteri (FloraActive™) 12246 in infant colic: A randomized dietary study. *Nutrients* **2018**, *10*, 1975. [CrossRef] [PubMed]
13. Sung, V.; D'Amico, F.; Cabana, M.D.; Chau, K.; Koren, G.; Savino, F.; Szajewska, H.; Deshpande, G.; Dupont, C.; Indrio, F.; et al. Lactobacillus reuteri to treat infant colic: A meta-analysis. *Pediatrics* **2018**, *141*, e20171811. [CrossRef] [PubMed]
14. Baldassarre, M.E.; Di Mauro, A.; Tafuri, S.; Rizzo, V.; Gallone, M.S.; Mastromarino, P.; Capobianco, D.; Laghi, L.; Zhu, C.; Capozza, M.; et al. Effectiveness and safety of a probiotic-mixture for the treatment of infantile colic: A double-blind, randomized, placebo-controlled clinical trial with fecal real-time PCR and NMR-based metabolomics analysis. *Nutrients* **2018**, *10*, 195. [CrossRef] [PubMed]
15. Lo Vecchio, A.; Vandenplas, Y.; Benninga, M.; Broekaert, I.; Falconer, J.; Gottrand, F.; Lifschitz, C.; Lionetti, P.; Orel, R.; Papadopoulou, A.; et al. An international consensus report on a new algorithm for the management of infant diarrhoea. *Acta Paediatr.* **2016**, *105*, e384–e389. [CrossRef] [PubMed]
16. Maragkoudaki, M.; Chouliaras, G.; Moutafi, A.; Thomas, A.; Orfanakou, A.; Papadopoulou, A. Efficacy of an oral rehydration solution enriched with Lactobacillus reuteri DSM 17938 and zinc in the management of acute diarrhoea in infants: A randomized, double-blind, placebo-controlled trial. *Nutrients* **2018**, *10*, 1189. [CrossRef] [PubMed]
17. Freedman, S.B.; Williamson-Urquhart, S.; Farion, K.J.; Gouin, S.; Willan, A.R.; Poonai, N.; Hurley, K.; Sherman, P.M.; Finkelstein, Y.; PERC PROGUT Trial Group; et al. Multicenter trial of a combination probiotic for children with gastroenteritis. *N. Engl. J. Med.* **2018**, *379*, 2015–2026. [CrossRef] [PubMed]
18. Schnadower, D.; Tarr, P.I.; Casper, T.C.; Gorelick, M.H.; Dean, J.M.; O'Connell, K.J.; Mahajan, P.; Levine, A.C.; Bhatt, S.R.; Roskind, C.G.; et al. Lactobacillus rhamnosus GG versus placebo for acute gastroenteritis in children. *N. Engl. J. Med.* **2018**, *379*, 2002–2014. [CrossRef] [PubMed]
19. Ianiro, G.; Rizzatti, G.; Plomer, M.; Lopetuso, L.; Scaldaferri, F.; Franceschi, F.; Cammarota, G.; Gasbarrini, A. Bacillus clausii for the treatment of acute diarrhea in children: A systematic review and meta-analysis of randomized controlled trials. *Nutrients* **2018**, *10*, 1074. [CrossRef]
20. Sudha, M.R.; Jayanthi, N.; Pandey, D.C.; Verma, A.K. Bacillus clausii UBBC-07 reduces severity of diarrhoea in children under 5 years of age: A double blind placebo controlled study. *Benef. Microbes* **2019**, 1–6. [CrossRef]
21. Aceti, A.; Beghetti, I.; Maggio, L.; Martini, S.; Faldella, G.; Corvaglia, L. Filling the Gaps: Current Research Directions for a Rational Use of Probiotics in Preterm Infants. *Nutrients* **2018**, *10*, 1472. [CrossRef]

22. Aceti, A.; Maggio, L.; Beghetti, I.; Gori, D.; Barone, G.; Callegari, M.L.; Fantini, M.P.; Indrio, F.; Meneghin, F.; Italian Society of Neonatology; et al. Probiotics prevent late-onset sepsis in human milk-fed, very low birth weight preterm infants: Systematic review and meta-analysis. *Nutrients* **2017**, *9*, 904. [CrossRef]
23. Van den Akker, C.H.P.; van Goudoever, J.B.; Szajewska, H.; Embleton, N.D.; Hojsak, I.; Reid, D.; Shamir, R.; ESPGHAN Working Group for Probiotics, Prebiotics & Committee on Nutrition; et al. Probiotics for preterm infants: A strain-specific systematic review and network meta-analysis. *J. Pediatr. Gastroenterol. Nutr.* **2018**, *67*, 103–122. [PubMed]
24. Vandenplas, Y.; Berger, B.; Carnielli, V.P.; Ksiazyk, J.; Lagström, H.; Sanchez Luna, M.; Migacheva, N.; Mosselmans, J.M.; Picaud, J.C.; Possner, M.; et al. Human milk oligosaccharides: 2′-Fucosyllactose (2′-FL) and Lacto-N-Neotetraose (LNnT) in infant formula. *Nutrients* **2018**, *10*, 1161. [CrossRef] [PubMed]
25. Triantis, V.; Bode, L.; van Neerven, R.J.J. Immunological effects of human milk oligosaccharides. *Front. Pediatr.* **2018**, *6*, 190. [CrossRef] [PubMed]
26. Bering, S.B. Human milk oligosaccharides to prevent gut dysfunction and necrotizing enterocolitis in preterm neonates. *Nutrients* **2018**, *10*, 1461. [CrossRef] [PubMed]
27. Wejryd, E.; Martí, M.; Marchini, G.; Werme, A.; Jonsson, B.; Landberg, E.; Abrahamsson, T.R. Low diversity of human milk oligosaccharides is associated with necrotising enterocolitis in extremely low birth weight infants. *Nutrients* **2018**, *10*, 1556. [CrossRef] [PubMed]
28. Souza, D.D.S.; Tahan, S.; Weber, T.K.; Araujo-Filho, H.B.; de Morais, M.B. Randomized, double-blind, placebo-controlled parallel clinical trial assessing the effect of fructooligosaccharides in infants with constipation. *Nutrients* **2018**, *10*, 1602. [CrossRef]
29. Feruś, K.; Drabińska, N.; Krupa-Kozak, U.; Jarocka-Cyrta, E. A randomized, placebo-controlled, pilot clinical trial to evaluate the effect of supplementation with prebiotic Synergy 1 on iron homeostasis in children and adolescents with celiac disease treated with a gluten-free diet. *Nutrients* **2018**, *10*, 1818. [CrossRef]

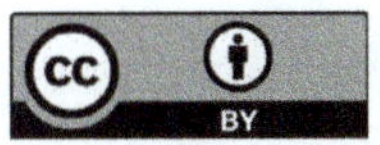

© 2019 by the authors. Licensee MDPI, Basel, Switzerland. This article is an open access article distributed under the terms and conditions of the Creative Commons Attribution (CC BY) license (http://creativecommons.org/licenses/by/4.0/).

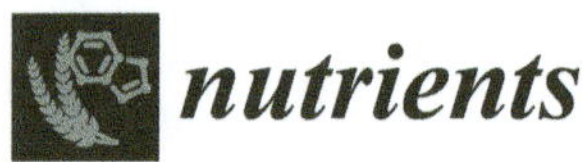

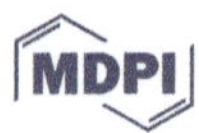

Review

Bacillus clausii for the Treatment of Acute Diarrhea in Children: A Systematic Review and Meta-Analysis of Randomized Controlled Trials

Gianluca Ianiro [1,*], Gianenrico Rizzatti [1], Manuel Plomer [2], Loris Lopetuso [1], Franco Scaldaferri [1], Francesco Franceschi [1], Giovanni Cammarota [1] and Antonio Gasbarrini [1]

[1] Fondazione Policlinico Universitario A. Gemelli IRCCS-Università Cattolica del Sacro Cuore, 00143 Roma, Italy; gianenrico.rizzatti@gmail.com (G.R.); lopetusoloris@libero.it (L.L.); francoscaldaferri@gmail.com (F.S.); francesco.franceschi@unicatt.it (F.F.); giovanni.cammarota@unicatt.it (G.C.); antonio.gasbarrini@unicatt.it (A.G.)

[2] Medical Affairs CHC Germany, Sanofi-Aventis Deutschland GmbH, Industriepark Höchst, D-65926 Frankfurt am Main, Germany; Manuel.Plomer@sanofi.com

* Correspondence: gianluca.ianiro@hotmail.it; Tel.: +39-(0)-63-0156265; Fax: +39-(0)-63-5502775

Received: 26 June 2018; Accepted: 8 August 2018; Published: 12 August 2018

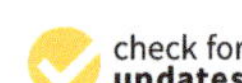

Abstract: Acute diarrhea is a burdensome disease with potentially harmful consequences, especially in childhood. Despite its large use in clinical practice, the efficacy of the probiotic *Bacillus clausii* in treating acute childhood diarrhea remains unclear. Our objective was to systematically review the efficacy of *Bacillus clausii* in the treatment of acute childhood diarrhea. The following electronic databases were systematically searched up to October 2017: MEDLINE (via PubMed/OVID), EMBASE (via OVID), Cochrane Central Database of Controlled Trials (via CENTRAL), Google Scholar, and ClinicalTrials.gov. Only randomized controlled trials were included. The overall effect for the meta-analysis was derived by using a random effects model. Six randomized controlled trials (1298 patients) met the eligibility criteria. Data arising from pooled analysis showed that *Bacillus clausii* significantly reduced the duration of diarrhea (mean difference = −9.12 h; 95% confidence interval [CI]: −16.49 to −1.75, $p = 0.015$), and the duration of hospitalization (mean difference = −0.85 days; 95% CI: −1.56 to −0.15, $p = 0.017$), compared with control. There was a trend of decreasing stool frequency after *Bacillus clausii* administration compared with the control group (mean difference = −0.19 diarrheal motions; 95% CI: −0.43 to −0.06, $p = 0.14$). *Bacillus clausii* may represent an effective therapeutic option in acute childhood diarrhea, with a good safety profile.

Keywords: acute diarrhea; children; *Bacillus clausii*; efficacy; randomized controlled trials

1. Introduction

Diarrhea refers to the abrupt onset of three or more loose or liquid stools per day [1]. More specifically, acute diarrhea is defined as an abnormally frequent discharge of semi-solid or fluid fecal matter from the bowel, lasting less than 14 days [2]. Although it is a preventable disease, acute diarrhea remains a major cause of morbidity and mortality in children worldwide, resulting in 525,000 deaths per year among those younger than five years. Most of these mortalities occur in developing countries [1]. Other direct consequences of diarrhea in children include growth faltering, malnutrition, and impaired cognitive development [3]. Acute diarrhea in children is caused by a wide range of pathogens—including viral, bacterial, and protozoal pathogens—which makes overcoming the high disease burden a large challenge [4].

Currently, the World Health Organization (WHO) recommends treatment of acute childhood diarrhea with oral rehydration salts (ORS) and continued feeding for the prevention and treatment of dehydration, as well as zinc supplementation to shorten the duration and severity of the diarrheal episode [1]. Probiotics are living micro-organisms that, upon ingestion in certain numbers, exert health benefits beyond inherent general nutrition [5]. It has been suggested that probiotics modulate the immune response, produce antimicrobial agents, and compete in nutrient uptake and adhesion sites with pathogens [6–8].

Bacillus clausii is a rod-shaped, non-pathogenic, spore-forming, aerobic, Gram-positive bacterium that is able to survive transit through the acidic environment of the stomach and colonize the intestine even in the presence of antibiotics [9]. Prospective clinical trials conducted in adult subjects found *Bacillus clausii* to be effective and safe in the treatment and prevention of acute diarrhea [10,11]. In a prospective, Phase II clinical trial of *Bacillus clausii* in 27 adult patients with acute diarrhea, the mean $\pm$ standard deviation (SD) duration of diarrhea decreased from 34.81 $\pm$ 4.69 min at baseline to 9.26 $\pm$ 3.05 ($p < 0.0001$) minutes per day after 10 days of *Bacillus clausii* therapy. The mean $\pm$ SD frequency of defecation also decreased from 6.96 $\pm$ 1.05 to 1.78 $\pm$ 0.50 ($p < 0.0001$) times per day, abdominal pain decreased from 3.22 $\pm$ 0.93 (severe) to 0.74 $\pm$ 0.71 (absent) ($p < 0.0001$), and stool consistency improved from 3.93 $\pm$ 0.38 (watery) to 1.22 $\pm$ 0.42 (soft) ($p < 0.0001$). No significant change in safety parameters was observed during treatment with *Bacillus clausii*. Thus, the study concluded that *Bacillus clausii* can potentially be effective in alleviating the symptoms of diarrhea without causing any adverse effects [11].

The European Society for Pediatric Gastroenterology, Hepatology, and Nutrition (ESPGHAN) and the European Society of Pediatric Infectious Diseases (ESPID) currently recommend the use of *Lactobacillus rhamnosus* GG and *Saccharomyces boulardii* in the management of children with acute diarrhea as an adjunct to rehydration therapy, whereas a recommendation for *Bacillus clausii* is missing due to limited data [12]. The aim of this paper is to systematically review randomized controlled trials that assessed the efficacy and safety of *Bacillus clausii* in the treatment of acute childhood diarrhea. According to our knowledge, no systematic reviews with meta-analyses addressing the effectiveness of *Bacillus clausii* in acute pediatric diarrhea have yet been published. We will focus only on studies using *Bacillus clausii* as a probiotic, because critics of using a meta-analytical approach to assess the efficacy of probiotics argue that beneficial effects of probiotics seem to be strain-specific.

2. Methods

2.1. Criteria for Considering Studies for this Review

We included randomized controlled trials conducted among children under 18 years of age with acute diarrhea ($\leq$14 days). Patients in the experimental groups had to receive *Bacillus clausii* at any dose and in the following four bacterial stains: O/C, SIN, N/R, and T. Patients in the control groups had to receive either a placebo, an appropriate standard of care for acute diarrhea in lieu of the probiotic, or no treatmentcontrol. The designations of these bacterial strains are derived from their resistance to diverse antibiotics: O/C is resistant to chloramphenicol, SIN to neomycin and streptomycin, N/R to novobiocin and rifampin, and T to tetracycline [13].

The primary outcome measures were duration of diarrhea, stool frequency after intervention, and hospitalization duration. The secondary outcome measures were vomiting episodes, quality of life, and adverse events. All randomized controlled trials regardless of language or publication date or state (published, unpublished, in press, and in progress) were included in the review. Studies investigating probiotics other than *Bacillus clausii* (including synthetic microbiota suspensions), as well as those conducted in adult subjects or in children receiving *Bacillus clausii* for indications other than acute diarrhea were excluded. In vitro/vivo studies, observational studies, narrative/systematic reviews, case reports, letters, editorials, and commentaries were also excluded, but read to identify potential additional studies.

2.2. Search Strategy for Identification of Studies

The following electronic databases were systematically searched up to October 2017 for relevant studies: MEDLINE (via PubMed/OVID), EMBASE (via OVID), Cochrane Central Database of Controlled Trials (via CENTRAL), Google Scholar, and ClinicalTrials.gov (https://clinicaltrials.gov). The last literature search was conducted on 23 October 2017. The text word terms used were: *Bacillus clausii*; Enterogermina; probiotic; probiotics; diarrhea; diarrhoea; acute diarrhea; acute diarrhoea; diarrh *; children; child *; pediatric; and pediatr *. In addition, we hand-searched the bibliographies of papers of interest to provide additional references. Relevant meeting abstracts via EMBASE and the International Probiotic Conference were also hand-searched. When needed, we contacted the authors for additional data and clarification of study methods. Finally, the pharmaceutical company Sanofi-Aventis Group (Paris, France), which manufactures *Bacillus clausii* was contacted to identify further published and unpublished studies. No limit was imposed regarding the language of publication, and both studies published as full text or as abstracts at conferences/proceedings of scientific meetings were included in the review.

2.3. Study Selection

Titles and abstracts of publications identified according to the above described search strategy were independently screened by two reviewers (G.I. and G.R.). All potentially relevant articles were retained and the full text of these studies were examined to determine which studies satisfied the inclusion criteria. In the case of any differences of opinion or disagreements between the two reviewers, an adjudicator (A.G.) was consulted.

2.4. Data Extraction

Data extraction was carried out independently by two reviewers (G.I. and G.R.), using a data collection form designed for this review prepared in Microsoft Excel 2013 (Microsoft, Redmond, WA, USA). Discrepancies between the two reviewers were resolved by discussion. Information about the study design and outcomes was verified by all reviewers. Authors' names, publication year, study design, study location, study duration, inclusion and exclusion criteria, interventions, type of comparator, number of patients, age and gender of included patients, outcomes, and adverse events were extracted from each study. To keep track of study references, EndNote version X7.71 (Thomson Reuters, New York, NY, USA) was used.

2.5. Quality Assessment

To assess the methodological quality of each study included in the review, two reviewers (G.I. and G.R.) independently performed a risk of bias assessment using the criteria (generation of allocation sequence; allocation concealment; blinding of investigators, participants, outcome assessors, and data analysts; intention-to-treat (ITT) analysis; and comprehensive follow-up) described by the Center for Reviews and Dissemination (CRD)'s guidance for undertaking reviews in health care (2009) [14]. For each criterion, the risk of bias was assessed answering the respective questions with 'yes', 'no', or 'unclear' and the overall quality of each study was rated « good », « fair » or «poor ».

2.6. Statistical Methods

Mean values and SDs of diarrhea duration, number of stools, and hospitalization duration were extracted to calculate the mean difference between the treatment and control groups for each of these outcomes. Overall effect for each meta-analysis was derived by using a random effects model, which takes between-study variation into account [15]. We also reported the corresponding 95% confidence intervals (CI) and *p*-values. Statistical heterogeneity between studies was assessed by using Cochran's Q test and I-squared [16]. An I^2 value of 0% indicates no observed heterogeneity, and larger values show increasing heterogeneity.

The risk of publication bias was assessed by visual inspection of Begg's funnel plots. Formal statistical assessment of funnel plot asymmetry was also done using Egger's regression asymmetry test and Begg's adjusted rank correlation test [17]. All statistical analyses were conducted by using the metafor package (Maastricht University, Maastricht, NL, USA) [18]. *p*-Values < 0.05 were considered statistically significant.

3. Results

3.1. Characteristics of Included Studies

The literature search retrieved 2165 potential relevant citations. After carefully reviewing the titles and abstracts, 2154 citations were excluded. For the remaining 11 citations, full papers were obtained and reviewed. After a full-text assessment, six citations were included in the final database, and five excluded for the following reasons: two studies were non-randomized, one study was conducted in an adult population, one was a review article, and one was a commentary. The flow diagram of the study selection process is given in Figure 1.

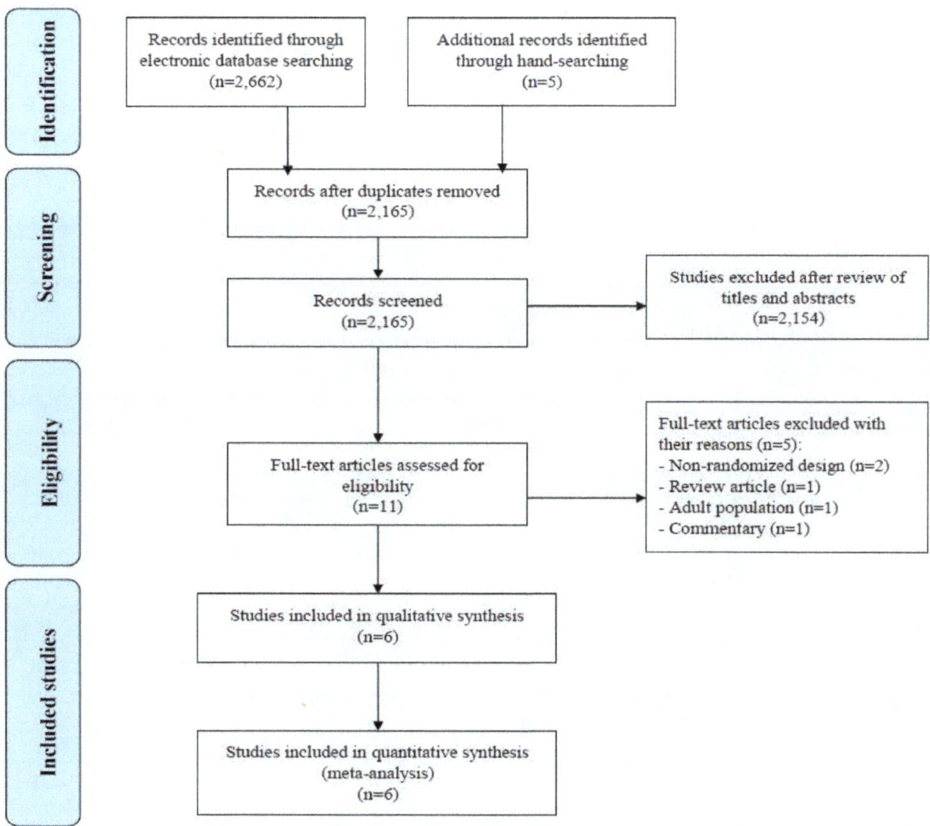

Figure 1. Flow diagram of the study selection process.

Table 1 summarizes the characteristics of the six randomized controlled trials included in the review, which were published between 2007 and 2015. Of these, one was performed in Italy [19], one in Kenya [20], one in the Philippines [21], and three in India [22–24]. Three of the included studies were published as original articles [19,23,24], one as a meeting abstract [21], one as a Master's dissertation [20], and one as a clinical study report [22]. Of the six studies, two were conducted in a multicentric setting [19,22]. All six studies included an outcome for diarrhea duration, four included an outcome for stool frequency [19,20,22,24], and three included an outcome for duration of hospitalization [20,21,23].

Overall, 1298 patients were enrolled in the six selected studies. Among these, 467 patients were treated with *Bacillus clausii*. In the Canani et al. (2007) study [19], patients were allocated to six different groups: a control group ($n = 92$), a group treated with *Bacillus clausii* ($n = 100$), a group treated with *Lactobacillus casei* ($n = 100$), a group treated with *Saccharomyces boulardii* (n=91), a group treated with *Lactobacillus delbrueckii var bulgaricus, Lactobacillus acidophilus, Streptococcus thermophilus, Bifidobacterium bifidum* ($n = 97$), and a group treated with *Enterococcus faecium* ($n = 91$). All groups, with the exception of the control group and the group receiving *Bacillus clausii* were excluded from this meta-analysis. Thus, in total, 919 patients were included in the meta-analysis (467 in the experimental group and 452 in the control group). The age of the patients ranged from 3 months to 12 years. Four studies enrolled inpatients [20,21,23,24], whereas two enrolled outpatients [19,22].

In all six clinical trials, the control group was treated with ORS. In the Canani et al. (2007) study [19], the control group ($n = 92$) was given an oral rehydration solution for 3 to 6 h and then fed with a full-strength milk formula containing lactose or cows' milk, depending on age. In the three Indian studies, the control group ($n = 132$ in the Lahiri trial [22]; $n = 80$ in the Lahiri, D'Souza et al. trial [24]; and $n = 62$ in the Lahiri, Jadhav et al. trial [23]) received ORS with zinc supplementation. The control group in the Urtula and Dacula (2008) study ($n = 35$) received ORS alone [21]. Finally, the control group in the Maugo (2012) study ($n = 51$) received in addition to zinc sulfate and ORS, one vial twice daily of a placebo packaged in identical looking vials containing sterile water [20]. Concerning the interventions in the experimental group, in one study, the daily dosage of *Bacillus clausii* was 1×10^9 colony-forming units (CFU) administrated twice daily [19], while in four other studies, children were administered 2×10^9 CFU of *Bacillus clausii* twice daily [20,22–24], and in the Urtula and Dacula (2008) trial, 2×10^9 or 4×10^9 CFU of *Bacillus clausii* were administrated per day, depending on the age of the children [21]. In all studies, the experimental group received ORS in addition to *Bacillus clausii* therapy. Moreover, zinc supplementation was also added to the treatment of the experimental group in four studies [20,22–24]. The duration of the interventions was five days in all clinical trials, with the exception of the Urtula and Dacula (2008) trial [21] which treated patients for three days.

3.2. Risk of Bias within Included Studies

The methodological quality of the clinical trials varied (Table 2). Three studies [19–21] were rated as adequate for both generation of the allocation sequence and allocation concealment. In the remaining three studies, the method used for allocation sequence and allocation concealment was unclear [22–24]. In only one study [20], care providers, participants, and outcome assessors were blind to treatment allocation. In the Canani et al. (2007) study [19] and in the Lahiri (2008) trial [22], analyses were conducted on an ITT basis. Three studies [21,23,24] were unclear for an ITT analysis, and the Maugo (2012) trial [20] did not include an ITT analysis. Loss to follow-up was adequate in two studies [20,22], and was unclear in the remaining four studies [19,21,23,24]. The overall quality was assessed, with two studies [19,20] rated as 'good' (low risk for bias), two other studies [21,22] which were susceptible to some bias rated as 'fair', and the remaining two studies [23,24] were rated as 'poor' (high risk for bias).

Table 1. Characteristics and results of included studies.

Authors, Publication Year (Country)	Study Design	Number of Treated Patients (I/C)	M/F (In %)	Age	Intervention vs. Comparator (Dosage and Duration)	Outcome Measures	Follow-Up	Main Results
Canani et al., 2007 (Italy) [19]	Prospective, multicenter, single-blind, randomized, controlled	100/92	47/53	Median: 18 months	1×10^9 CFU of *Bacillus clausii* bid for 5 days + ORS for 3 to 6 h vs. ORS for 3 to 6 h (followed by full strength formula of lactose or cows' milk, depending on age, in both groups)	Total duration of diarrhea, number of stools/day and their consistency, incidence and median duration of vomiting, fever (>37.5 °C), number of hospital admissions, safety and tolerability	Day 1 to day 7	Median duration of diarrhea in patients receiving *Bacillus clausii* (118 h) similar to control group (115 h), with an estimated difference of 1 h between both groups ($p = 0.76$). All other outcomes were also similar in both groups. *Bacillus clausii* was well tolerated, with no observed adverse events.
Lahiri, 2008 (India) [22]	Phase III, controlled, open-label, randomized, parallel-group, multicenter, comparative	132/132	54.5/45.5	Mean (SD): 1.6 (1.0) years	2×10^9 CFU of *Bacillus clausii* bid + ORS + 20 mg/day of zinc supplement, for 5 days vs. ORS + 20 mg/day of zinc supplement, for 5 days	Duration of diarrhea, mean number of daily stools, effect on consistency of stools, vomiting episodes per day, reported adverse events, parents' overall global assessment of tolerability at end of treatment period	Day 6 to day 10 (after end of study treatment)	Mean (SD) duration of diarrhea lower in the experimental group (48.6 (38.2) h), vs. control group (56.1 (40) h; $p = 0.13$). Difference in the mean (SD) number of stools until recovery statistically not significant ($p = 0.19$); trend favoring the experimental group (7.4 (6.5) motions vs. 8.6 (6.5) motions in control group).
Lahiri, Jadhav et al., 2015 (India) [23]	Open-label, prospective, randomized, controlled	69/62	63.4/36.6	6 months to 12 years	2×10^9 CFU of *Bacillus clausii* bid + ORS + zinc, for 5 days vs. ORS + zinc for 5 days	Mean duration of diarrhea, mean duration of hospitalization, frequency of diarrhea, direct and indirect costs	At 6, 12, 24, 36, 48, 60, and 72 h	Mean duration of diarrhea 22.64 h and mean duration of hospital stay 2.78 days in the *Bacillus clausii* group vs. 47.05 h and 4.30 days, respectively, in the control group ($p < 0.01$ for diarrhea duration). Treatment with *Bacillus clausii* reduced total treatment costs by 472 Indian rupees compared to ORS alone.

Table 1. Characteristics and results of included studies.

Authors, Publication Year (Country)	Study Design	Number of Treated Patients (I/C)	M/F (In %)	Age	Intervention vs. Comparator (Dosage and Duration)	Outcome Measures	Follow-Up	Main Results
Lahiri, D'Souza et al., 2015 (India) [24]	Open-label, prospective, randomized, controlled	80/80	52.5/47.5	Up to 6 years	2×10^9 CFU of *Bacillus clausii* bid + ORS + zinc, for 5 days vs. ORS + zinc for 5 days	Mean duration of diarrhea, mean stool frequency, % of children with no dehydration, % of children benefiting from breastfeeding	At 6, 12, 24, 36, 48, 60, and 72 h	Mean (SD) duration of diarrhea 22.26 h and mean stool frequency 1.15 in the *Bacillus clausii* group vs. 34.16 h and 1.70, respectively in control group ($p < 0.05$).
Maugo, 2012 (Kenya) [20]	Randomized, double-blind, placebo-controlled	51/51	51.1/48.9	Mean (SD): *Bacillus clausii* group: 11.3 (5.3) and control group: 11.9 (6.4) months	2×10^9 CFU of *Bacillus clausii* bid + ORS + zinc sulfate, for 5 days vs. zinc sulfate + ORS + 1 vial bid of a placebo packaged in identical looking vials containing sterile water, for 5 days	Mean duration of diarrhea, mean duration of hospitalization, mean reduction of the number of diarrheal episodes per day	Day 1 to day 7	Mean (SD) duration of diarrhea in *Bacillus clausii* group was shorter (77.59 (34.10) h) than placebo group (86.74 (40.16) h), with mean absolute difference between groups of 9.15 h ($p = 0.248$). Significant decrease in mean number of diarrheal motions on day 3 (2.74 (1.81) motions in the *Bacillus clausii* group vs. 3.80 (2.70) motions in placebo group, mean absolute difference = 1.05 motions; $p = 0.033$) and day 4 (1.45 (1.13) motions in the *Bacillus clausii* group vs. 2.35 (2.19) motions in placebo group, mean absolute difference = 0.9 motions; $p = 0.018$) in the *Bacillus clausii* group vs. placebo group.
Urtula and Dacula, 2008 (The Philippines) [21]	Monocentric, randomized, controlled	35/35	NR	NR	2×10^9 or 4×10^9 CFU of *Bacillus clausii* per day, depending on the age of the children + ORS, for 3 days vs. ORS for 3 days	Mean duration of diarrhea, mean duration of hospitalization, mean frequency of stools	After day 3 of therapy, and upon discharge	Mean (SD) duration of diarrhea significantly shorter in the *Bacillus clausii* group (69.84 (16.84) h) than in control group (83.76 (22.05) h) ($p = 0.005$), with absolute difference of duration of diarrhea between groups of 13.92 h. Mean duration of hospital stay was also shorter favoring *Bacillus clausii* group (59.0 h vs. 76.8 h) ($p = 0.063$).

bid, twice daily; C, control; CFU, colony-forming units; F, female; h, hour; I, intervention; M, male; NR, not reported; ORS, oral rehydration salts; SD, standard deviation; vs., versus.

Table 2. Risk of bias assessment.

Authors and Publication Year	Was Randomization Carried Out Appropriately?	Was the Concealment of Treatment Allocation Adequate?	Were the Groups Similar at the Outset of the Study in Terms of Prognostic Factors?	Were the Care Providers, Participants and Outcome Assessors Blind to Treatment Allocation?	Were There any Unexpected Imbalances in Drop-Outs between Groups?	Is There any Evidence to Suggest that the Authors Measured More Outcomes than They Reported?	Did the Analysis Include an Intention-To-Treat Analysis? If So, Was This Appropriate and Were Appropriate Methods Used to Account for Missing Data?	Overall Study Quality
Canani et al., 2007 [19]	Yes	Yes	Yes	No	No	No	Yes/Yes	Good
Lahiri, 2008 [22]	Unclear	Unclear	Unclear	No	No	Unclear	Yes/Yes	Fair
Lahiri, Jadhav et al., 2015 [23]	Unclear	Unclear	Unclear	No	Unclear	No	Unclear	Poor *
Lahiri, D'Souza et al., 2015 [24]	Unclear	Unclear	Unclear	No	Unclear	No	Unclear	Poor *
Maugo, 2012 [20]	Yes	Yes	Yes	Yes	No	No	No	Good
Urtula and Dacula, 2008 [21]	Yes	Yes	Yes	Unclear	Unclear	No	Unclear	Fair

* Risk of bias was classified according to the Centre for Reviews and Dissemination (CRD) [14], based on the information available in the publications. However, the principle investigator was contacted directly and confirmed the validity of the data quality, providing the authors with confidence that the risk for bias can be considered as 'fair'.

3.3. Primary Findings

All six studies contained data on the duration of diarrhea. Compared to the control group ($n = 441$), the change in diarrhea duration in patients treated with *Bacillus clausii* ($n = 457$) ranged from −24.4 to +2.5 h among included studies. In the Canani et al. (2007) trial [19], duration of diarrhea was expressed as median (interquartile range [IQR]) duration, whereas in three studies [20–22], it was expressed as mean (SD) duration, and in two studies [23,24], it was simply expressed as mean duration. According to the Cochrane Reviewers' Handbook 4.2.2 (2004) [25] and assuming normal distribution, median duration of diarrhea in the Canani et al. (2007) study [19] was treated as a mean value, and the width of IQR was considered as 1.35 × SD. After this conversion, a meta-analysis of the six randomized controlled trials (898 participants) showed a significant reduction in the duration of the diarrhea (mean difference = −9.12 h, 95% CI: −16.49 to −1.75) for those treated with *Bacillus clausii* compared to ORS with or without zinc supplementation ($p = 0.015$) (Figure 2). The heterogeneity test for diarrhea duration showed a substantial heterogeneity between the six studies (Cochrane's Q test, $p = 0.02$, $I^2 = 63.4\%$).

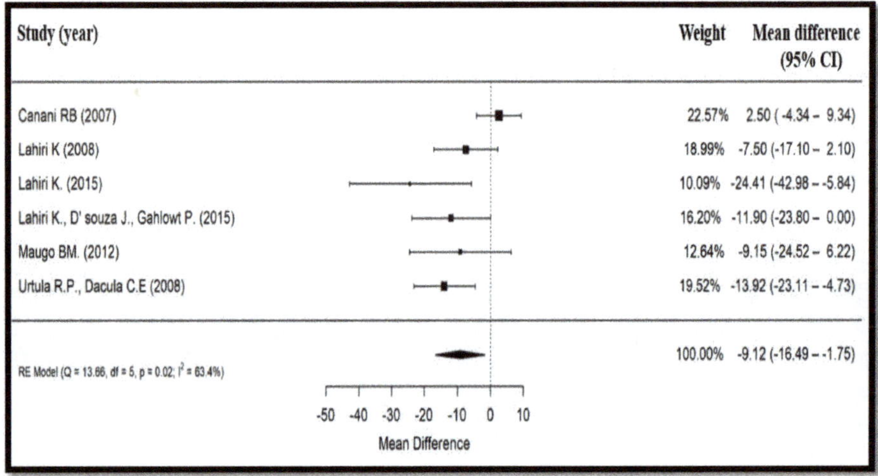

Figure 2. Forest plot showing effect of *Bacillus clausii* on mean duration of diarrhea. CI, confidence interval, RE, random effects.

Four studies (697 participants) evaluated stool frequency after intervention [19,20,22,24]. In the Canani et al. (2007) trial [19], daily stool frequency was expressed as median (IQR), and it was evaluated from the first day of *Bacillus clausii* administration up to day 7. In the Maugo (2012) study [20], daily diarrheal output was expressed as mean (SD), and it was also evaluated from day 1 of *Bacillus clausii* administration up to day 7. In the Lahiri (2008) trial [22], daily diarrheal output was expressed as both mean (SD) and median (range) values, and it was evaluated from day 1 of *Bacillus clausii* administration up to day 6. Finally, in the Lahiri, D'Souza et al. (2015) study [24], stool frequency was expressed as a mean value, and it was assessed before and after treatment with *Bacillus clausii*. Similarly to the duration of diarrhea, median stool frequency in the Canani et al. (2007) study [19] was treated as a mean value, and the width of IQR was considered as 1.35 × SD [25]. Pooling the results of the four trials showed that *Bacillus clausii* reduces the stool frequency after intervention (mean difference = −0.19 diarrheal motions, 95% CI: −0.43 to −0.06, $p = 0.14$) compared with the control group which received ORS with or without zinc supplementation (Figure 3). The heterogeneity test for stool frequency after intervention revealed a slight heterogeneity between the four trials (Cochrane's Q test, $p = 0.22$, $I^2 = 32.9\%$).

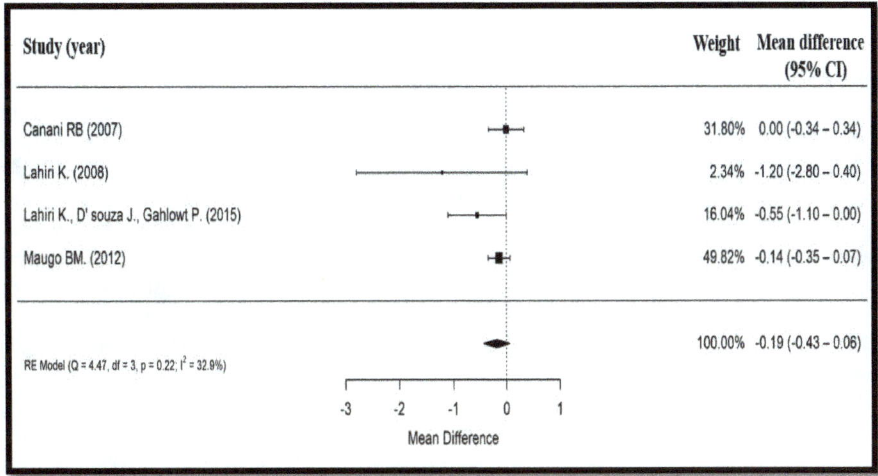

Figure 3. Forest plot showing effect of *Bacillus clausii* on mean stool frequency. CI, confidence interval, RE, random effects.

Finally, duration of hospitalization was assessed in three studies [20,21,23] among 291 patients. In the Maugo (2012) study [20], hospitalization duration was expressed as mean (SD), whereas in the two other trials [21,23], it was simply expressed as mean. Based on the results of these three clinical trials [20,21,23], there was a significant reduction in the duration of hospitalization (mean difference = −0.85 days, 95% CI: −1.56 to −0.15) for those treated with *Bacillus clausii* compared to ORS with or without zinc ($p = 0.017$) (Figure 4). The heterogeneity test for duration of hospital stay showed a substantial heterogeneity between the three studies (Cochrane's Q test, $p = 0.03$, $I^2 = 71.3\%$).

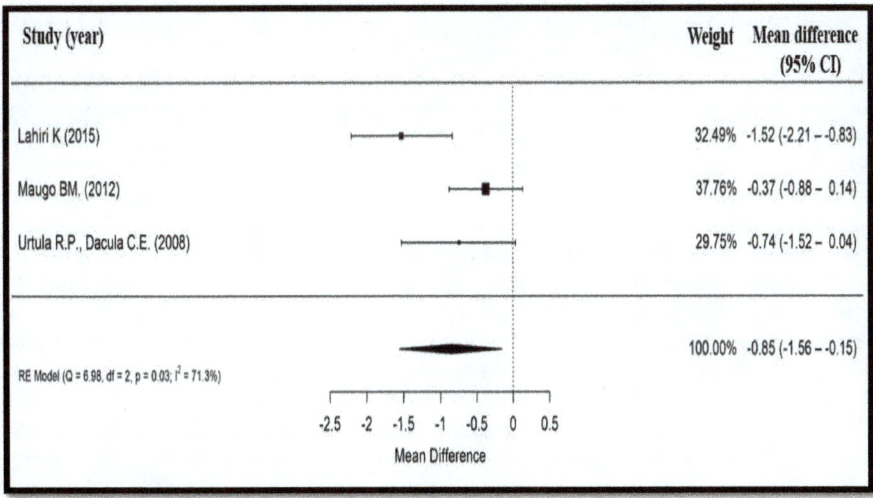

Figure 4. Forest plot showing effect of *Bacillus clausii* on mean duration of hospitalization. CI, confidence interval, RE, random effects.

3.4. Secondary Findings

Two clinical trials [19,22] included an outcome related to the incidence and/or duration of vomiting episodes among 447 patients. In the Canani et al. (2007) trial [19], both median (IQR) duration of vomiting and the number (%) of children experiencing vomiting episodes were similar in the group treated with *Bacillus clausii* (n = 100) and in the control group (n = 92). In the control group, 34 children (37%) experienced vomiting episodes versus 32 children (32%) in the *Bacillus clausii* group (p = 0.47). Similarly, the median (IQR) vomiting duration was 2 (1–2) days in the control group versus 1.5 (1–2) days in the group treated with *Bacillus clausii* (p = 0.25). In the Lahiri (2008) study [22], the mean $\pm$ SD number of vomiting episodes on day 4 of treatment was 0.1 $\pm$ 0.6 in the *Bacillus clausii* + ORS group (n = 129) versus 0.2 $\pm$ 0.6 in the ORS group (n = 126). Hence, the difference in the mean number of vomiting episodes was not statistically significant between the two groups (p = 0.79).

The studies [19,22] did not report any serious adverse effects related to *Bacillus clausii*. According to Canani and colleagues [19], treatment by *Bacillus clausii* was well tolerated, and no adverse events were observed. In the Lahiri (2008) trial [22], 40/129 patients (31%) from the *Bacillus clausii* + ORS group and 39/126 patients (31%) from the ORS group experienced undesirable side effects. There was no statistically significant difference in the number of patients experiencing adverse events between the two groups (p = 0.48). Vomiting was the most reported adverse event in both the *Bacillus clausii* + ORS group (20/129; 15.5%) and the ORS group (17/126; 13.5%).

Outcomes related to quality of life were not reported in any of the studies included in the meta-analysis.

3.5. Publication Bias

The publication bias was assessed by using a funnel plot depicting the mean differences in duration of diarrhea, stool frequency, and duration of hospital stay against their effect sizes as a measure of precision. A slight asymmetry was seen in Begg's funnel plot for duration of diarrhea, resulting in evidence of publication bias (Egger's test, p = 0.02). In contrast, duration of hospital stay and stool frequency showed neither asymmetry nor evidence for publication bias (Egger's test, p = 0.55 for hospitalization duration and p = 0.11 for stool frequency).

4. Discussion

We conducted a systematic review and a meta-analysis of randomized controlled trials to estimate the efficacy of *Bacillus clausii* in the treatment of acute diarrhea in children. Results of this systematic review indicate that *Bacillus clausii* combined with ORS might significantly reduce the duration of acute childhood diarrhea and the duration of hospital stay compared to ORS alone.

To our knowledge, this is the first systematic review focusing on randomized controlled trials of *Bacillus clausii* in acute childhood diarrhea. In this review, the duration of diarrhea was reduced by a mean of 9.12 h with *Bacillus clausii* treatment compared to controls (p = 0.015). These findings were replicated in a prospective, phase II, Indian clinical study conducted among 27 adult patients with acute diarrhea treated with 2×10^9 CFU of *Bacillus clausii* twice daily for a duration of 10 days, in which mean $\pm$ SD duration of diarrhea decreased from 34.81 $\pm$ 4.69 min at baseline to 9.26 $\pm$ 3.05 ($p < 0.0001$) minutes per day after 10 days of *Bacillus clausii* administration [11]. In contrast, in the Canani et al. (2007) trial [19], it was found that the duration of diarrhea in patients receiving *Bacillus clausii* was similar to that in the group receiving only oral rehydration, with an estimated difference of one hour between the control group and the group treated with *Bacillus clausii* (p = 0.76). The difference between the overall results of our meta-analysis and the results of the Canani et al. (2007) trial [19] may be due to the difference in the prescribed dosage of *Bacillus clausii* in the different randomized controlled trials and the zinc supplementation provided in some study protocols [20,22–24]. In the other studies, children were administered 4×10^9 CFU of *Bacillus clausii* per day [20,22–24], while in the Canani et al.

(2007) trial [19], children received 2×10^9 CFU of *Bacillus clausii* per day, which also corresponds to the prescribed dosage of *Bacillus clausii* in the younger children of the Urtula and Dacula (2008) study [21].

Our results also showed that administration of *Bacillus clausii* preparations significantly reduced the duration of hospitalization by a mean of 0.85 days compared to controls ($p = 0.017$). The reduction of hospital stay by *Bacillus clausii* is important considering that in low-income countries, children under three years old experience on average three episodes of diarrhea every year [1]. Moreover, a 2008 study set in in Vellore, India, in 439 children under the age of five years found that median household expenditures incurred per diarrheal episode ranged from 2.2% to 5.8% of the household's annual income [26]. Similarly, a 2013 cross-sectional study set in Bolivia and conducted among 1107 caregivers of pediatric patients (<5 years of age) with diarrhea found that 45% of patients' families paid ≥1% of their annual household income for a single diarrheal episode [27]. Thus, diarrheal disease in children constitutes a considerable worldwide economic burden. The results of this systematic review are of particular importance, since these reductions in the length of hospital stay and duration of diarrhea that were obtained with *Bacillus clausii* in our analysis may offer significant social and economic benefit in the treatment of acute childhood diarrhea, particularly in low- and middle-income countries. In addition, in the Lahiri, Jadhav et al. (2015) study [23], treatment with *Bacillus clausii* reduced total treatment costs by 472 Indian rupees compared to ORS alone. Further studies may be needed to clarify the cost-effectiveness of *Bacillus clausii* preparations in treating children with acute diarrhea.

The effect of *Bacillus clausii* on stool frequency reduction compared to ORS alone did not reach statistical significance after pooling the results of four clinical trials ($p = 0.14$). This result could have different explanations. First, assessing such a specific outcome, as stool frequency can be challenging. Moreover, these four studies [19,20,22,24] differed in sample size, study design, and treatment protocols. Consequently, large studies might be needed to clarify the efficacy of *Bacillus clausii* on stool frequency reduction in acute pediatric diarrhea.

Our systematic review suggested that treatment with *Bacillus clausii* is well tolerated, without causing serious adverse events. This finding is consistent with the safety results of the prospective, Phase II clinical trial conducted in 27 adult patients with acute diarrhea which found no significant change in safety parameters during treatment with *Bacillus clausii* [11]. Additionally, in a 2004 single-center, double-blind, prospective, randomized, placebo-controlled study performed in 120 consecutive *Helicobacter pylori*-positive adult patients free from gastrointestinal symptoms, it was found that *Bacillus clausii* treatment during and after a standard seven-day anti-*Helicobacter pylori* regimen was also associated with lower incidence of self-reported side-effects and a better tolerability to multiple antibiotic treatment when compared with placebo ($p < 0.05$) [10].

Between-trial heterogeneity was detected for diarrhea duration and duration of hospital stay. This heterogeneity among the included studies could be partially explained by trials at high/unclear risk of bias for sequence generation, allocation concealment, and/or blinding. Indeed, only one included study was double-blinded [20], whereas the five other studies were either single-blinded [19], open-label [22–24], or had unclear blinding [21]. However, a slight heterogeneity for stool frequency after intervention was detected, reflecting an apparent effect of *Bacillus clausii* administration on stool frequency reduction compared with the control group.

Several mechanisms have been proposed to explain the effect of *Bacillus clausii* against acute childhood diarrhea. Urdaci and colleagues found *Bacillus clausii* to possess antimicrobial and immunomodulatory activities. Moreover, *Bacillus clausii* strains were found to release antimicrobial substances in the medium, and this was observed during stationary growth phase and coincided with sporulation. These substances were active against Gram-positive bacteria, in particular against *Staphylococcus aureus*, *Enterococcus faecium*, and *Clostridium difficile*. The antimicrobial activity of *Bacillus clausii* was resistant to subtilisin, proteinase K, and chymotrypsin treatment, whereas it was sensitive to pronase treatment [28]. The ability of *Bacillus clausii* spores to germinate during gastrointestinal transit and grow as vegetative cells both in the presence of bile and under limited oxygen availability was also described in an experimental study by Cenci et al. (2006) [29]. Additionally, *Bacillus clausii* O/C supernatant was found to reduce the cytotoxic effects of *Clostridium difficile* and *Bacillus cereus* toxins through the secreted alkaline serine M-protease [30]. Finally, the production of vitamin B2 by *Bacillus clausii* (strains O/C, N/R, SIN, and T) was compared with that of other probiotics in an in vitro agar-diffusion assay, and it was found that only *Bacillus clausii* and *Bacillus subtilis* permitted the growth of MS0057, a riboflavin-auxotrophic mutant of *Bacillus cereus*, which indicates secretion and diffusion of vitamin B2 in the solid medium [31]. These results are consistent with the beneficial effects evidenced for *Bacillus clausii* preparations in our study.

Our review had limitations that must be considered while interpreting our results. Three studies had unclear sequence generation and allocation concealment, five had inadequate or unclear blinding, and four were unclear for or had no ITT analysis. In addition, the definition of diarrhea, the termination of diarrhea, and inclusion and exclusion criteria varied among the included studies. In our meta-analysis, we also noticed publication bias detected for diarrhea duration. A key strength of the study comes from the fact that only a clearly defined probiotic micro-organism mix of four *Bacillus clausii* strains was assessed. Moreover, all treatments received by the control groups in the included studies were standardized consisting of ORS with or without zinc supplementation. Only the control group in the Maugo (2012) study received a placebo [20].

In summary, our results indicate that *Bacillus clausii* might represent an effective therapeutic option in acute childhood diarrhea, with a good safety profile. One limitation of this meta-nalysis is represented by the heterogeneity we found among studies, that prevent us from drawing definitive conclusions. Further, well designed studies are needed to confirm our findings.

Author Contributions: G.I. took the lead in writing the manuscript. G.R., M.P., L.L., F.S., F.F., G.C., and A.G. provided critical feedback and helped shape the research, analysis, and manuscript. All authors discussed the results and contributed to and approved the final manuscript.

Funding: This study was funded in full by Sanofi-Aventis Deutschland GmbH.

Acknowledgments: The authors would like to thank Thomas Rohban (Partner 4 Health, France) for providing medical writing support which was funded by Sanofi-Aventis Deutschland GmbH in accordance with Good Publication Practice (GPP3) guidelines.

Conflicts of Interest: Manuel Plomer is an employee of Sanofi-Aventis Deutschland GmbH.

References

1. World Health Organization (WHO). Diarrhoeal Disease: Fact Sheet. 2017. Available online: http://www.who.int/mediacentre/factsheets/fs330/en/ (accessed on 2 March 2018).
2. Beaugerie, L.; Sokol, H. Acute infectious diarrhea in adults: Epidemiology and management. *Presse Med.* **2013**, *42*, 52–59. [CrossRef] [PubMed]
3. Farthing, M.; Salam, M.A.; Lindberg, G.; Dite, P.; Khalif, I.; Salazar-Lindo, E.; Ramakrishna, B.S.; Goh, K.L.; Thomson, A.; Khan, A.G.; et al. Acute diarrhea in adults and children: A global perspective. *J. Clin. Gastroenterol.* **2013**, *47*, 12–20. [CrossRef] [PubMed]
4. Navaneethan, U.; Giannella, R.A. Mechanisms of infectious diarrhea. *Nat. Clin. Pract. Gastroenterol. Hepatol.* **2008**, *5*, 637–647. [CrossRef] [PubMed]
5. Guarner, F.; Schaafsma, G.J. Probiotics. *Int. J. Food Microbiol.* **1998**, *39*, 237–238. [CrossRef]
6. Matsuzaki, T.; Chin, J. Modulating immune responses with probiotic bacteria. *Immunol. Cell. Biol.* **2000**, *78*, 67–73. [CrossRef] [PubMed]
7. Cheikhyoussef, A.; Pogori, N.; Chen, W.; Zhang, H. Antimicrobial proteinaceous compounds obtained from bifidobacteria: From production to their application. *Int. J. Food Microbiol.* **2008**, *125*, 215–222. [CrossRef] [PubMed]
8. Abedi, D.; Feizizadeh, S.; Akbari, V.; Jafarian-Dehkordi, A. In vitro anti-bacterial and antiadherence effects of Lactobacillus delbrueckii subsp bulgaricus on *Escherichia coli. Res. Pharm. Sci.* **2013**, *8*, 260–268. [PubMed]
9. Duc, L.H.; Hong, H.A.; Barbosa, T.M.; Henriques, A.O.; Cutting, S.M. Characterization of Bacillus probiotics available for human use. *Appl. Environ. Microbiol.* **2004**, *70*, 2161–2171. [CrossRef]

10. Nista, E.C.; Candelli, M.; Cremonini, F.; Cazzato, I.A.; Zocco, M.A.; Franceschi, F.; Cammarota, G.; Gasbarrini, G.; Gasbarrini, A. *Bacillus clausii* therapy to reduce side-effects of anti-Helicobacter pylori treatment: Randomized, double-blind, placebo controlled trial. *Aliment. Pharmacol. Ther.* **2004**, *20*, 1181–1188. [CrossRef] [PubMed]
11. Sudha, M.R.; Bhonagiri, S.; Kumar, M.A. Efficacy of *Bacillus clausii* strain UBBC-07 in the treatment of patients suffering from acute diarrhoea. *Benef. Microbes* **2013**, *4*, 211–216. [CrossRef] [PubMed]
12. Guarino, A.; Ashkenazi, S.; Gendrel, D.; Lo Vecchio, A.; Shamir, R.; Szajewska, H. European Society for Pediatric Gastroenterology, Hepatology, and Nutrition; European Society for Pediatric Infectious Diseases. European Society for Pediatric Gastroenterology, Hepatology, and Nutrition/European Society for Pediatric Infectious Diseases evidence-based guidelines for the management of acute gastroenteritis in children in Europe: Update 2014. *J. Pediatr. Gastroenterol. Nutr.* **2014**, *59*, 132–152. [PubMed]
13. Ciffo, F. Determination of the spectrum of antibiotic resistance of the "*Bacillus subtilis*" strains of Enterogermina. *Chemioterapia* **1984**, *3*, 45–52. [PubMed]
14. Centre for Reviews and Dissemination, University of York. CRD's Guidance for Undertaking Reviews in Health Care. 2009. Available online: https://www.york.ac.uk/media/crd/Systematic_Reviews.pdf (accessed on 2 March 2018).
15. DerSimonian, R.; Laird, N. Meta-analysis in clinical trials. *Control. Clin. Trials* **1986**, *7*, 177–188. [CrossRef]
16. Higgins, J.P.; Thompson, S.G. Quantifying heterogeneity in a meta-analysis. *Stat. Med.* **2002**, *21*, 1539–1558. [CrossRef] [PubMed]
17. Egger, M.; Smith, G.D.; Altman, D.G. *Systematic Reviews in Health Care: Meta-Analysis in Context*, 2nd ed.; BMJ: London, UK, 2001.
18. Viechtbauer, W. Conducting Meta-Analyses in R with the metafor Package. *J. Stat. Softw.* **2010**, *36*, 1–48. [CrossRef]
19. Canani, R.B.; Cirillo, P.; Terrin, G.; Cesarano, L.; Spagnuolo, M.I.; De Vincenzo, A.; Albano, F.; Passariello, A.; De Marco, G.; Manguso, F.; et al. Probiotics for treatment of acute diarrhoea in children: Randomised clinical trial of five different preparations. *BMJ* **2007**, *335*, 340. [CrossRef] [PubMed]
20. Maugo, B.M. Effectiveness of *Bacillus clausii* in Reducing Duration of Illness in Acute Diarrhoea in Children 6–59 Months of Age Admitted With Severe Dehydration. Available online: http://erepository.uonbi.ac.ke/bitstream/handle/11295/8325/DR._MAUGO_BRIAN_MAUGO_M.MED_PAEDS_2012.pdf?sequence=1 (accessed on 19 April 2018).
21. Urtula, R.P.; Dacula, C.E. *Bacillus clausii* an Adjunct Treatment for Pediatric Patients with Acute Non-Bloody Diarrhea: A Randomized, Controlled Clinical Trial [Abstract]. Available online: http://arl4.library.sk/arl-sllk/en/detail-sllk_un_cat-0013574-Bacillus-clausii-an-adjunct-treatment-for-pediatric-patients-with-acute-nonbloody-diarrhea-a-rando/ (accessed on 19 April 2018).
22. Lahiri, K.R. GMA-CO Clinical Study Report: ENTER_L_01486. Sanofi-Aventis. Available online: https://www.sanofi.com/media/Project/One-Sanofi-Web/sanofi-com/common/docs/clinical-study-results/ENTER_L._01486_summary.pdf (accessed on 19 April 2018).
23. Lahiri, K.; Jadhav, K.; Gahlowt, P.; Najmuddin, F. *Bacillus Clausii* As An Adjuvant Therapy In Acute Childhood Diarrhoea. *IOSR-JDMS* **2015**, *14*, 74–76. Available online: http://www.iosrjournals.org/iosr-jdms/papers/Vol14-issue5/Version-1/S014517476.pdf (accessed on 19 April 2018).
24. Lahiri, K.; D'Souza, J.; Gahlowt, P. Beneficial Role of Probiotic in Acute Childhood Diarrhea. *J. Harmoniz. Res. Med. Health Sci.* **2015**, *2*, 26–30. Available online: https://www.johronline.com/issue/20150614-174258.724.pdf (accessed on 19 April 2018).
25. The Cochrane Collaboration. Cochrane Reviewers' Handbook 4.2.2. Available online: https://www.iecs.org.ar/cochrane/guias/Handbook_4-2-2.pdf (accessed on 19 April 2018).
26. Mendelsohn, A.S.; Asirvatham, J.R.; Mkaya Mwamburi, D.; Sowmynarayanan, T.V.; Malik, V.; Muliyil, J.; Kang, G. Estimates of the economic burden of rotavirus-associated and all-cause diarrhoea in Vellore, India. *Trop. Med. Int. Health* **2008**, *13*, 934–942. [CrossRef] [PubMed]
27. Burke, R.M.; Rebolledo, P.A.; Embrey, S.R.; Wagner, L.D.; Cowden, C.L.; Kelly, F.M.; Smith, E.R.; Iñiguez, V.; Leon, J.S. The burden of pediatric diarrhea: A cross-sectional study of incurred costs and perceptions of cost among Bolivian families. *BMC Public Health* **2013**, *13*, 708. [CrossRef] [PubMed]
28. Urdaci, M.C.; Bressollier, P.; Pinchuk, I. *Bacillus clausii* probiotic strains: Antimicrobial and immunomodulatory activities. *J. Clin. Gastroenterol.* **2004**, *38*, S86–S90. [CrossRef] [PubMed]

29. Cenci, G.; Trotta, F.; Caldini, G. Tolerance to challenges miming gastrointestinal transit by spores and vegetative cells of *Bacillus clausii*. *J. Appl. Microbiol.* **2006**, *101*, 1208–1215. [CrossRef] [PubMed]
30. Ripert, G.; Racedo, S.M.; Elie, A.M.; Jacquot, C.; Bressollier, P.; Urdaci, M.C. Secreted Compounds of the Probiotic *Bacillus clausii* Strain O/C Inhibit the Cytotoxic Effects Induced by *Clostridium difficile* and *Bacillus cereus* Toxins. *Antimicrob. Agents Chemother.* **2016**, *60*, 3445–3454. [CrossRef] [PubMed]
31. Salvetti, S.; Celandroni, F.; Ghelardi, E.; Baggiani, A.; Senesi, S. Rapid determination of vitamin B2 secretion by bacteria growing on solid media. *J. Appl. Microbiol.* **2003**, *95*, 1255–1260. [CrossRef] [PubMed]

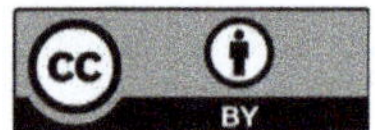

© 2018 by the authors. Licensee MDPI, Basel, Switzerland. This article is an open access article distributed under the terms and conditions of the Creative Commons Attribution (CC BY) license (http://creativecommons.org/licenses/by/4.0/).

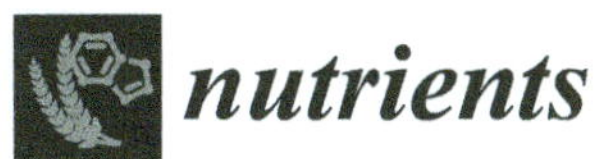

MDPI

Review

Human Milk Oligosaccharides: 2′-Fucosyllactose (2′-FL) and Lacto-N-Neotetraose (LNnT) in Infant Formula

Yvan Vandenplas [1,*], Bernard Berger [2], Virgilio Paolo Carnielli [3], Janusz Ksiazyk [4], Hanna Lagström [5], Manuel Sanchez Luna [6], Natalia Migacheva [7], Jean-Marc Mosselmans [8], Jean-Charles Picaud [9], Mike Possner [10], Atul Singhal [11] and Martin Wabitsch [12]

1 KidZ Health Castle, UZ Brussel, Vrije Universiteit Brussel, 1090 Brussels, Belgium
2 Department of Gastro-Intestinal Health, Nestlé Institute of Health Sciences, Nestlé Research, Nestec Ltd., 1015 Lausanne, Switzerland; bernard.berger@rdls.nestle.com
3 Neonatal Pediatrics, Polytechnic University of Marche, 60121 Ancona, Italy; v.carnielli@univpm.it
4 Department of Paediatrics, Nutrition and Metabolic Diseases, The Children's Memorial Health Institute, 04-730 Warsaw, Poland; J.Ksiazyk@IPCZD.Pl
5 Department of Public Health, University of Turku and Turku University Hospital, 20014 Turku, Finland; hanlag@utu.fi
6 Neonatology Division, Research Institute University Hospital Gregorio Marañón, Complutense University, 28009 Madrid, Spain; msluna@salud.madrid.org
7 Department of Pediatrics, Samara State Medical University, 443084 Samara, Russia; nbmigacheva@gmail.com
8 Citadelle For Life, 1000 Brussels, Belgium; jmm.mosselmans@gmail.com
9 Neonatology, Croix-Rousse Hospital, Lyon and CarMen Unit, INSERM U1060, INRA U197, Claude Bernard University, 69100 Lyon 1, France; jean-charles.picaud@chu-lyon.fr
10 Nestlé Nutrition Institute, 60528 Frankfurt/Main, Germany; Mike.Possner@de.nestle.com
11 Paediatric Nutrition, UCL Great Ormond Street Institute of Child Health, London WC1N 1EH, UK; a.singhal@ucl.ac.uk
12 Department of Paediatrics and Adolescent Medicine, Division of Paediatric Endocrinology and Diabetes, Centre for Hormonal Disorders in Children and Adolescents, Ulm University Hospital, 89075 Ulm, Germany; Martin.Wabitsch@uniklinik-ulm.de
* Correspondence: yvan.vandenplas@uzbrussel.be; Tel.: +32-(0)24775794

Received: 23 July 2018; Accepted: 14 August 2018; Published: 24 August 2018

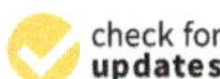

Abstract: The authors reviewed the published evidence on the presence of oligosaccharides in human milk (HMO) and their benefits in in vitro and in vivo studies. The still limited data of trials evaluating the effect of mainly 2′-fucosyllactose (2′-FL) on the addition of some of HMOs to infant formula were also reviewed. PubMed was searched from January 1990 to April 2018. The amount of HMOs in mother's milk is a dynamic process as it changes over time. Many factors, such as duration of lactation, environmental, and genetic factors, influence the amount of HMOs. HMOs may support immune function development and provide protection against infectious diseases directly through the interaction of the gut epithelial cells or indirectly through the modulation of the gut microbiota, including the stimulation of the bifidobacteria. The limited clinical data suggest that the addition of HMOs to infant formula seems to be safe and well tolerated, inducing a normal growth and suggesting a trend towards health benefits. HMOs are one of the major differences between cow's milk and human milk, and available evidence indicates that these components do have a health promoting benefit. The addition of one or two of these components to infant formula is safe, and brings infant formula closer to human milk. More prospective, randomized trials in infants are need to evaluate the clinical benefit of supplementing infant formula with HMOs.

Keywords: breast feeding; formula feeding; human milk oligosaccharide; 2′-fucosyllactose; Lacto-N-neotetraose; microbiota; bifidobacteria

1. Introduction

Breast milk is the natural and ideal food for infants, providing the energy and nutrients that every infant needs during the first four to six months of life in the correct quality and amount. Infants who are breastfed for shorter periods or are not breastfed suffer more infectious diseases, such as gastroenteritis and acute otitis media, more immune-mediated diseases, have a lower intelligent quotient (IQ) and are likely to have a higher risk of being overweight and type 2 diabetes in later life [1,2]. However, any breastfeeding is beneficial. In a pooled analysis of 24 studies from the USA and Europe, for example, any form of breastfeeding was found to be protective for acute otitis media in the first two years of life, but exclusive breastfeeding for the first six months was associated with the greatest protection [3].

The composition of breast milk is unique. Aside from nutrients for the infant's healthy growth and development, it contains thousands of bioactive substances [4], including human milk oligosaccharides (HMOs) [5]. HMOs are non-digestible carbohydrates [6]. Although they have little nutritional value for the infant, HMOs are the third largest solid component in human milk after lactose and lipids [7,8]. More than 200 free oligosaccharide structures have so far been identified from human milk samples [9]. Compared to human milk, oligosaccharide concentrations in the milk of farm animals, such as cows, goats, and sheep are 100–1000-fold lower. In fact, these unique complex carbohydrate structures in human milk are virtually absent in cow's milk or any other farmed animal milk, and their variety is much lower [10]. The difference in oligosaccharide content on human milk and cow milk, and, thus, cow milk-based infant formula, is likely to explain, at least in part, the differences in health outcomes between formula and breastfed infants.

2. Human Milk Oligosaccharides

Around 1900, infant mortality rate (deaths in the first year of life per 1000 live births) in Europe was very high at up to and above 20% [11,12]. Mortality was especially high in non-breastfed infants and was seven times greater in bottle-fed than breastfed infants [11,13]. It was around this time that differences in stool bacterial composition were discovered between breastfed and formula-fed infants and both breastfeeding and the resulting gut microbiota were linked to the better health of the infants [11,13]. In the 1930s, oligosaccharides were identified as the most important bifidogenic factor in human milk [11]. The most abundant oligosaccharides in human milk were discovered in 1954. However, it was only recently that scientists and industry were able to produce the first oligosaccharides structurally identical to those in human milk [14]. It is important to note that HMOs resist cold and heat and are not affected by pasteurization and freeze-drying [15,16].

The amount of HMOs is 20–25 g/L in colostrum and 10–15 gram per liter (g/L) in mature milk, or 1.5–2.3 g/100 kcal assuming an energy density of human milk of 64 kcal/100 mL [13,17]. Three major HMO categories are present in breast milk: (i) fucosylated neutral HMOs (35–50%); (ii) sialylated acidic HMOs (12–14%), and (iii) non-fucosylated neutral HMOs (42–55%) [18,19]. Neutral HMOs account for more than 75% of the total HMOs in human breast milk. 2′-fucosyllactose (2′-FL) is part of the fucosylated, while Lacto-N-neotetraose (LNnT) is part of the non-fucosylated neutral HMOs. In women who are "secretors", 2′-FL is by far the most abundant HMO and constitutes nearly 30% of all HMOs.

All HMOs are synthesized in the mammary gland [20]. The amount and composition of HMOs vary between women and over the course of lactation. HMO concentration is higher during the early stages of lactation and decreases gradually over time [21–23]. The Lewis antigen system is a human blood group system based upon two genes on chromosome 19: fucosyltransferase-3 (*FUT3)*, or Lewis gene; and *FUT2*, or Secretor gene. *FUT2* has a dominant allele which codes for an enzyme and a recessive allele which does not produce a functional enzyme. Similarly, *FUT3* has a functional dominant allele and a non-functional recessive allele. A recent study could not confirm the observation that the content of HMOs is also higher after a term than preterm delivery [24]. The most extreme intra individual variation in HMO fucosylation is based on the maternal secretor and Lewis blood group status [13,20,24]. Both the *FUT2* or secretor gene and the *FUT3* or Lewis gene are expressed in glandular epithelia. The secretor (*Se*) gene encodes for the *FUT2* which is necessary for the synthesis of 2′-FL and other Fucosyl-HMOs and is expressed in the lactating mammary gland. The milk of secretor (*Se*+) women is, therefore, characterized by an abundance of α1-2-fucosylated HMOs, especially 2′-FL [6,13,24]. Non-secretors, by contrast, lack the *FUT2* enzyme and, therefore, their milk does not contain 2′-FL and other α1-2-fucosylated HMOs, or is in only minimal amounts [6,25]. The absence of 2′-FL and other α1-2-fucosylated HMOs explains the lower total amount of HMOs in "non-secretor" milk [20]. For example, a recent study found approximately 35% to 45% less total HMOs in the milk of non-secretor Lewis-positive women than in the milk of Lewis-positive secretor women [20]. The acidic HMOs do not depend on secretor status [20].

Based on the expression of *FUT2* and *FUT3*, breast milk can be assigned to one of four groups (Table 1) [13]:

Group 1: Secretors, Lewis-positive, (Se+Le+) (*FUT2* active, *FUT3* active)
Group 2: Non-secretors, Lewis-positive, (Se−Le+) (*FUT2* inactive, *FUT3* active)
Group 3: Secretors, Lewis-negative (Se+Le−) (*FUT2* active, *FUT3* inactive)
Group 4: Non-secretors, Lewis-negative (Se−Le−) (*FUT2* inactive, *FUT3* inactive)

Table 1. Diversity of human milk oligosaccharides (HMO) based on genetic background of the mother.

Gene	Lewis Gene +	Lewis Gene −
Secretor gene +	Lewis positive secretors	Lewis negative secretors
	Secrete all HMOs	Secrete 2′-FL, 3′-FL, LNFP-I, LNFP-III
Secretor gene −	Lewis positive non-secretors	Lewis negative non-secretors
	Secrete 3′-FL, LNFP-II and LNFP III	Secrete 3′-FL, LNFP-III and LNFP-V

2′-FL: 2′-fucosyllactose; 3′-FL: 3′-fucosyllactose; LNFP: Lacto-N-fucopentaose.

About 80% of the European and American women are secretors [26]. About 70% of the populations are Lewis-positive secretors (Se+Le+) and around 5–10% are Lewis-negative secretors (Se+Le−) [27].

However, other factors also influence HMO synthesis. A recent study showed that HMO content and profiles vary geographically, even when secretor and Lewis blood group genes were considered [20,28]. Findings on HMO concentrations over time of lactation and clusters bas ed on 2′-FL concentrations suggest that LNnT and Lacto-N-Tetraose (LNT) are 'co-regulated' with the FUT2 dependent 2′-FL concentration, with LNnT showing a positive and LNT a negative relation to the amount of 2′-FL [6]. Mothers' milk with low levels of 2′-FL also contains low levels of LNnT but high levels of LNT [6]. The clinical impact of these findings still needs to be unraveled.

The European Union (EU) considers two HMOs, 2′-FL and LNnT, novel foods (Commission Implemented Regulation (EU) 2017/2470). Today, the USA's FDA considers three HMOs to be Generally Regarded as Safe (GRAS notice no 650). On 29 June 2015, the European Food Safety Authority (EFSA), based on the scientific and technical information provided, concluded that 2′-FL is safe for infants up to one year of age when added to infant and follow-on formulae, in combination with LNnT, at concentrations up to 1.2 g/L of 2′-FL and up to 0.6 g/L of LNnT, at a ratio of 2:1 in the reconstituted formulae. 2′-FL is safe for young children (older than one year of age) when added to follow-on and young-child formulae, at concentrations up to 1.2 g/L of 2′-FL (alone or in combination with LNnT, at concentrations up to 0.6 g/L, at a ratio of 2:1) (EFSA-Q-2015-00052, EFSA Journal 2015).

3. Health Benefit of Human Milk Oligosaccharides

Secretor milk (due to its high levels of 2′-FL and other Fucosyl-HMOs) may have advantages for the infant because it more effectively promotes an early high Bifidobacteria-dominated gut microbiota [29] and provides better protection against specific diarrheal diseases [30] than non-secretor milk.

Several studies have documented beneficial effects of HMOs, including modification of the intestinal microbiota, anti-adhesive antimicrobial effects, modulation of intestinal epithelial cell response, effects on immune development and on brain development.

4. Preclinical and Observational Studies

4.1. Modification of the Intestinal Microbiota

In vitro studies have shown that HMOs promote the growth of certain, but not all, bifidobacteria [13]. *Bifidobacterium longum subsp. infantis (B. infantis)* grows well on HMOs (including 2′-FL) as the sole source of carbohydrates [31–34]. Compared to *B. infantis*, *Bifidobacterium bifidum* grows slightly slower on HMOs [33]. Recent literature showed in strains from other bifidobacterial species that the metabolic capacity to utilize HMOs is not restricted to *B. infantis* [35–37].

Observational studies showed that 2′-Fucosyl-HMOs are associated with bifidobacteria dominated early gut microbiota in breastfed infants [29,35,38].

The fact that HMOs are a preferred substrate for *B. infantis* and other bifidobacteria strains may reduce the nutrients available for potentially harmful bacteria and keep their growth under control. In addition, *B. infantis* produces short-chain fatty acids (SCFA), which help create an environment favoring the growth of commensal bacteria instead of potential pathogens [39].

An in vitro study evaluated HMOs′ utilization by *Enterobacteriaceae*, which has been linked to the onset of necrotizing enterocolitis (NEC) in preterm infants [40]. The study showed that none of the *Enterobacteriaceae* strains grow on 2′-FL, 6-siallylactose (6′-SL), and LNnT, whereas several *Enterobacteriacea* strains, including pathogens, grew well on galacto-oligosaccharides (GOS) [40]. The influence of secretor status and breastfeeding on gut microbiota composition persists up to two to three years [38].

4.2. Anti-Adhesive Antimicrobial

Many viruses, bacterial pathogens or toxins need to adhere to mucosal surfaces to colonize or invade the host and cause disease [13,41,42]. Some HMOs are structurally similar to the intestinal epithelial cell surface glycan receptors and serve as decoy receptors to prevent pathogen binding and enhance pathogen clearance [13]. This unique beneficial effect of HMOs is highly dependent on their structure.

Evidence for an anti-adhesive effect of specific HMOs comes from in vitro and ex vivo studies. For instance, Ruiz-Palacios et al. demonstrated that human milk oligosaccharides inhibited *Campylobacter jejuni (C. jejuni)* adherence to epithelial cells in vitro [43], one of the major causes of bacterial diarrhea worldwide. A second study conducted by the same group confirmed that fucosylated human milk oligosaccharides inhibit *Campylobacter* colonization of human intestinal mucosa ex vivo [43]. Yu et al. tested the ability of 2′-FL to inhibit *C. jejuni* infection of the intestinal epithelium and *C. jejuni*-associated mucosal inflammation [44]. In an in vitro model, 2′-FL attenuated 80% of *C. jejuni* invasion ($p < 0.05$) and decreased the release of mucosal pro-inflammatory signals. In a mouse model, ingestion of 2′-FL reduced *C. jejuni* colonization by 80%, weight loss by 5%, intestinal inflammation (shown by histologic features), and induction of inflammatory signaling molecules ($p < 0.05$) [44].

In infants, observations from a prospective study conducted by Morrow et al. suggested a beneficial effect of α1-2-fucosylated HMO on reducing episodes of *C. jejuni*-associated diarrhea [30]. In Mexican breastfed infants, *Campylobacter* diarrhea occurred less often in those infants whose mother′s milk contained a high percentage of milk oligosaccharides of 2′-FL than in those infant whose mother's milk contained a lower percentage of 2′-FL oligosaccharides. There was a dose-dependent association with higher rates of moderate-to-severe diarrhea of all causes. The association between milk oligosaccharides measured during the first months and diarrhea in breastfed infants persisted through the course of lactation but not after cessation of breastfeeding [30].

Other observational studies of breastfed infants also suggested beneficial effects of fucosyl-HMOs in breast milk. They showed that fucosyl-HMOs in breast milk are related to lower morbidity in Gambian infants at four months of age [45] and fewer respiratory and enteric problems in US infants at three months of age [46].

The influence of 2′-FL and 6′-SL on adhesion of *Escherichia coli* and *Salmonella fyris* to Caco-2 cells was tested with positive results for *E. coli* but not for *Salmonella* [47].

HMOs have also been suggested to possibly protect against important systemic infections of the newborn. For instance, LNnT reduces *Streptococcus (S.) pneumoniae* load in lungs in a rabbit model [48]. A clinical study with infants older than six months, however, could not achieve a reduction in the colonization of the oropharynx with *S. pneumoniae* through a synthetic LNnT-supplemented infant formula [49].

HMOs may function as an alternative substrate to modify a group B *Streptococcus* component in a manner that impairs growth kinetics [50]. There is a unique antibacterial role for HMOs against this leading neonatal pathogen [50].

There is increasing evidence that HMOs could reduce infant mortality and morbidity in preterm infants, for example by shaping a favorable gut microbiome protecting against NEC, candidiasis, and several other immune-related diseases [51]. In support of this, a lower concentration of the HMO disialyllacto-N-tetraose (DSNLT) was shown to predict the risk of NEC in preterm infants. This finding has been demonstrated by a recent multicenter clinical cohort study including 200 mothers and their very low birthweight infants who were predominantly human milk-fed [52]. DSLNT concentrations were significantly lower in almost all milk samples in NEC cases compared with controls, and its abundance could identify NEC cases before onset, i.e., DSLNT content in breast milk is a potential non-invasive marker to identify infants at risk of developing NEC, and screen high-risk donor milk. Beneficial effects on NEC have also been reported for 2′-FL. Good et al. demonstrated that 2′-FL attenuates the severity of the experimental NEC by enhancing mesenteric perfusion in the neonatal intestine on an experimental mouse model of NEC [53].

4.3. Modulators of Intestinal Epithelial Cell Response

HMOs are able to reduce cell growth, induce differentiation, apoptosis and maturation, and increase the barrier function in vitro [54–57]. Intestinal health and intestinal barrier function constitute the first defense line in innate immunity.

Zehra et al. demonstrated that the HMOs 6′-siallyllactose and 2′-FL modulate human epithelial cell responses related to allergic disease in different ways [58]. 6′-Sialyllactose inhibited chemokine (Interleukin (IL)-8 and CCL20) release from T-84 and HT-29 cells stimulated with antigen-antibody complex tumor necrosis factor-alfa (TNF-α) or prostaglandin-E2 (PGE-2); an effect that was PPARγ dependent and associated with decreased activity of the transcription factors AP-1 and nuclear factor kappa-light-chain-enhancer of activated B cells) NF-κB. In contrast, 2′-FL selectively inhibited CCL20 release in response to the antigen-antibody complex in PPARγ dependent manner. These findings reinforce the concept that structurally different oligosaccharides have distinct biological activities and identifies, and for the first time, that the HMOs, 6′-SL, and 2′-FL, modulate human epithelial cell responses related to allergic diseases. This encourages further investigation of the therapeutic potential of specific HMOs in food allergy [58].

4.4. Immune Modulators

Among the multiple functions of HMOs, immunomodulation is one of the most remarkable [59]. HMOs directly affect intestinal epithelial cells and modulate their gene expression, which leads to changes in cell surface glycans and other cell responses. HMOs modulate lymphocyte cytokine production, potentially leading to a more balanced TH1/TH2 response.

An increasing number of in vitro studies suggest that HMOs not only affect the infant's immune system indirectly by changing gut microbiota but also directly modulate immune responses by affecting immune cell populations and cytokine secretion [5]. HMOs may either act locally on cells of the mucosa-associated lymphoid tissues or on a systemic level [13].

Dietary HMOs were more effective than non-human prebiotic oligosaccharides in altering systemic and gastrointestinal immune cells in pigs [60]. These altered immune cell populations may mediate the effects of dietary HMOs on rotavirus infection susceptibility [60]. Daily oral treatment with 2′-FL attenuated food allergy symptoms in a mouth model by induction of IL-10+ T-regulatory cells and indirect stabilization of mast cells [61].

In vitro studies have shown that 2′-FL directly inhibits lypopolysaccharide-mediated inflammation during enterotoxigenic *E. coli* (ETEC) invasion of T84 (modeling mature) and H4 (modeling immature) intestinal epithelial cells through attenuation of CD14 induction [62]. CD14 expression mediates lypoplysaccharide-TLR4 (toll-like receptor 4) stimulation of portions of the 'macrophage migration inhibitory factors' inflammatory pathway via suppressors of cytokine signaling 2/signal transducer and activator of transcription 3/NF-κB.

In an animal model, early life provision for a period of 6 weeks of 1% authentic HMOs delayed and suppressed Type 1 diabetes development in non-obese diabetic mice and reduced the development of severe pancreatic insulitis in later life [63]. In a murine influenza vaccination model dietary 2′-FL improved both humoral and cellular immune responses to vaccination in mice, enhancing vaccine specific delayed-type hypersensitivity responses accompanied by increased serum levels of vaccine-specific immunoglobulin proliferation. Vaccine-specific CD4+ and CD8+ T-cells, as well as interferon-gamma production, were significantly increased in spleen cells of mice receiving 2′-FL leading to the conclusion that dietary intervention with 2′-FL improved both humoral and cellular immune responses to vaccination in mice [64].

4.5. Brain Development

Metabolic products of HMOs such as sialic acid promote brain development, neuronal transmission, and synaptogenesis. HMOs provide sialic acid as potentially essential nutrients for brain development and cognition [65,66]. Application of L-fucose and 2′-FL increases the potentiation of the population spike amplitude (POP-spike) and the field excitatory postsynaptic potential (fEPSP) after tetanization of the Schaffer collaterals of the rat hippocampus [67]. Dietary 2′-FL interferes with cognitive domains and improves learning and memory in rodents [68]. HMOs, 3′-Sialyllactose and 6′-Sialyllactose, support normal microbial communities and behavioral responses during stressor exposure, potentially through effects on the gut microbiota–brain axis [69].

4.6. Improved Gut Adaptation after Resection

Patients with short bowel syndrome require parental nutrition and may require frequent treatment with antibiotics that modify intestinal microbiota and have an adverse effect on gastrointestinal function [70]. The hypothesis that 2′-FL contributes to the adaptive response after intestinal resection was confirmed on the basis of a murine model of intestinal adaptation. Modulating of gut microbiota following intestinal resection improved the outcome of short bowel syndrome in an experimental setting. Supplementation with 2′-FL increased weight gain following ileo-cecal resection and promoted histological changes in gut mucosa suitable for adaptation [71].

5. Clinical Studies with 2′-fucosyllactose

One prospective, randomized, controlled study tested the tolerance and safety in relation to growth of an infant formula containing 2′-FL (0.2 g/L or 1.0 g/L) in combination with galacto-oligosaccahrides (2.2 g/L or 1.4 g/L) in healthy full-term infants from 28 sites across USA [72].

No differences in growth parameters and adverse events were found between the infants fed the formula with 2′-FL from enrolment (0–5 days of age) up to the age of four months compared to infants fed a control formula containing only galacto-oligosaccharides and between both formula-fed groups and the breastfed reference group. This study was the first publication showing that growth of infants consuming a formula containing 2′-FL was similar to that of human milk-fed infants [72]. Both formulas with 2′-FL and galacto-oligosaccharides were well tolerated and did not influence stool frequency or consistency.

The effects of feeding formulas supplemented with 2′-FL on biomarkers of immune function were investigated in a subgroup of this study population [73]. Infants fed formulas with 2′-FL and galacto-oligosaccharides had 29–83% lower concentrations of plasma inflammatory cytokines and TNF-α than infants fed the control formula with galacto-oligosaccharides only [73]. There were no differences in plasma inflammatory cytokines and TNF-α between infants fed formulas with 2′-FL and galacto-oligosaccharides and infants breastfed. These findings indicate that supplementation of infant formula with 2′-FL supports aspects of immune development and regulation similar to that of breastfed infants; while supplementation with galacto-oligosachairdes alone does not [73].

Another prospective, randomized, controlled study tested the gastrointestinal tolerance of an infant formula containing 2′-FL (0.2 g/L) in combination with fructo-oligosaccharides (2 g/L) compared to a control formula without oligosaccharides [74]. The formula with 2′-FL and fructo-oligosaccharides fed from less than eight days of age for approximately one month was well tolerated; stool consistency, anthropometric data, and frequency of feedings with spitting up/vomiting and was similar to that of infants given formula without oligosaccharides or to infants breastfed [74].

Puccio et al. conducted the first clinical trial with an infant formula supplemented with two HMOs [75]. In this prospective, randomized, controlled multicenter study, healthy term infants received a formula with 2′-FL and LNnT or the same formula without HMOs from enrolment at $\leq$14 days of age to age six months and for at least four months as the exclusive diet [75]. The formula with 2′-FL and LNnT was well-tolerated and supported age-appropriate growth. Gastrointestinal symptoms (flatulence, spitting up, and vomiting) were similar between the groups. Infants receiving formula with 2′-FL and LNnT had significantly softer stools and fewer episodes of night-time wake-ups at age two months, and infants born by caesarian section also had a lower incidence of colic at four months of age. Puccio et al. also analyzed the incidence of different health outcomes as secondary outcomes. Infants fed the formula with 2′-FL and LNnT compared to infants fed the formula without HMOs had significantly fewer parental reports of bronchitis (at 4, 6, and 12 months), reduced incidence of lower respiratory tract infections (through 12 months), reduced use of antipyretics (through four months) and reduced use of antibiotics (through 6 and 12 months) with protective effects that continued after the six months intervention period [75].

In the same trial, infants fed the formula with 2′-FL and LNnT developed a gut microbiota that was closer to the microbiota observed in breastfed infants [76]. At three months of age, the stool microbiota was characterized by an increased quantity of beneficial bifidobacteria and decreased abundances of taxa with potentially pathogenic members. Moreover, the supplementation of infant formula with these two HMOs promoted the growth of a distinct fecal bacteria community, typical of breastfed infants and showing a very high density of bacteria. Formula-fed infants carrying this fecal community type had a two times decreased risk of requiring antibiotics during the first year of life [76]. Therefore, this study suggests that the association between consuming formula with 2′-FL and LNnT and lower parent-reported morbidity and medication use may be linked to gut microbiota community types [76].

Today, the amount of data available on HMO supplementation in infant formula from clinical trials in infants is still limited. More data are definitely needed. According to the data from the few studies, differences in clinical outcome of supplemented vs. non-supplemented formula are not yet conclusive [72–76]. The different primary outcomes of the different trials contribute to a lack of coherent results. The cost-benefit ratio also needs further evaluation. In addition, the optimal concentration of

HMO added needs further adjustment. And of course, there is the fact that only one or two HMOs are added to infant formula, while mother's milk contains 200 different oligosaccharides. Supplementation with more HMOs could result in further evidence of benefit.

6. Conclusions

HMOs act as soluble decoy receptors that block the attachment of specific viral, bacterial or protozoan parasite pathogens to epithelial cell surface sugars, which may, in turn, help prevent infectious diseases in the gut, respiratory, and urinary tracts. In addition, HMOs alter host epithelial and immune cell responses with potential benefits for the neonate, beyond protection against infectious diseases.

Although the functions of HMOs have been known for many years, it was not possible to synthesize them on an industrial scale until recently. With the goal of imitating their effect, non-human milk oligosaccharides, mainly fructo and galacto-oligosaccharides have been added to infant formula. In recent years it has, to a certain extent, become technically possible to add 2′-FL and LNnT to infant formula.

The addition of one HMO, namely 2′-FL, is a step forward in bringing formula feeding closer to the gold standard: Mother's milk. No adverse effects have been reported for 2′-FL and in vitro and animal studies have shown benefits of supplementation of infant formula with 2′-FL. The first clinical data in infants show a normal growth pattern and normal defecation and suggest clinical benefit. More prospective, randomized trials in infants comparing formula without and with HMOs are still needed to evaluate the clinical effects of this supplementation. It can, therefore, be concluded that 2′-FL is a safe supplementation of infant formula.

Author Contributions: Y.V. participated as a clinical investigator, and/or advisory board member, and/or consultant, and/or speaker for Abbott Nutrition, Biocodex, Danone, Nestle Health Science, Nestle Nutrition Institute, Nutricia, Mead Johnson, United Pharmaceuticals. B.B. is an employee of Nestec Ltd., a subsidiary company of the Nestlé group. V.P.C. participated as an advisory board member for Nestle Nutrition Institute. J.K. was a speaker for Danone, Nutricia, Nestle, Fresenius Kabi and participated in the meetings of Nestle Nutrition Institute. H.L. participated as an advisory board member, consultant, and speaker for Nestlé Nutrition Institute and Nestlé Finland. M.S.L. participated as a clinical investigator, and/or advisory board member, and/or consultant, and/or speaker for Abbvie, Dräger, Nestle Nutrition Institute, Linde Healthcare. N.M. declares no conflict of interest. J.-M.M. is an advisory board moderator for Nestle Nutrition Institute. J.-C.P. participated as a clinical investigator, and/or advisory board member, and/or speaker for Nestle Nutrition Institute, Modilac France, Bledina France and Nestlé Health Science. M.P. is employed by Nestlé Nutrition Institute. A.S. participated as a clinical investigator, and/or advisory board member, and/or speaker for Abbott Nutrition, Wyeth Nutrition, Nestle Health Science, Nestle Nutrition Institute, Danone and Phillips. M.W. participated as an advisory board member for Nestle Nutrition Institute.

Funding: This research received no external funding.

Conflicts of Interest: The authors declare no conflict of interest.

References

1. ESPGHAN Committee on Nutrition; Agostoni, C.; Braegger, C.; Decsi, T.; Kolacek, S.; Koletzko, B.; Michaelsen, K.F.; Mihatsch, W.; Moreno, L.A.; Puntis, J.; et al. Breast-feeding: A commentary by the ESPGHAN Committee on Nutrition. *J. Pediatr. Gastroenterol. Nutr.* **2009**, *49*, 112–125. [CrossRef] [PubMed]
2. Victora, C.G.; Bahl, R.; Barros, A.J.; França, G.V.; Horton, S.; Krasevec, J.; Murch, S.; Sankar, M.J.; Walker, N.; Rollins, N.C. Lancet Breastfeeding Series Group. Breastfeeding in the 21st century: Epidemiology, mechanisms, and lifelong effect. *Lancet* **2016**, *387*, 475–490. [CrossRef]
3. Bowatte, G.; Tham, R.; Allen, K.J.; Tan, D.J.; Lau, M.; Dai, X.; Lodge, C.J. Breastfeeding and childhood acute otitis media: A systematic review and meta-analysis. *Acta Paediatr.* **2015**, *104*, 85–95. [CrossRef] [PubMed]
4. Mosca, F.; Giannì, M.L. Human milk: Composition and health benefits. *Pediatr. Med. Chir.* **2017**, *39*, 155. [CrossRef] [PubMed]
5. Donovan, S.M.; Comstock, S.S. Milk oligosaccharides influence neonatal mucosal and systemic immunity. *Ann. Nutr. Metab.* **2016**, *69* (Suppl. 2), 42–51. [CrossRef] [PubMed]

6. Sprenger, N.; Lee, L.Y.; De Castro, C.A.; Steenhout, P.; Thakkar, S.K. Longitudinal change of selected human milk oligosaccharides and association to infants' growth, an observatory, single center, longitudinal cohort study. *PLoS ONE* **2017**, *12*, e0171814. [CrossRef] [PubMed]
7. Ballard, O.; Morrow, A.L. Human milk composition: Nutrients and bioactive factors. *Pediatr. Clin. North Am.* **2013**, *60*, 49–74. [CrossRef] [PubMed]
8. Austin, S.; De Castro, C.A.; Bénet, T.; Hou, Y.; Sun, H.; Thakkar, S.K.; Vinyes-Pares, G.; Zhang, Y.; Wang, P. Temporal change of the content of 10 oligosaccharides in the milk of Chinese urban mothers. *Nutrients* **2016**, *8*, 346. [CrossRef] [PubMed]
9. Ruhaak, L.R.; Lebrilla, C.B. Advances in analysis of human milk oligosaccharides. *Adv. Nutr.* **2012**, *3*, 406S–414S. [CrossRef] [PubMed]
10. Urashima, T.; Taufik, E.; Fukuda, K.; Asakuma, S. Recent advances in studies on milk oligosaccharides of cows and other domestic farm animals. *Biosci. Biotechnol. Biochem.* **2013**, *77*, 455–466. [CrossRef] [PubMed]
11. Kunz, C. Historical aspects of human milk oligosaccharides. *Adv. Nutr.* **2012**, *3*, 430S–439S. [CrossRef] [PubMed]
12. Elwood, J.H. Infant mortality in Belfast and Dublin—1900–1969. *Irish J. Med. Sci.* **1973**, *142*, 166–173. [CrossRef] [PubMed]
13. Bode, L. Human milk oligosaccharides: Every baby needs a sugar mama. *Glycobiology* **2012**, *22*, 1147–1162. [CrossRef] [PubMed]
14. Petschacher, B.; Nidetzky, B. Biotechnological production of fucosylated human milk oligosaccharides: Prokaryotic fucosyltransferases and their use in biocatalytic cascades or whole cell conversion systems. *J. Biotechnol.* **2016**, *235*, 61–83. [CrossRef] [PubMed]
15. Hahn, W.H.; Kim, J.; Song, S.; Park, S.; Kang, N.M. The human milk oligosaccharides are not affected by pasteurization and freeze-drying. *J. Matern.-Fetal Neonatal Med.* **2017**, *6*, 1–7. [CrossRef] [PubMed]
16. Daniels, B.; Coutsoudis, A.; Autran, C.; Amundson Mansen, K.; Israel-Ballard, K.; Bode, L. The effect of simulated flash heating pasteurisation and Holder pasteurisation on human milk oligosaccharides. *Paediatr. Int. Child Health* **2017**, *37*, 204–209. [CrossRef] [PubMed]
17. Zivkovic, A.M.; German, J.B.; Lebrilla, C.B.; Mills, D.A. Human milk glycobiome and its impact on the infant gastrointestinal microbiota. *Proc. Natl. Acad. Sci. USA* **2011**, *108* (Suppl. 1), 4653–4658. [CrossRef] [PubMed]
18. Smilowitz, J.T.; Lebrilla, C.B.; Mills, D.A.; German, J.B.; Freeman, S.L. Breast milk oligosaccharides: Structure-function relationships in the neonate. *Ann. Rev. Nutr.* **2014**, *34*, 143–169. [CrossRef] [PubMed]
19. Van Niekerk, E.; Autran, C.A.; Nel, D.G.; Kirsten, G.F.; Blaauw, R.; Bode, L. Human milk oligosaccharides differ between HIV-infected and HIV-uninfected mothers and are related to necrotizing enterocolitis incidence in their preterm very-low-birth-weight infants. *J. Nutr.* **2014**, *144*, 1227–1233. [CrossRef] [PubMed]
20. Akkerman, R.; Faas, M.M.; de Vos, P. Non-digestible carbohydrates in infant formula as substitution for human milk oligosaccharide functions: Effects on microbiota and gut maturation. *Crit. Rev. Food Sci. Nutr.* **2018**, *15*, 1–12. [CrossRef] [PubMed]
21. Xu, G.; Davis, J.C.; Goonatilleke, E.; Smilowitz, J.T.; German, J.B.; Lebrilla, C.B. Absolute quantitation of human milk oligosaccharides reveals phenotypic variations during lactation. *J. Nutr.* **2017**, *147*, 117–124. [CrossRef] [PubMed]
22. Chaturvedi, P.; Warren, C.D.; Altaye, M.; Morrow, A.L.; Ruiz-Palacios, G.; Pickering, L.K.; Newburg, D.S. Fucosylated human milk oligosaccharides vary between individuals and over the course of lactation. *Glycobiology* **2001**, *11*, 365–372. [CrossRef] [PubMed]
23. Thurl, S.; Munzert, M.; Henker, J.; Boehm, G.; Muller-Werner, B.; Jelinek, J. Varation of human milk oligosaccharides in relation to milk groups and lactational periods. *Br. J. Nutr.* **2010**, *104*, 1261–1271. [CrossRef] [PubMed]
24. Kunz, C.; Rudloff, S. Compositional analysis and metabolism of human milk oligosaccharides in infants. *Nestle Nutr. Inst. Workshop Ser.* **2017**, *88*, 137–147. [PubMed]
25. Jantscher-Krenn, E.; Bode, L. Human milk oligosaccharides and their potential benefits for the breast-fed neonate. *Minerva Pediatr.* **2012**, *64*, 83–99. [PubMed]
26. Goehring, K.C.; Kennedy, A.D.; Prieto, P.A.; Buck, R.H. Direct evidence for the presence of human milk oligosaccharides in the circulation of breastfed infants. *PLoS ONE* **2014**, *9*, e101692. [CrossRef] [PubMed]
27. Rudloff, S.; Kunz, C. Milk oligosaccharides and metabolism in infants. *Adv. Nutr.* **2012**, *3*, 398S–405S. [CrossRef] [PubMed]

28. McGuire, M.K.; Meehan, C.L.; McGuire, M.A.; Williams, J.E.; Foster, J.; Sellen, D.W.; Kamau-Mbuthia, E.W.; Kamundia, E.W.; Mbugua, S.; Moore, S.E.; et al. What's normal? Oligosaccharide concentrations and profiles in milk produced by healthy women vary geographically. *Am. J. Clin. Nutr.* **2017**, *105*, 1086–1100. [CrossRef] [PubMed]
29. Lewis, Z.T.; Totten, S.M.; Smilowitz, J.T.; Popovic, M.; Parker, E.; Lemay, D.G.; Van Tassell, M.L.; Miller, M.J.; Jin, Y.S.; German, J.B.; et al. Maternal fucosyltransferase 2 status affects the gut bifidobacterial communities of breastfed infants. *Microbiome* **2015**, *3*, 13. [CrossRef] [PubMed]
30. Morrow, A.L.; Ruiz-Palacios, G.M.; Altaye, M.; Jiang, X.; Guerrero, M.L.; Meinzen-Derr, J.K.; Farkas, T.; Chaturvedi, P.; Pickering, L.K.; Newburg, D.S. Human milk oligosaccharide blood group epitopes and innate immune protection against *Campylobacter* and calicivirus diarrhea in breastfed infants. *Adv. Exp. Med. Biol.* **2004**, *554*, 443–446. [PubMed]
31. Lo Cascio, R.G.; Ninonuevo, M.R.; Freeman, S.L.; Sela, D.A.; Grimm, R.; Lebrilla, C.B.; Mills, D.A.; German, J.B. Glycoprofiling of bifidobacterial consumption of human milk oligosaccharides demonstrates strain specific, preferential consumption of small chain glycans secreted in early human lactation. *J. Agric. Food Chem.* **2007**, *55*, 8914–8919. [CrossRef] [PubMed]
32. Marcobal, A.; Barboza, M.; Froehlich, J.W.; Block, D.E.; German, J.B.; Lebrilla, C.B.; Mills, D.A. Consumption of human milk oligosaccharides by gut-related microbes. *J. Agric Food Chem.* **2010**, *58*, 5334–5340. [CrossRef] [PubMed]
33. Asakuma, S.; Hatakeyama, E.; Urashima, T.; Yoshida, E.; Katayama, T.; Yamamoto, K.; Kumagai, H.; Ashida, H.; Hirose, J.; Kitaoka, M. Physiology of consumption of human milk oligosaccharides by infant gut-associated bifidobacteria. *J. Biol. Chem.* **2011**, *286*, 34583–34592. [CrossRef] [PubMed]
34. Bunesova, V.; Lacroix, C.; Schwab, C. Fucosyllactose and L-fucose utilization of infant *Bifidobacterium longum* and *Bifidobacterium kashiwanohense*. *BMC Microbiol.* **2016**, *16*, 248. [CrossRef] [PubMed]
35. Matsuki, T.; Yahagi, K.; Mori, H.; Matsumoto, H.; Hara, T.; Tajima, S.; Ogawa, E.; Kodama, H.; Yamamoto, K.; Yamada, T.; et al. A key genetic factor for fucosyllactose utilization affects infant gut microbiota development. *Nat. Commun.* **2016**, *7*, 11939. [CrossRef] [PubMed]
36. James, K.; Motherway, M.O.; Bottacini, F.; van Sinderen, D. *Bifidobacterium breve* UCC2003 metabolises the human milk oligosaccharides lacto-N-tetraose and lacto-N-neo-tetraose through overlapping, yet distinct pathways. *Sci. Rep.* **2016**, *6*, 38560. [CrossRef] [PubMed]
37. Garrido, D.; Ruiz-Moyano, S.; Kirmiz, N.; Davis, J.C.; Totten, S.M.; Lemay, D.G.; Ugalde, J.A.; German, J.B.; Lebrilla, C.B.; Mills, D.A. A novel gene cluster allows preferential utilization of fucosylated milk oligosaccharides in *Bifidobacterium longum* subsp. longum SC596. *Sci. Rep.* **2016**, *6*, 35045. [CrossRef] [PubMed]
38. Smith-Brown, P.; Morrison, M.; Krause, L.; Davies, P.S. Mothers secretor status affects development of childrens microbiota composition and function: A pilot study. *PLoS ONE* **2016**, *11*, e0161211. [CrossRef] [PubMed]
39. Gibson, G.R.; Wang, X. Regulatory effects of bifidobacteria on the growth of other colonic bacteria. *J. Appl. Bacteriol.* **1994**, *77*, 412–420. [CrossRef] [PubMed]
40. Hoeflinger, J.L.; Davis, S.R.; Chow, J.; Miller, M.J. In vitro impact of human milk oligosaccharides on *Enterobacteriaceae* growth. *J. Agric. Food Chem.* **2015**, *63*, 3295–3302. [CrossRef] [PubMed]
41. Bode, L. The functional biology of human milk oligosaccharides. *Early Hum. Dev.* **2015**, *9*, 619–622. [CrossRef] [PubMed]
42. Hu, L.; Crawford, S.E.; Czako, R.; Cortes-Penfield, N.W.; Smith, D.F.; Le Pendu, J.; Estes, M.K.; Prasad, B.V. Cell attachment protein VP8* of a human rotavirus specifically interacts with A-type histo-blood group antigen. *Nature* **2012**, *485*, 256–259. [CrossRef] [PubMed]
43. Ruiz-Palacios, G.M.; Cervantes, L.E.; Ramos, P.; Chavez-Munguia, B.; Newburg, D.S. *Campylobacter jejuni* binds intestinal H(O) antigen (Fucα1, 2Galβ1, 4GlcNAc), and fucosyloligosaccharides of human milk inhibit its binding and infection. *J. Biol. Chem.* **2003**, *278*, 14112–14120. [CrossRef] [PubMed]
44. Yu, Z.T.; Nanthakumar, N.N.; Newburg, D.S. The human milk oligosaccharide 2′-fucosyllactose quenches *Campylobacter jejuni*-induced inflammation in human epithelial cells HEp-2 and HT-29 and in mouse intestinal mucosa. *J. Nutr.* **2016**, *146*, 1980–1990. [CrossRef] [PubMed]
45. Davis, J.C.; Lewis, Z.T.; Krishnan, S.; Bernstein, R.M.; Moore, S.E.; Prentice, A.M.; Mills, D.A.; Lebrilla, C.B.; Zivkovic, A.M. Growth and morbidity of Gambian infants are influenced by maternal milk oligosaccharides and infant gut microbiota. *Sci. Rep.* **2017**, *7*, 40466. [CrossRef] [PubMed]

46. Stepans, M.B.; Wilhelm, S.L.; Hertzog, M.; Rodehorst, T.K.; Blaney, S.; Clemens, B.; Polak, J.J.; Newburg, D.S. Early consumption of human milk oligosaccharides is inversely related to subsequent risk of respiratory and enteric disease in infants. *Breastfeed. Med.* **2006**, *1*, 207–215. [CrossRef] [PubMed]
47. Facinelli, B.; Marini, E.; Magi, G.; Zampini, L.; Santoro, L.; Catassi, C.; Monachesi, C.; Gabrielli, O.; Coppa, G.V. Breast milk oligosaccharides: Effects of 2′-fucosyllactose and 6′-sialyllactose on the adhesion of *Escherichia coli* and *Salmonella fyris* to Caco-2 cells. *J. Matern. Fetal Neonatal Med.* **2018**, *21*, 1–3. [CrossRef] [PubMed]
48. Idänpään-Heikkilä, I.; Simon, P.M.; Zopf, D.; Vullo, T.; Cahill, P.; Sokol, K.; Tuomanen, E. Oligosaccharides interfere with the establishment and progression of experimental pneumococcal pneumonia. *J. Infect. Dis.* **1997**, *176*, 704–712. [CrossRef] [PubMed]
49. Prieto, P.A. In vitro and clinical experiences with a human milk oligosaccharide, Lacto-N-neoTetraose, and Fructooligosaccharides. *Foods Food Ingred. J. Jpn.* **2005**, *210*, 1018–1030.
50. Lin, A.E.; Autran, C.A.; Szyszka, A.; Escajadillo, T.; Huang, M.; Godula, K.; Prudden, A.R.; Boons, G.J.; Lewis, A.L.; Doran, K.S.; et al. Human milk oligosaccharides inhibit growth of group B *Streptococcus*. *J. Biol. Chem.* **2017**, *292*, 11243–11249. [CrossRef] [PubMed]
51. Moukarzel, S.; Bode, L. Human milk oligosaccharides and the preterm infant: A journey in sickness and in health. *Clin. Perinatol.* **2017**, *44*, 193–207. [CrossRef] [PubMed]
52. Autran, C.A.; Kellman, B.P.; Kim, J.H.; Asztalos, E.; Blood, A.B.; Spence, E.C.; Patel, A.L.; Hou, J.; Lewis, N.E.; Bode, L. Human milk oligosaccharide composition predict risk of necrotizing entecolitis in preterm infants. *Gut* **2018**, *67*, 1064–1070. [CrossRef] [PubMed]
53. Good, M.; Sodhi, C.P.; Yamaguchi, Y.; Jia, H.; Lu, P.; Fulton, W.B.; Martin, L.Y.; Prindle, T.; Nino, D.F.; Zhou, Q.; et al. The human milk oligosaccharide 2′-fucosyllactose attenuates the severity of experimental NEC by enhancing mesenteric perfusion in the neonatal intestine. *Br. J. Nutr.* **2016**, *116*, 1175–1187. [CrossRef] [PubMed]
54. Kuntz, S.; Rudloff, S.; Kunz, C. Oligosaccharides from human milk influence growth-related characteristics of intestinally transformed and non-transformed intestinal cells. *Br. J. Nutr.* **2008**, *99*, 462–471. [CrossRef] [PubMed]
55. Kuntz, S.; Kunz, C.; Rudloff, S. Oligosaccharides from human milk induce growth arrest via G2/M by influencing growth-related cell cycle genes in intestinal epithelial cells. *Br. J. Nutr.* **2009**, *101*, 1306–1315. [CrossRef] [PubMed]
56. Holscher, H.D.; Davis, S.R.; Tappenden, K.A. Human milk oligosaccharides influence maturation of human intestinal Caco-2Bbe and HT-29 cell lines. *J. Nutr.* **2014**, *144*, 586–591. [CrossRef] [PubMed]
57. Holscher, H.D.; Bode, L.; Tappenden, K.A. Human milk oligosaccharides influence intestinal epithelial cell maturation in vitro. *J. Pediatr. Gastroenterol. Nutr.* **2017**, *64*, 296–301. [CrossRef] [PubMed]
58. Zehra, S.; Khambati, I.; Vierhout, M.; Mian, M.F.; Buck, R.; Forsythe, P. Human milk oligosaccharides attenuate antigen-antibody complex induced chemokine release from human intestinal epithelial cell lines. *J. Food Sci.* **2018**, *83*, 499–508. [CrossRef] [PubMed]
59. Kulinich, A.; Liu, L. Human milk oligosaccharides: The role in the fine-tuning of innate immune responses. *Carbohydr. Res.* **2016**, *432*, 62–70. [CrossRef] [PubMed]
60. Comstock, S.S.; Li, M.; Wang, M.; Monaco, M.H.; Kuhlenschmidt, T.B.; Kuhlenschmidt, M.S.; Donovan, S.M. Dietary human milk oligosaccharides but not prebiotic oligosaccharides increase circulating natural killer cell and mesenteric lymph node memory T-cell populations in non-infected and rotavirus-infected neonatal piglets. *J. Nutr.* **2017**, *147*, 1041–1047. [CrossRef] [PubMed]
61. Castillo-Courtade, L.; Han, S.; Lee, S.; Mian, F.M.; Buck, R.; Forsythe, P. Attenuation of food allergy symptoms following treatment with human milk oligosaccharides in a mouse model. *Allergy* **2015**, *70*, 1091–1102. [CrossRef] [PubMed]
62. He, Y.; Liu, S.; Leone, S.; Newburg, D.S. Human colostrum oligosaccharides modulate major immunologic pathways of immature human intestine. *Mucosal Immunol.* **2014**, *7*, 1326–1339. [CrossRef] [PubMed]
63. Xiao, L.; Van't Land, B.; Engen, P.A.; Naqib, A.; Green, S.J.; Nato, A.; Leusink-Muis, T.; Garssen, J.; Keshavarzian, A.; Stahl, B.; et al. Human milk oligosaccharides protect against the development of autoimmune diabetes in NOD-mice. *Sci. Rep.* **2018**, *8*, 3829. [CrossRef] [PubMed]
64. Xiao, L.; Leusink-Muis, T.; Kettelarij, N.; van Ark, I.; Blijenberg, B.; Hesen, N.A.; Stahl, B.; Overbeek, S.A.; Garssen, J.; Folkerts, G.; et al. Human milk oligosaccharide 2′-Fucosyllactose improves innate and adaptive immunity in an influenza-specific murine vaccination model. *Front. Immunol.* **2018**, *9*, 452. [CrossRef] [PubMed]
65. Bienenstock, J.; Buck, R.H.; Linke, H.; Forsythe, P.; Stanisz, A.M.; Kunze, W.A. Fucosylated but not sialylated milk oligosaccharides diminish colon motor contractions. *PLoS ONE* **2013**, *8*, e76236. [CrossRef] [PubMed]

66. Jacobi, S.K.; Yatsunenko, T.; Li, D.; Dasgupta, S.; Yu, R.K.; Berg, B.M.; Chichlowski, M.; Odle, J. Dietary isomers of sialyllactose increase ganglioside sialic acid concentrations in the corpus callosum and cerebellum and modulate the colonic microbiota of formula-fed piglets. *J. Nutr.* **2016**, *146*, 200–208. [CrossRef] [PubMed]
67. Matthies, H.; Staak, S.; Krug, M. Fucose and fucosyllactose enhance in-vitro hippocampal long-term potentiation. *Brain Res.* **1996**, *725*, 276–280. [CrossRef]
68. Vázquez, E.; Barranco, A.; Ramírez, M.; Gruart, A.; Delgado-García, J.M.; Martínez-Lara, E.; Blanco, S.; Martín, M.J.; Castanys, E.; Buck, R.; et al. Effects of a human milk oligosaccharide, 2′-fucosyllactose, on hippocampal long-term potentiation and learning capabilities in rodents. *J. Nutr. Biochem.* **2015**, *26*, 455–465. [CrossRef] [PubMed]
69. Tarr, A.J.; Galley, J.D.; Fisher, S.E.; Chichlowski, M.; Berg, B.M.; Bailey, M.T. The prebiotics 3′Sialyllactose and 6′Sialyllactose diminish stressor-induced anxiety-like behavior and colonic microbiota alterations: Evidence for effects on the gut-brain axis. *Brain Behav. Immun.* **2015**, *50*, 166–177. [CrossRef] [PubMed]
70. Sommovilla, J.; Zhou, Y.; Sun, R.C.; Choi, P.M.; Diaz-Miron, J.; Shaikh, N.; Sodergren, E.; Warner, B.B.; Weinstock, G.M.; Tarr, P.; et al. Small bowel resection induces long-term changes in the enteric microbiota of mice. *J. Gastrointest. Surg.* **2015**, *19*, 56–64. [CrossRef] [PubMed]
71. Mezoff, E.A.; Hawkins, J.A.; Ollberding, N.J.; Karns, R.; Morrow, A.L.; Helmrath, M.A. The human milk oligosaccharide 2′-fucosyllactose augments the adaptive response to extensive intestinal resection. *Am. J. Physiol. Gastrointest. Liver Physiol.* **2016**, *310*, G427–G438. [CrossRef] [PubMed]
72. Marriage, B.J.; Buck, R.H.; Goehring, K.C.; Oliver, J.S.; Williams, J.A. Infants fed a lower calorie formula with 2′-fucosyllactose (2′-FL2′-FL) show growth and 2′-FL2′-FL uptake like breast-fed infants. *J. Pediatr. Gastroenterol. Nutr.* **2015**, *61*, 649–658. [CrossRef] [PubMed]
73. Goehring, K.C.; Marriage, B.J.; Oliver, J.S.; Wilder, J.A.; Barrett, E.G.; Buck, R.H. Similar to those who are breastfed, infants fed a formula containing 2′-fucosyllactose have lower inflammatory cytokines in a randomized controlled trial. *J. Nutr.* **2016**, *146*, 2559–2566. [CrossRef] [PubMed]
74. Kajzer, J.; Oliver, J.; Marriage, B. Gastrointestinal tolerance of formula supplemented with oligosaccharides. *FASEB J.* **2016**, *30* (Suppl. 1), 671–674.
75. Puccio, G.; Alliet, P.; Cajozzo, C.; Janssens, E.; Corsello, G.; Sprenger, N.; Wernimont, S.; Egli, D.; Gosoniu, L.; Steenhout, P. Effects of infant formula with human milk oligosaccharides on growth and morbidity: A randomized multicenter trial. *J. Pediatr. Gastroenterol. Nutr.* **2017**, *64*, 624–631. [CrossRef] [PubMed]
76. Berger, B.; Grathwohl, D.; Porta, N.; Foata, F.; Delley, M.; Moine, D.; Charpagne, A.; Descombes, P.; Mercenier, A.; Alliet, P.; Puccio, G.; Steenhout, P.; Sprenger, N. Infant formula with two human milk oligosaccharides promotes a microbial fecal community typical of breastfed infants and associated to a lower risk of antibiotic use. *Microbiome*. under review.

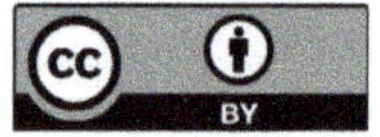

© 2018 by the authors. Licensee MDPI, Basel, Switzerland. This article is an open access article distributed under the terms and conditions of the Creative Commons Attribution (CC BY) license (http://creativecommons.org/licenses/by/4.0/).

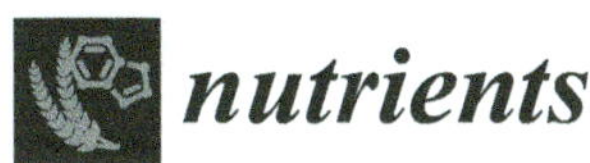

Article

Efficacy of an Oral Rehydration Solution Enriched with *Lactobacillus reuteri DSM 17938* and Zinc in the Management of Acute Diarrhoea in Infants: A Randomized, Double-Blind, Placebo-Controlled Trial

Maria Maragkoudaki, George Chouliaras, Antonia Moutafi, Athanasios Thomas, Archodoula Orfanakou and Alexandra Papadopoulou *

Division of Gastroenterology and Hepatology, First Department of Pediatrics, University of Athens Children's Hospital "Agia Sofia", Thivon and Papadiamantopoulou, 11527 Athens, Greece; mariamariaki@gmail.com (M.M.); georgehouliaras@msn.com (G.C.); tania.moutafi@yahoo.com (A.M.); nassos.thomas@gmail.com (A.T.); adaorfanakou@yahoo.gr (A.O.)

* Correspondence: a.papadopoulou@paidon-agiasofia.gr

Received: 5 August 2018; Accepted: 27 August 2018; Published: 1 September 2018

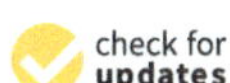

Abstract: The efficacy of oral rehydration solution (ORS) enriched with *Lactobacillus reuteri DSM 17938* and zinc in infants with acute gastroenteritis, is poorly defined. The aim of this double-blind, randomized, placebo-controlled study, was to assess the efficacy of an ORS enriched with *Lactobacillus reuteri DSM 17938* and zinc (ORS^+Lr&Z) in well-nourished, non-hospitalized infants with acute diarrhoea. Fifty one infants with acute diarrhoea were randomly assigned to receive either ORS^+Lr&Z (28 infants, mean $\pm$ SD age 1.7 $\pm$ 0.7 years, 21 males), or standard ORS (ORS^-Lr&Z; 23 infants, mean $\pm$ SD age 1.8 $\pm$ 0.7 years, 16 males). Stools volume and consistency were recorded pre- and posttreatment using the Amsterdam Infant Stool Scale and were compared between the two groups, as well as lost work/day care days, drug administration and need for hospitalization. Both groups showed reduction in the severity of diarrhoea on day two ($p < 0.001$) while, all outcomes showed a trend to be better in the ORS^+Lr&Z group, without reaching statistical significance, probably due to the relatively small number of patients. No adverse effects were recorded. In conclusion, both ORS were effective in managing acute diarrhoea in well-nourished, non-hospitalized infants. ORS enriched with *L. reuteri DSM 17938* and zinc was well tolerated with no adverse effects.

Keywords: acute gastroenteritis; children; *Lactobacillus reuteri*; oral rehydration solution; probiotics; zinc

1. Introduction

Oral rehydration solution (ORS) is recommended in infants and children with acute diarrhoea for the treatment or the prevention of dehydration [1]. Zinc supplementation is beneficial in infants and children with acute diarrhoea living in developing countries [2], however, its efficacy in those living in developed countries is poorly defined. Furthermore, selected strains of probiotics have been shown to reduce the duration and the severity of diarrhoea in children with acute diarrhoea and the effect is greater if the probiotics are given within 60 hours from the onset of symptoms [3–8]. *Lactobacillus reuteri* (*L. reuteri*) *ATCC 55730* was reported to have a beneficial effect in reducing the duration and severity of acute gastroenteritis of both bacterial and viral (rotavirus) origin in infants and toddlers aged 6–36 months [6–8]. However, the above strain was found to carry transferable resistance traits for tetracycline and lincomycin, and for this reason it was replaced by a new strain—*L. reuteri DSM 17938*—by removal of two potentially transferable plasmid-borne resistances.

Furthermore, *L. reuteri DSM 17938* was assessed in hospitalized and non-hospitalized children with acute diarrhoea with varied results. The administration of *L. reuteri DSM 17938* at a dose of 4×10^8 CFU in hospitalized 69 Italian children aged six months to three years for acute diarrhoea, reduced significantly the frequency and the duration of diarrhoea on days 2 and 3, and also the number of children with diarrhoea on days 2 and 3, compared to the placebo without though affecting the duration of hospital stay [9]. In another multicenter, randomized, single-blinded, case control clinical trial [10] in 64 hospitalized children with acute watery diarrhoea, the administration of *L. reuteri DSM 17938* at a dose of 1×10^8 CFU for five days was associated with reduction of the duration of diarrhoea and of the hospital stay as well as with better success rate on day 2 compared to 63 controls while, the same strain at a subsequent study in 60 children with acute diarrhoea presented at outpatients clinics, showed reduced duration of diarrhoea and better success rate on day two but no differences from the third day between the two groups [11]. Although the above strain has been solitary studied in childhood acute diarrhoea, the efficacy of the combined supplementation of ORS with *L. reuteri DSM 17938* and zinc in infants with acute diarrhoea, has not been studied so far.

The aim of the present study therefore, was to assess whether an ORS enriched with *L. reuteri DSM 17938* and zinc (ORS^+Lr&Z) would be superior or equivalent to ORS without added probiotic and zinc (ORS^-Lr&Z) in managing acute diarrhoea in well-nourished non-hospitalized infants and toddlers, and its effects on child's and family's normal activities

2. Patients and Methods

2.1. Study Design

The study was a randomized, double-blind, placebo-controlled study, conducted in patients with acute diarrhoea who were followed up at outpatient paediatric clinics in Athens, Greece during 30 months. The study protocol was approved by the ethics committee of the hospital and the study was registered at ClinicalTrials.gov (NCT 01886755), before the enrolment of the first patient. Informed consent was obtained from at least one parent or legal guardian prior to study inclusion.

2.2. Patients

Infants aged 6–36 months with acute diarrhoea defined as three or more watery or soft stools per day for the past 24–48 h and with mild to moderate degree of dehydration defined as one to four scores on Baily's clinical dehydration scale [12], seen as outpatients were recruited. The exclusion criteria included the following: diarrhoea lasting more than 48 hours, clinical signs of severe dehydration defined as Bailey scale scores = or > 5, malnutrition defined as weight/height ratio below the 5th percentile, clinical signs of a coexisting severe acute systemic illness (meningitis, sepsis, pneumonia), immunodeficiency, severe chronic disease including cystic fibrosis, food allergy diagnosed by physician or other chronic gastrointestinal diseases, use of pre-/probiotics in the previous two weeks, use of antibiotics or any anti-diarrhoeal medication in the previous four weeks.

2.3. Methods

The patients were randomly assigned to receive either ORS^+Lr&Z or ORS^-Lr&Z of similar composition and osmolality (Table 1) both provided by BioGaia AB, Sweden. Oral rehydration took place over the first four hours while ongoing losses were replaced by administering 10 mL/kg of ORS using a graduated bottle provided by the sponsor, after each loose/watery stool or vomit until diarrhoea ceased or up to five days from the enrolment. Patients were allocated to each group according to a computer—generated randomisation using Random Allocation Software version 2.3.8 (StatsDirect Ltd., Chesire, UK). Treatment allocation was concealed to maintain the double-blind status.

Table 1. Composition of the study products.

	ORS Enriched with *L. reuteri DSM 17938* and Zinc (1 Sachet)	ORS without *L. reuteri DSM 17938* and Zinc (1 Sachet)
Protein	<0.1 g	<0.1 g
Carbohydrates	3.75 g	3.75 g
of which glucose	3.75 g	3.75 g
Fat	<0.1 g	<0.1 g
Sodium	0.35 g/15 mmol	0.35 g/15 mmol
Chloride	0.4 g/11 mmol	0.4 g/11 mmol
Potassium	0.2 g/5 mmol	0.2 g/5 mmol
Citrate	0.5 g/3 mmol	0.5 g/3 mmol
Zinc	1.5 mg/0.02 mmol	0 mg/0 mmol
Osmolality	220 mOsm/kg H_2O	220 mOsm/kg H_2O
L. reuteri DSM 17938	1×10^9 CFU (Colony Forming Units)	0

The parents/legal guardians of the enrolled children were instructed to make daily records of the stools in a specific form using the Amsterdam stool scale (ISS) [13], the vomiting episodes, the volume of ORS consumed by the child on each day, other treatments or medications during the study period, adverse events, missed number of workdays for the parents and days at day care/nursery for the child, as well as any hospital admissions.

2.4. Outcome Measures

The primary outcome measures included the proportion of children without watery or soft (type A3–4 or B3–4 ISS) stools on day 2 of treatment, as well the time from the start of treatment up to the day of recording the last watery or soft stool. The secondary outcome measures included the reduction in the severity of diarrhoea assessed by the following: (a) the number of watery and soft (type A3–4 or B3–4 ISS) stools on each of the days during the study period; (b) the percentage of patients with watery or soft (type A3–4 or B3–4 ISS) stools on each day during the study period; and (c) the decrease in the diarrhoea severity score consisting of the sum of the points of three variables according to ISS: (i) number of bowel movements; (ii) type (A, B, C, and D) of stools and (iii) volume (1, 2, 3 and 4) of stools (Table 2); the number of vomiting episodes; the volume of ORS intake during the first day of treatment; the need for hospitalization; the loss of workdays for the parents; the loss of days from the day care/nursery for the children as well the need for medication administration due to diarrhoea.

Table 2. Total score of severity of diarrhoea based on Amsterdam stool scale.

	Variable								
		Consistency				Volume			
Category		A	B	C	D	1	2	3	4
Points	1 point for each bowel movement	2	1	0	0	1	2	3	4

The total score consists of the sum of the product of the points of three variables: (i) number of bowel movements; (ii) Type (A, B, C, and D) of stools and iii) Volume (1, 2, 3, and 4) of stools.

2.5. Statistical Analysis

Continuous parameters are presented as mean and standard deviation (SD) and compared by non-parametric tests (Mann-Whitney) due to the small sample sizes and the extremely skewed distributions of outcome variables which are discrete and with relatively narrow range. Categorical variables are presented as absolute (n) and relative (%) frequencies and compared by the Fisher exact test. Mean differences (MD) of continuous outcomes between the two groups and 95% confidence intervals (CI) are reported, whereas absolute risk difference (ARD) with 95% CI were estimated for categorical outcomes. The level of statistical significance was set to 0.05. In cases of multiple comparisons, the Bonferroni correction was applied (0.05 divided by the number of comparisons). Data were analysed with Stata 11.2 MP statistical software (StataCorp, TX, USA).

3. Results

Fifty-eight children were randomly allocated to receive either ORS$^+$Lr&Z (n = 30) or ORS$^-$Lr&Z (n = 28) seven of whom (two from the ORS$^+$Lr&Z and five from the ORS$^-$Lr&Z group) were lost from follow up. A total of 51 children mean ± SD age 1.8 ± 0.7, 1.7 (1.3, 2.3), 37 males, 14 females, received either ORS$^+$Lr&Z (n = 28, aged 1.7 ± 0.7, 21 males, seven females) or ORS$^-$Lr&Z (n = 23, mean ± SD age 1.8 ± 0.7, 16 males, seven females) and were included in the analysis. The CONSORT flow diagram of the study is shown in Figure 1.

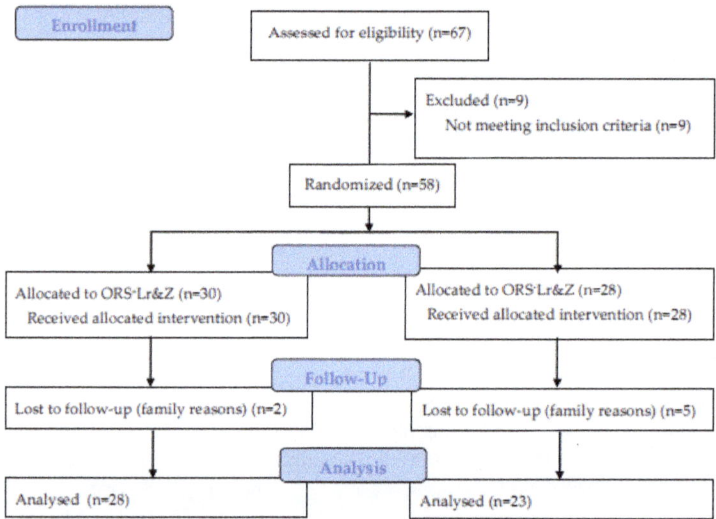

Figure 1. CONSORT flow diagram.

Age and gender were comparable between the two groups at baseline, as well as the severity of diarrhoea before recruitment (Table 3).

Table 3. Baseline characteristics in the two study arms.

	ORS$^-$Lr&Z	ORS$^+$Lr&Z	p-Value
Age (years) *	1.8 ± 0.7, 1.8 (1.3, 2.4)	1.7 ± 0.7, 1.6 (1.3, 2.1)	0.5 **
Severity of diarrhoea (score) *	4.7 ± 3.6, 5 (2, 6)	4.3 ± 3.1, 3.5 (2.0, 6.5)	0.6 **
Gender, males/females, n (%)	16/7 (69.6%/30.4%)	21/7 (75.0%/25%)	0.8 ***

* Mean ± SD, median (IQR); ** Mean (95% confidence interval); *** Mann-Whitney test, level of significance after Bonferroni correction: 0.01.

The proportion of children without diarrhoea on day two after the start of treatment did not differ significantly between the two groups: ORS$^-$Lr&Z 13/23 (56.5%), ORS$^+$Lr&Z 18/28 (64.3%), p = 0.8, ARD: 7.7% (−19.2%, 34.7%).

All of the outcomes in the intention to treat analysis showed a trend to be better in the ORS$^+$Lr&Z group, however statistical significance was not reached in any of them. Both groups showed comparable improvement in the severity of diarrhoea on day two following the start of treatment (Table 4, Figure 2) as well as during the study period (Table 4, Figure 3).

Table 4. Resolution of diarrhoea during the study period.

	Number of Watery or Soft (type A3–4 or B3–4 ISS [#]) Stools *				Proportion of Patients without Diarrhoea			
	$ORS^-Lr\&Z$	$ORS^+Lr\&Z$	MD ($ORS^+Lr\&Z$ vs. $ORS^-Lr\&Z$ **	*p*-Value ***	$ORS^-Lr\&Z$	$ORS^+Lr\&Z$	ARD ** ($ORS^+Lr\&Z$ vs. $ORS^-Lr\&Z$)	*p*-Value ****
Day 1	1.17 ± 1.85 0 (0, 2)	0.96 ± 1.13 1 (0, 2)	−0.21 (−1.05, 0.63)	0.9	12/23 (52.2%)	13/28 (46.4%)	−5.7% (−33.2%, 21.8%)	0.8
Day 2	0.74 ± 1.00 0 (0, 1)	0.64 ± 1.00 0 (0, 1)	−0.10 (−0.66, 0.46)	0.6	13/23 (56.5%)	18/28 (64.3%)	7.7% (−19.2%, 34.7%)	0.8
Day 3	0.69 ± 0.87 0 (0, 2)	0.46 ± 0.83 0 (0, 1)	−0.23 (−0.71, 0.25)	0.3	13/23 (56.5%)	20/28 (71.4%)	14.9% (−11.1%, 41.2%)	0.4
Day 4	0.34 ± 0.71 0 (0, 1)	0.39 ± 0.62 0 (0, 1)	0.05 (−0.33, 0.42)	0.6	17/23 (73.9%)	19/28 (67.9%)	6.1% (−31.0%, 18.9%)	0.8
Day 5	0.30 ± 0.47 0 (0, 1)	0.14 ± 0.52 0 (0, 0)	−0.16 (−0.44, 0.12)	0.05	16/23 (69.6%)	26/28 (92.9%)	23.3% (2.0%, 44.5%)	0.06

[#] Infant Stool Scale; * Mean ± SD, median (IQR); ** Mean (95% confidence interval); *** Mann-Whitney test, level of significance after Bonferroni correction: 0.01; **** Fisher's exact test, level of significance after Bonferroni correction: 0.01.

Both ORS with or without supplementation with *L. reuteri DSM 17938* and zinc managed to decrease significantly the severity of diarrhoea on day 2, based on the severity score that took into account both stool consistency and volume according to ISS (Figure 2).

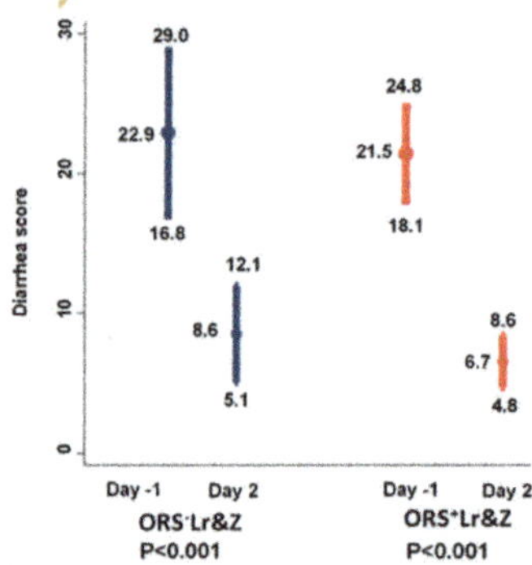

Figure 2. Improvement of the severity score of diarrhoea at day 2 compared to baseline (day^{-1}). At each time point, the results are presented with means and 95% confidence intervals. Comparisons within groups were performed by the Wilcoxon signed-rank test for paired data, whereas data between groups were compared by the Mann-Whitney U test. Comparisons in the ORS^{+}Lr&Z arm on day two versus day^{-1} ($p < 0.001$). Comparisons in the ORS^{-}Lr&Z arm on day two versus day^{-1} ($p < 0.001$).

Furthermore, although the ORS supplemented with *L. reuteri DSM 17938* and zinc had a tendency to achieve a greater decrease in the 6-day severity score of diarrhoea, the difference between the two groups did not reach statistical significance (Figure 3).

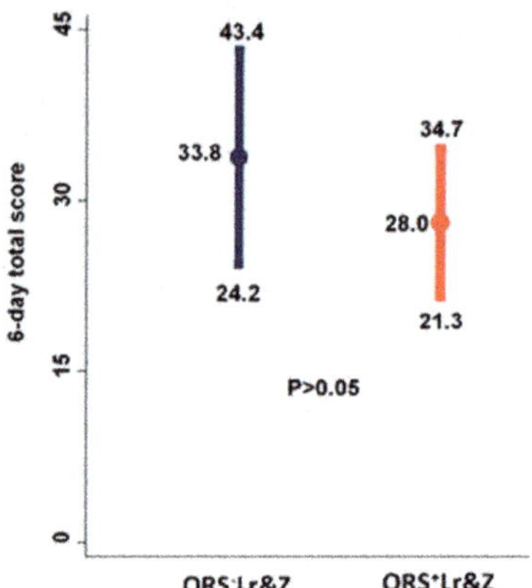

Figure 3. Total six-day severity score of diarrhoea. Results are presented with means and 95% confidence intervals. Comparisons between the ORS^{+}Lr&Z and the ORS^{-}Lr&Z arms were performed by the Mann-Whitney U test ($p > 0.5$).

Similarly, although a tendency was seen in the group receiving ORS supplemented with *L. reuteri DSM 17938* and zinc to have smaller duration of watery diarrhoea as well as of soft stools compared to the group which received non-supplemented ORS, again, the difference did not reach statistical significance (Figure 4A,B).

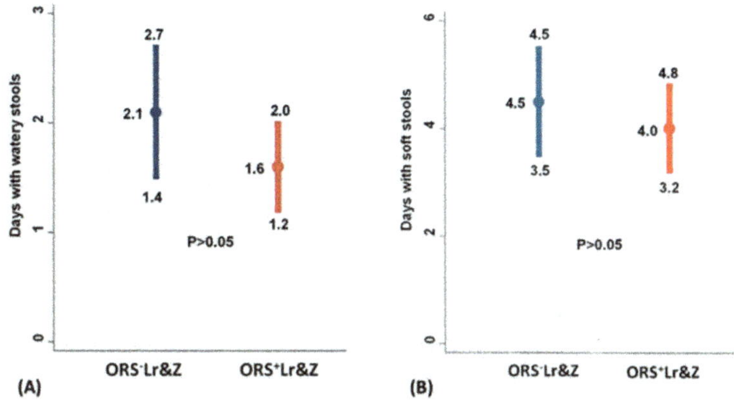

Figure 4. (**A**): Number of days with watery stools. (**B**): Number of days with soft stools. Results are presented with means and 95% confidence intervals. Comparisons between the ORS$^+$Lr&Z and the ORS$^-$Lr&Z arms were performed by the Mann-Whitney U test ($p > 0.5$).

The same was true for the number of days lost from the day care for the infants and from work for the parents, which tended to be less in the group which received ORS supplemented with *L. reuteri DSM 17938* and zinc, but again, the differences did not reach statistical significance (Figure 5A,B).

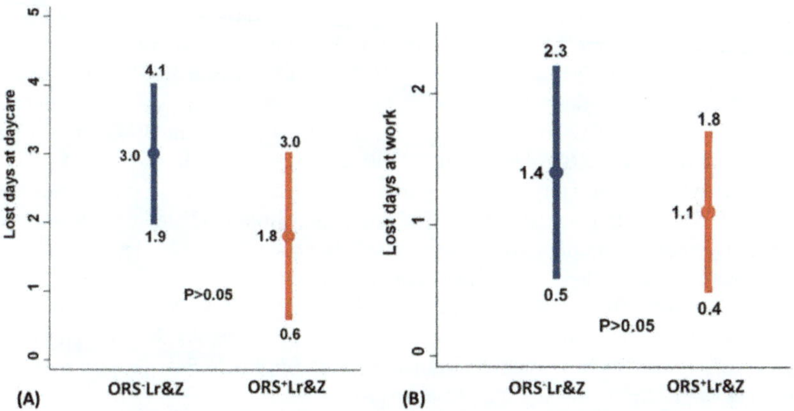

Figure 5. (**A**): Number of lost day care/nursery days for patients. (**B**): Number of lost work days for parents. Results are presented with means and 95% confidence intervals. Comparisons between the ORS$^+$Lr&Z and the ORS$^-$Lr&Z arms were performed by the Mann-Whitney U test ($p > 0.5$).

The number of vomiting episodes was comparable between the ORS$^-$Lr&Z and the ORS$^+$Lr&Z groups at baseline: mean ± SD, median (IQR) 0.09 ± 0.28, 0 (0, 0) vs. 0.07 ± 0.26, 0 (0, 0) respectively, $p = 0.4$, while no vomiting episodes were recorded during the study period in any of the two groups.

The consumed volume of ORS during the first 24 h did not differ between the ORS$^+$Lr&Z and the ORS$^-$Lr&Z groups: mean ± SD, median (IQR) 309.8 ± 235.3, 265 (120, 415) vs. 326.5 ± 195.9 respectively, 300 (170, 490), $p = 0.5$.

None of the patients was hospitalized during the study period and no other medications for diarrhoea or antibiotics were administered by any of the patients.

4. Discussion

This study is the first study assessing the efficacy of an ORS supplemented with *L. reuteri DSM 17938* and zinc in infants with acute diarrhoea. Furthermore, this is the first study that uses for the assessment of the efficacy of the above ORS supplementation, an objective measure (ISS), that takes into account both consistency and volume of the infant's stools. In addition, this is the first study assessing the effects of the above combination, on child's and family's normal activities during acute diarrhoea. We showed that ORS^{+}Lr&Z and ORS^{-}Lr&Z were both associated with reduction in the severity of diarrhoea two days following the start of treatment in a group of well-nourished, non-hospitalized infants and toddlers with acute gastroenteritis. Furthermore, we showed that all of the outcomes including the severity of diarrhoea based on ISS, the duration of watery diarrhoea, the percentages of infants with no diarrhoea on days 3 and 5 as well as the number of absences from the day care for the infants and the parents from the work, all showed a trend to be better in the ORS^{+}Lr&Z group without though reaching statistical significance, probably due to the relatively small number of recruited patients.

Other studies using probiotic strains such as *L. reuteri ATCC 55730*, *Lactobacillus rhamnosus 19070-2* and *L. reuteri DSM 12246*, reported beneficial effects in children with acute gastroenteritis [3–7,14]. *Lactobacillus rhamnosus 19070-2* and *L. reuteri DSM 12246* were both effective in reducing the duration of diarrhoea after intervention in hospitalized and non-hospitalized children with mild diarrhoea while, a greater efficacy was noted in case of early (<60 hours after the start of diarrhoea) intervention [4,5]. Furthermore, *L. reuteri DSM 17938* and *L. reuteri ATCC 55730* were reported in one meta-analysis in hospitalized children 3 to 60 months (n = 196 and n = 156 respectively), to reduce significantly the duration of diarrhoea compared to placebo or no treatment respectively [15].

The mechanisms of the effect of *L. reuteri* in acute diarrhoea are not fully understood. It has been shown that *L. reuteri* can produce reuterin, a broad-spectrum antimicrobial agent [16], which may be responsible for the inhibition of pathogenic microorganisms in the gastrointestinal tract, but also, it can decrease intestinal permeability [17,18] and stimulate the intestinal immune responses [19,20]. Furthermore, *L. reuteri DSM 17938* and *ATCC PTA 6475* were shown in a model of rotavirus infection in new-born mice, to increase the early mucosal rotavirus-specific IgA as well as the diversity of the distal gut microbiome, attenuating rotavirus induced enteritis and reducing the duration of diarrhoea by one day. In our study, we did not perform gut microbiome analysis in the recruited infants with acute diarrhoea. Therefore, we cannot draw any conclusions from this study on the possible effects of the supplemented ORS with *L. reuteri DSM 17938* and zinc on infants distal gut microbiome during acute diarrhoea. Other preliminary studies suggested that *L. reuteri 17938* increased the number of villus goblet cells bearing markers of intestinal stem cell activity [21–23].

Based on the available evidence, the European Society for Pediatric Gastroenterology, Hepatology and Nutrition recommended the use of *Lactobacillus rhamnosus GG*, *Saccharomyces boulardii*, *L. reuteri DSM 17938*, and the heat-inactivated *Lactobacillus acidophilus LB* as a supplement of the ORS for the management of childhood acute gastroenteritis [24].

With regards to zinc supplementation of ORS in children with acute diarrhoea, it has been shown to be beneficial in malnourished children [25] but has been poorly studied in well-nourished ones. The postulated mechanisms include improved absorption of water and electrolytes by the intestine [26–28], regeneration of gut epithelium [29], increased levels of enterocyte brush-border enzymes [30], and enhanced immunologic mechanisms. Therefore, WHO recommended early oral rehydration therapy and zinc supplementation to treat acute diarrhoea in children [1]. Our study failed to show superiority of the enriched with zinc ORS in the study group consisting of well-nourished infants with mild diarrhoea not requiring hospitalization, probably due to the fact that the study was underpowered due to the relatively small number of recruited patients.

The main limitation of the study was, therefore, the relatively small number of the recruited children. The fact, however, that the study was a well-designed, double blind, placebo-controlled trial, the first that assessed an ORS enriched with *L. reuteri DSM 17938* and zinc in infants with acute gastroenteritis, and also used for the assessment of the severity of diarrhoea an objective method

(ISS), make the results a valuable contribution to the meta-analyses on the topic, which has clinical importance for health professionals, including general practitioners, general pediatricians, pediatric gastroenterologists, and nutritionists.

5. Conclusions

This randomised, double blind, placebo-controlled trial showed that ORS supplemented with *L. reuteri DSM 17938* and zinc had comparable efficacy with ORS of similar composition and osmolality without added probiotic and zinc, in managing acute diarrhoea, in well-nourished, non-hospitalised infants and toddlers with acute diarrhoea. ORS enriched with *L. reuteri DSM 17938* and zinc was well tolerated without adverse effects.

Author Contributions: M.M. made substantial contributions to the data acquisition, as well as drafting the manuscript and revising it critically. G.C. made substantial contributions to the data analysis and interpretation, as well as revising the manuscript critically. A.M. made substantial contributions to the recruitment of patients and data acquisition, as well as revising the manuscript critically. A.O. made substantial contributions to the recruitment of patients and data acquisition as well as revising the manuscript critically. A.T. made substantial contributions to the recruitment of patients and data acquisition as well as revising the manuscript critically. A.P. made substantial contributions to the design of the study, data acquisition and interpretation, drafting the manuscript, and revising it critically.

Funding: The study was funded by BioGaia AB, Sweden. The sponsor was not involved in the data collection, analysis and interpretation, in the writing of the manuscript, as well as in the decision to submit the article for publication.

Conflicts of Interest: M.M., G.C., A.M., A.O. and A.P. received research grants from BioGaia, the manufacturer of the ORS enriched with *Lactobacillus reuteri DSM 17938* and zinc and the ORS without enrichment. A.T. had nothing to declare.

Abbreviations

ORS	Oral rehydration solution
L. reuteri	Lactobacillus reuteri
ORS^{+}Lr&Z	ORS enriched with *L. reuteri DSM 17938* and zinc
ORS^{-}Lr&Z	ORS of similar composition and osmolality without added probiotic and zinc
MD	Mean differences
SD	Standard deviation
95% CI	95% confidence intervals

References

1. World Health Organization, Dept. of Child and Adolescent Health and Development & UNICEF. *Clinical Management of Acute Diarrhoea: WHO/UNICEF Joint Statement*; World Health Organization: Geneva, Switzerland, 2004.
2. Castillo Duran, C.; Vial, P.; Uauy, R. Trace mineral balance during acute diarrhea in infants. *J. Pediatr.* **1988**, *113*, 452–457. [CrossRef]
3. Allen, S.J.; Martinez, E.G.; Gregorio, G.V.; Dans, L.F. Probiotics for treating acute infectious diarrhoea. *Cochrane Database Syst. Rev.* **2010**. [CrossRef] [PubMed]
4. Rosenfeldt, V.; Michaelsen, K.F.; Jakobsen, M.; Larsen, C.N.; Møller, P.L.; Pedersen, P.; Tvede, M.; Weyrehter, H.; Valerius, N.H.; Paerregaard, A. Effect of probiotic *Lactobacillus* strains in young children hospitalized with acute diarrhea. *Pediatr. Infect. Dis. J.* **2002**, *21*, 411–416. [CrossRef] [PubMed]
5. Rosenfeldt, V.; Michaelsen, K.F.; Jakobsen, M.; Larsen, C.N.; Møller, P.L.; Tvede, M.; Weyrehter, H.; Valerius, N.H.; Paerregaard, A. Effect of probiotic *Lactobacillus* strains on acute diarrhea in a cohort of non-hospitalized children attending day-care centers. *Pediatr. Infect. Dis. J.* **2002**, *21*, 417–419. [CrossRef] [PubMed]
6. Shornikova, A.V.; Casas, I.A.; Isolauri, E.; Mykkanen, N.; Vesikari, T. *Lactobacillus reuteri* as a therapeutic agent in acute diarrhoea in young children. *J. Pediatr. Gastroenterol. Nutr.* **1997**, *24*, 399–404. [CrossRef] [PubMed]

7. Shornikova, AV.; Casas, I.A.; Mykkanen, N.; Salo, E.; Vesikari, T. Bacteriotherapy with *Lactobacillus reuteri* in rotavirus gastroenteritis. *Pediatr. Infect. Dis. J.* **1997**, *16*, 1103–1107. [CrossRef] [PubMed]
8. Eom, T.H.; Oh, E.Y.; Kim, Y.H.; Lee, H.S.; Yang, P.S.; Kim, D.U.; Kim, J.-T.; Lee, B.-C. The therapeutic effect of *Lactobacillus reuteri* in acute diarrhea in infants and toddlers. *Korean J. Pediatr.* **2005**, *48*, 986–989.
9. Francavilla, R.; Lionetti, E.; Castellaneta, S.; Ciruzzi, F.; Indrio, F.; Masciale, A.; Fontana, C.; La Rosa, M.M.; Cavallo, L.; Francavilla, A. Randomised clinical trial: Lactobacillus reuteri DSM 17938 vs. Placebo in children with acute diarrhea—A double-blind study. *Aliment. Pharmacol. Ther.* **2012**, *36*, 362–369. [CrossRef] [PubMed]
10. Dinleyici, E.C.; PROBAGE Study Group; Vandenplas, Y. Lactobacillus reuteri DSM 17938 effectively reduces the duration of acute diarrhoea in hospitalised children. *Acta Paediatr.* **2014**, *103*, e300–e305. [PubMed]
11. Dinleyici, E.C.; Dalgic, N.; Guven, S.; Metin, O.; Yasa, O.; Kurugol, Z.; Turel, O.; Tanir, G.; Yazar, A.S.; Arica, V.; et al. *Lactobacillus reuteri* DSM 17938 shortens acute infectious diarrhea in a pediatric outpatient setting. *J. Pediatr.* **2015**, *91*, 392–396. [CrossRef] [PubMed]
12. Bailey, B.; Gravel, J.; Goldman, R.D.; Friedman, J.N.; Parkin, P.C. External validation of the clinical dehydration scale for children with acute gastroenteritis. *Acad. Emerg. Med.* **2010**, *17*, 583–588. [CrossRef] [PubMed]
13. Bekkali, N.; Hamers, S.L.; Reitsma, J.B.; Van Toledo, L.; Benninga, M.A. Infant stool form scale: Development and results. *J. Pediatr.* **2009**, *154*, 521–526. [CrossRef] [PubMed]
14. Chmielewska, A.; Ruszczynski, M.; Szajewska, H. Lactobacillus reuteri strain ATCC 55730 for the treatment of acute infectious diarrhea in children: A meta-analysis of randomized controlled trials. *Pediatr. Wspolczesna* **2008**, *10*, 33–37.
15. Szajewska, H.; Urbanska, M.; Chmielewska, A.; Weizman, Z.; Shamir, R. Meta-analysis. *Lactobacillus reuteri* strain DSM 17938 (and the original strain ATCC 55730) for treating acute gastroenteritis in children. *Benef. Microbes* **2014**, *5*, 285–293. [PubMed]
16. Brunser, O.; Araya, M.; Espinoza, J.; Guesry, P.R.; Secretin, M.C.; Pacheco, I. Effect of an acidified milk on diarrhea and the carrier state in infants of low socio-economic stratum. *Acta Paediatr. Scand.* **1989**, *78*, 259–264. [CrossRef] [PubMed]
17. Isolauri, E.; Majamaa, H.; Arvola, T.; Rantala, I.; Virtanen, E.; Arvilommi, H. *Lactobacillus casei* strain GG reverses increased intestinal permeability induced by cow milk in suckling rats. *Gastroenterology* **1993**, *105*, 1643–1650. [CrossRef]
18. Isolauri, E.; Kaila, M.; Arvola, T.; Majamaa, H.; Rantala, I.; Virtanen, E.; Arvilommi, H. Diet during rotavirus enteritis affects jejunal permeability to macromolecules in suckling rats. *Pediatr. Res.* **1993**, *33*, 548–553. [CrossRef] [PubMed]
19. Perdigon, G.; Alvarex, S.; Nader De Macias, M.; Roux, M.; Pesce de Ruiz Holgado, A. The oral administration of lactic acid bacteria increases the mucosal intestinal immunity in response to enteropathogens. *J. Food Prot.* **1990**, *53*, 404–410. [CrossRef]
20. Perdigon, G.; Medici, M.; BibasBonet de Jorrat, M.E.; Valverde de Budeguer, M.; Pesce de Ruiz Holgado, A. Immunomodulating effects of lactic acid bacteria on mucosal and humoral immunity. *Int. J. Immunother.* **1993**, *9*, 29–52.
21. Preidis, G.A.; Saulnier, D.M.; Blutt, S.E.; Mistretta, T.A.; Riehle, K.P.; Major, A.M.; Venable, S.F.; Finegold, M.J.; Petrosino, J.F.; Conner, M.E.; et al. Probiotics stimulate enterocyte migration and microbial diversity in the neonatal mouse intestine. *FASEB J.* **2012**, *26*, 1960–1969. [CrossRef] [PubMed]
22. Preidis, G.A.; Saulnier, D.M.; Blutt, S.E.; Mistretta, T.A.; Riehle, K.P.; Major, A.M.; Venable, S.F.; Barrish, J.P.; Finegold, M.J.; Petrosino, J.F.; et al. Host response to probiotics determined by nutritional status of rotavirus-infected neonatal mice. *J. Pediatr. Gastroenterol. Nutr.* **2012**, *55*, 299–307. [CrossRef] [PubMed]
23. Preidis, G. Mechanisms of probiosis by *Lactobacillus reuteri* in Acute Rotaviral Gastroenteritis. Translational Biology and Molecular Medicine. Ph.D. Thesis, Baylor College of Medicine, Houston, TX, USA, 2011.
24. Szajewska, H.; Guarino, A.; Hojsak, I.; Indrio, F.; Kolacek, S.; Shamir, R.; Vandenplas, Y.; Weizman, Z.; European Society for Pediatric Gastroenterology, Hepatology, and Nutrition. Use of probiotics for management of acute gastroenteritis: A position paper by the ESPGHAN Working Group for Probiotics and Prebiotics. *J. Pediatr. Gastroenterol. Nutr.* **2014**, *58*, 531–539.
25. Ghishan, F.K. Transport of electrolytes, water, and glucose in zinc deficiency. *J. Pediatr. Gastroenterol. Nutr.* **1984**, *3*, 608–612. [CrossRef] [PubMed]

26. Patrick, J.; Golden, B.E.; Golden, M.H. Leucocyte sodium transport and dietary zinc in protein energy malnutrition. *Am. J. Clin. Nutr.* **1980**, *33*, 617–620. [CrossRef] [PubMed]
27. Patrick, J.; Michael, J.; Golden, M.N.; Golden, B.E.; Hilton, P.J. Effect of zinc on leucocyte sodium transport in vitro. *Clin. Sci. Mol. Med.* **1978**, *54*, 585–587. [PubMed]
28. Roy, S.K.; Behrens, R.H.; Haider, R.; Akramuzzaman, S.M.; Mahalanabis, D.; Wahed, M.A.; Tomkins, A.M. Impact of zinc supplementation on intestinal permeability in Bangladeshi children with acute diarrhoea and persistent diarrhoea syndrome. *J. Pediatr. Gastroenterol. Nutr.* **1992**, *15*, 289–296. [CrossRef] [PubMed]
29. Gebhard, R.L.; Karouani, R.; Prigge, W.F.; McClain, C.J. The effect of severe zinc deficiency on activity of intestinal disaccharidases and 3-hydroxy-3-methylglutaryl coenzyme A reductase in the rat. *J. Nutr.* **1983**, *113*, 855–859. [CrossRef] [PubMed]
30. Galvao, T.F.; Thees, M.; Pontes, R.F.; Silva, M.T.; Pereira, M.G. Zinc supplementation for treating diarrhea in children: A systematic review and meta-analysis. *Rev. Panam. Salud Publica* **2013**, *33*, 370–377. [CrossRef] [PubMed]

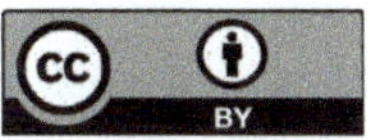

© 2018 by the authors. Licensee MDPI, Basel, Switzerland. This article is an open access article distributed under the terms and conditions of the Creative Commons Attribution (CC BY) license (http://creativecommons.org/licenses/by/4.0/).

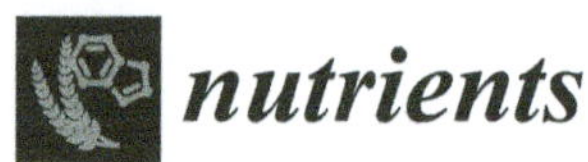
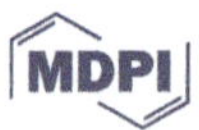

Review

Lactobacillus rhamnosus GG in the Primary Prevention of Eczema in Children: A Systematic Review and Meta-Analysis

Hania Szajewska * and Andrea Horvath

Department of Paediatrics, The Medical University of Warsaw, Żwirki i Wigury 63A, 02-091 Warsaw, Poland; andrea.hania@gmail.com

* Correspondence: hania@ipgate.pl; Tel.: +48-22-317-94-21

Received: 16 August 2018; Accepted: 14 September 2018; Published: 18 September 2018

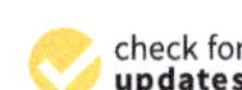

Abstract: Current guidelines recommend the use of probiotics to reduce the risk of eczema. It remains unclear which strain(s) to use. We systematically evaluated data on the efficacy of *Lactobacillus rhamnosus* GG (LGG) supplementation prenatally and/or postnatally for the primary prevention of eczema. The Cochrane Library, MEDLINE, and EMBASE databases were searched up to August 2018, with no language restrictions, for systematic reviews of randomized controlled trials (RCTs) and RCTs published afterwards. The primary outcome was eczema. For dichotomous outcomes, we calculated the risk ratio (RR) and 95% confidence interval (CI). A random-effects model was used to pool data. Heterogeneity was explored using the I^2 statistics. The GRADE criteria were used to assess the overall quality of evidence supporting the primary outcome. Seven publications reporting 5 RCTs (889 participants) were included. High to moderate certainty in the body of evidence suggests that LGG supplementation (regardless of the timing of administration) did not reduce the risk of eczema. There was also no consistent effect on other allergic outcomes. This meta-analysis shows that LGG was ineffective in reducing eczema. It does not support the general recommendation to use probiotics for preventing eczema, unless specific strains would be indicated.

Keywords: probiotics; allergy; infants; pediatrics

1. Introduction

Allergic diseases are a major public health concern in many countries [1]. Among other factors, disturbances in gut microbiota composition and/or activity (dysbiosis) may contribute to the pathogenesis of allergic diseases [2]. If so, gut microbiota may be a target for improving outcomes in subjects affected or at risk for allergic diseases. To date, modification of gut microbiota via the provision of probiotics and/or prebiotics is the most extensively studied strategy.

Probiotics are live microorganisms that, when administered in adequate amounts, confer a health benefit on the host [3]. The mechanisms of action of probiotics remain unclear. However, protolerogenic action of probiotics in the gastrointestinal tract has been suggested [4]. First, probiotics compete with pathogenic organisms for nutrients and binding sites on the intestinal epithelium. Second, they may secrete bacteriocins and induce intestinal epithelium to secrete defensins, natural antimicrobial peptides. Third, through fermenting fibers, probiotics stimulate the production of metabolites such as short-chain fatty acids, the majority of which are acetate, propionate, and butyrate. Short-chain fatty acids activate G protein-coupled receptors that stimulate colonic dendritic cells and macrophages to secrete interleukin-10 (IL-10) and promote development of regulatory T lymphocytes (Tregs) in the mesenteric lymph nodes. Tregs are a source of tolerogenic cytokines such as IL-10 and transforming growth factor-beta (TGF-beta) that inhibit allergic and inflammatory responses [4].

A 2014 guideline by the World Allergy Organization (WAO) [5] did not recommend use of probiotics for reducing the risk of allergy in children. However, the WAO considered that there is a likely net benefit from using probiotics for preventing eczema. Specifically, the WAO suggests: *"(a) using probiotics in pregnant women at high risk for having an allergic child; (b) using probiotics in women who breastfeed infants at high risk of developing allergy; and (c) using probiotics in infants at high risk of developing allergy"*. All recommendations were conditional and supported by a very low quality of evidence. Since the beginning, these guidelines raised a debate [6], mainly because of the lack of answers to practical questions such as: Which probiotic(s) should be used to reduce the risk of eczema? When should one start the administration of probiotics with proven efficacy? When should one stop? What is the dose of an effective probiotic [7]? Our aim was to systematically evaluate evidence on the efficacy of *Lactobacillus rhamnosus* GG (LGG) supplementation during the prenatal and/or postnatal period for the reducing the risk of eczema. The effect on other allergic diseases was also evaluated. LGG is widely available and commonly used in the pediatric population. It is also the first probiotic for which a reduction in the risk of atopic eczema has been documented [8].

2. Materials and Methods

The methodology was similar to one followed in our earlier systematic review on allergy prevention [9]. The guidelines from the Cochrane Collaboration for undertaking and reporting the results of this systematic review and meta-analysis were followed [10].

2.1. Criteria for Considering Studies for This Review

2.1.1. Type of Studies

Randomized controlled trials (RCTs) were considered for inclusion.

2.1.2. Type of Participants

Participants had to be healthy (1) pregnant women at high risk for having an allergic child; (2) breastfeeding mothers of infants at high risk of developing allergy; or (3) healthy term infants at high risk of developing allergy.

2.1.3. Type of Interventions

We included trials that compared use of the LGG compared with placebo or no intervention. If other experimental arms were available, they were not considered.

2.1.4. Type of Outcomes

Our primary outcome was eczema. However, we also focused on the other allergic manifestations such as wheezing/asthma, allergic rhinitis, food allergy (all as defined by the authors of the original publications), and adverse events. We report outcomes at time intervals reported by the authors of the original publications (or as close as possible).

2.2. Search Methods for Identification of Studies

First, we identified RCTs via reviewing previously completed systematic reviews [11,12]. As there was no discrepancy between two recent reviews with regard to LGG studies, we only searched for RCTs published subsequently to these reviews. The Cochrane Central Register of Controlled Trials (CENTRAL, the Cochrane Library), MEDLINE, and EMBASE databases were searched for relevant studies from December 2014 (end date of last search in the first systematic review [9]) to August 2018. There were no language restrictions. The search was carried out independently by two reviewers. In brief, the following search terms were used: ("infant, newborn"(MeSH Terms) OR ("infant"(All Fields) AND "newborn"(All Fields)) OR "newborn infant"(All Fields) OR "neonat*"(All Fields) OR "infant"(MeSH Terms) OR "infant"(All Fields) OR "pediatric"(All Fields) OR "paediatric"(All Fields))

AND ("hypersensitivity"(MeSH Terms) OR "hypersensitivity"(All Fields) OR "allergy"(MeSH Terms) OR "allergy"(All Fields) OR "allergy and immunology"(All Fields) OR "food allergy"(All Fields) OR "milk allergy"(All Fields) OR "eczema"(MeSH Terms) OR "eczema"(All Fields) OR "wheezing"(All Fields)) OR "asthma"(MeSH Terms) OR "asthma"(All Fields)) AND (*Lactobacillus* (All Fields)).

Additionally, we searched reference lists from identified studies and key review articles. Experts in the field were contacted for additional references.

2.2.1. Selection of Studies

Two reviewers initially screened the title, abstract, and keywords of every record identified with the search strategy, and they retrieved the full texts of potentially relevant trials and of records for which the relevance was unclear. The same reviewers independently applied the inclusion criteria to each potentially relevant trial to determine its eligibility. If differences in opinion existed, they were resolved by discussion until a consensus was reached.

2.2.2. Data Extraction and Management

Data extraction was performed using standard data-extraction forms. In addition to data such as methods, participants, interventions, and outcomes (including the definitions of the primary outcome of interest used in the study), we collected information about sample size calculation and the funding of each study. One reviewer extracted the data from the included studies, and the second author checked the extracted data. Discrepancies between the reviewers were resolved by discussion until a consensus was reached. Participants, interventions, comparisons, and outcomes were taken into consideration to determine whether they were similar enough to allow pooling of data.

2.2.3. Assessment of Risk of Bias in Included Studies

The Cochrane Collaboration's tool for assessing risk of bias was used. The risk of bias parameters included the type of randomization method (selection bias), allocation concealment (selection bias), blinding of participants and personnel (performance bias), blinding of outcome assessment (detection bias), and incomplete outcome data (attrition bias). Additionally, selective reporting (reporting bias) and other types of bias were considered. If an item could not be evaluated due to missing information, it was rated as having an unclear risk of bias [13].

2.2.4. Dealing with Missing Data

We assessed pooled data using intention-to-treat analysis, i.e., an analysis in which data are analyzed for every participant for whom the outcome was obtained (also known as available case analysis), rather than intention-to-treat analysis with imputation [14].

2.2.5. Assessment of Heterogeneity

Heterogeneity was quantified by χ^2 and I^2. A value for I^2 of 0% indicates no observed heterogeneity, and larger values show increasing heterogeneity. All analyses were based on the random effects model.

2.2.6. Assessment of Reporting Biases

To test for publication bias, a test for asymmetry of the funnel plot, as proposed by Egger et al. [15], was planned; however, sufficient ($\geq$10) eligible trials were not available for any given outcome.

2.2.7. Data Synthesis

The data were entered into Review Manager (RevMan), Computer program, Version 5.3. (The Nordic Cochrane Centre, The Cochrane Collaboration, Copenhagen, Denmark) for analysis. The results for individual studies and pooled statistics are reported as the risk ratio (RR) between the experimental and control groups with 95% confidence intervals (95% CI). RR is significant when the 95% CI does not include 1.0.

2.2.8. Subgroup Analysis

Subgroup analysis was based on the timing of the intervention (prenatally only, prenatally and postnatally, postnatally only).

2.2.9. Quality of Evidence

For assessing the quality of evidence (also known as certainty in the evidence or confidence in the effect estimates) for the primary outcome, we chose to use the GRADE methodology and GradePro software, GRADEpro GDT: GRADEpro Guideline Development Tool (Software). (McMaster University, Evidence Prime, Inc., Hamilton, ON, Canada). This software is available from gradepro.org. The GRADE system offers 4 categories of the quality of the evidence (i.e., high, moderate, low, and very low).

3. Results

3.1. Description of Studies

We identified seven publications [8,16–21] reporting on 5 RCTs (Table S1), which involved 889 participants at enrollment (443 in the LGG group and 446 in the control group). Compared to previously published systematic reviews that identified 8 publications on LGG, we excluded the study by Rautava et al. [22], as it reported data on a subset of the population from the study by Kalliomaki et al. [8]. For a flow diagram documenting the identification process for eligible trials, see Figure S1.

All studies were carried out in high-income countries such as Australia (one), Finland (one), Germany (one), Taiwan (one), and the US (one). One trial reported data on the administration of LGG during late pregnancy only [17]. Three trials [8,20,21] reported data on the administration of LGG during pregnancy and to infants (duration of intervention prior to delivery ranged from 14–18 weeks to 2–4 weeks, and in all trials was for 6 months after delivery). One RCT [18] reported data on the administration of LGG to infants only (the duration of intervention was 6 months). The risk of allergy was assessed in the included trials by a family history (the presence of allergy in at least one parent and/or sibling) and/or other markers.

The daily doses of LGG ranged from 1.0×10^9 colony forming units (CFU) to 1.8×10^{10} CFU. The sample size ranged from 105 to 250. Four RCTs were placebo-controlled. In one trial, inulin was administered in both study groups, thus, any effect, if it exists, may be attributable to LGG. All included RCTs evaluated eczema. However, various definitions were used. Atopic eczema IgE-associated was reported separately in one trial only [16]. Other allergic manifestations were reported inconsistently. In case of wheezing and asthma, the definitions were often overlapping, hence, our decision to present these data jointly.

Risk of Bias in Included Studies

The included studies are described with respect to their risk of bias across the included RCTs in Figures 1 and 2. Only one trial [17] had a low risk of bias. The remaining trials had some methodological limitations. Sample size calculations were performed in all 5 trials. Funding was reported in 4 trials.

The GRADE assessment for the primary outcome related to use of LGG is presented in Table S2. Using the GRADE methodology, the overall quality of evidence was rated as high to moderate.

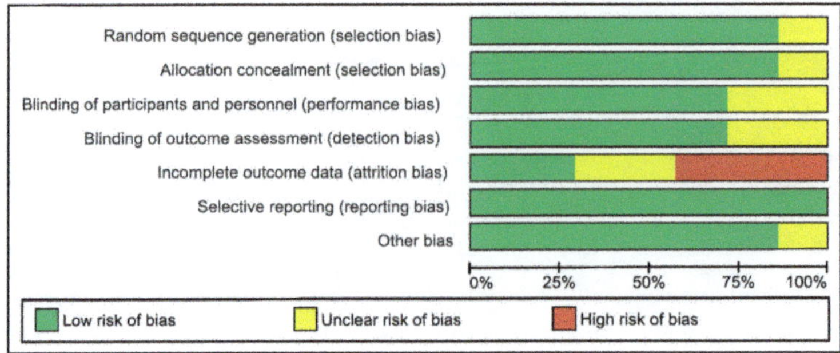

Figure 1. Risk of bias graph.

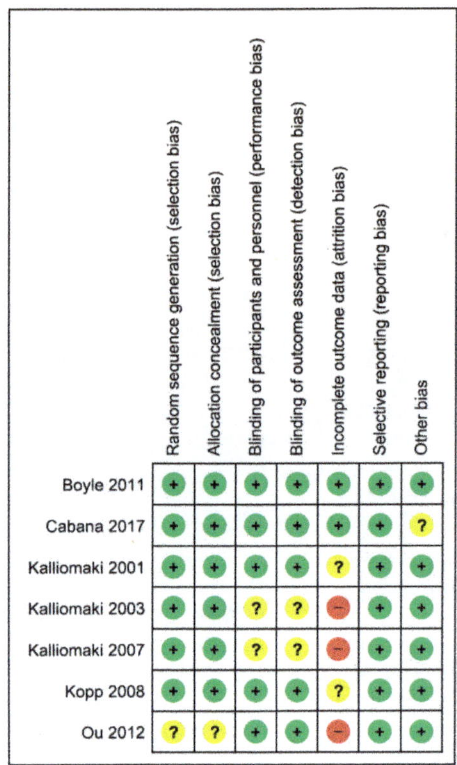

Figure 2. Risk of bias summary.

3.2. *Effects of Interventions*

3.2.1. Eczema

For data on eczema, see Figure 3.

LGG Administration during Late Pregnancy

Only 1 RCT (n = 242) [17] reported the effect of use of LGG administration during pregnancy on the cumulative incidence of eczema and found a similar risk in both study groups (RR 0.88 (95% CI: 0.63, 1.22)).

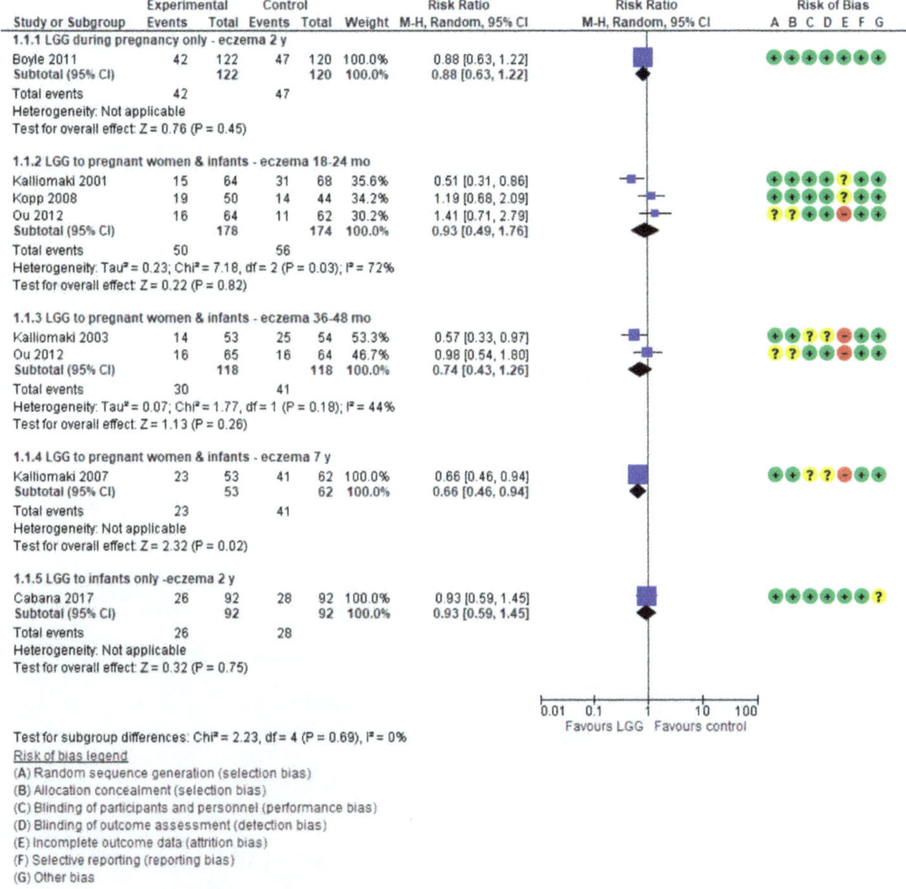

Figure 3. Primary outcome: Effect of LGG supplementation on eczema (data presented based on the timing of LGG administration and the timing of assessment).

LGG Administration during Pregnancy and after Delivery

Three RCTs [8,20,21] reported the effect of LGG administration during pregnancy and to infants on the cumulative incidence of eczema. The pooled results of data up to 2 years of age showed no reduction in the risk of eczema (3 RCTs, n = 352, RR. 0.93 (0.49, 1.76)). Significant heterogeneity was found (I^2 = 72%). There also was no difference between groups in the risk of eczema in children up to 3–4 years (2 RCTs, n = 236, RR 0.74 (0.43, 1.26); I^2 = 44%). Only one RCT (n = 115) reported a significant reduction in the risk of eczema in children up to 7 years in favor of the LGG group (RR 0.66 (0.46, 0.94)) [19]. However, only 72% (115 of 159) of participants were followed up at 7 years.

LGG Administration to Infants Only

One 1 RCT [18] in which LGG was administered to infants only reported no significant difference between groups in the risk of eczema up to 2 years of age (RR 0.93 (0.59, 1.45)).

The pooled results of 5 RCTs [8,17,18,20,21] (n = 778) showed no difference between the LGG-supplemented and control groups in the risk of eczema, regardless of the timing of LGG administration, up to 2 years (RR 0.90 (0.67, 1.21), I^2 = 45%).

3.2.2. Wheezing/Asthma

For data on wheezing/asthma, see Figure 4.

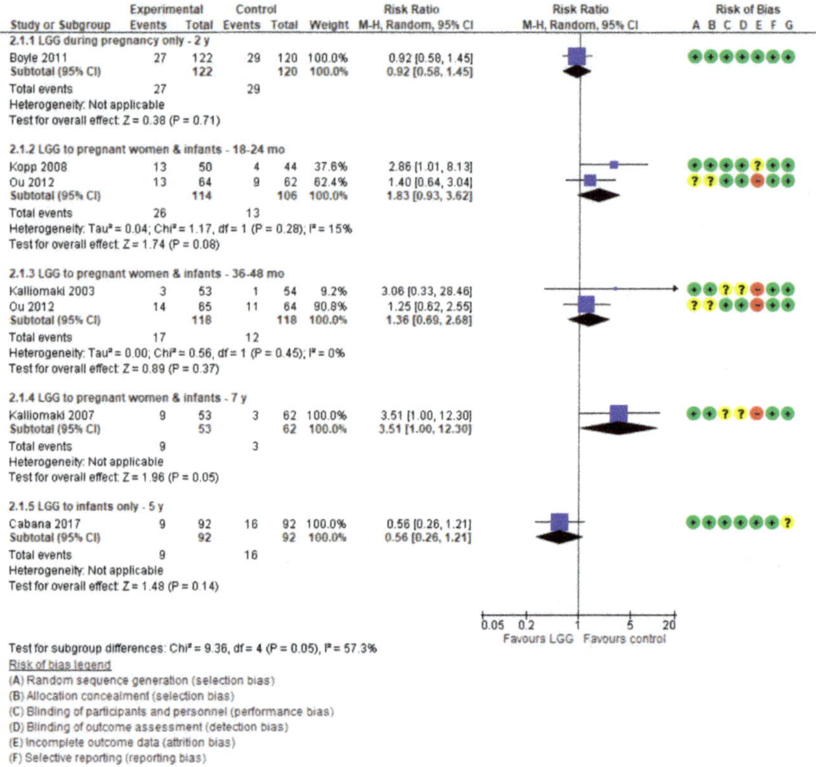

Figure 4. Secondary outcome: Effect of LGG supplementation on wheezing/asthma (data presented based on the timing of LGG administration and the timing of assessment).

LGG Administration during Late Pregnancy

One RCT [17] in which LGG was administered only during late pregnancy reported no effect of LGG administration on the risk of wheezing in children up to 2 years of age (RR 0.92 (0.58, 1.45)).

LGG Administration during Pregnancy and after Delivery

Four publications reporting on 3 RCTs [16,19–21] reported the effect of LGG administration during pregnancy and to infants on the cumulative incidence of wheezing/asthma at various time intervals. At 7 years, an increase in the risk of asthma in the LGG group compared with placebo group was observed; however, this difference was of a borderline significance (RR 3.51 (1.00, 12.30)). Furthermore, in addition to the previously stated high attrition rate in this trial (28%), the very wide confidence intervals call for caution when interpreting these findings. For other time intervals, there were no significant differences between the study groups.

LGG Administration to Infants Only

One RCT [18] in which LGG was administered only to infants reported no significant difference between groups in the risk of asthma at 5 years (RR 0.56 (0.26, 1.21)).

3.2.3. Allergic Rhinitis/Sneezing

For data on allergic rhinitis/sneezing, see Figure 5.

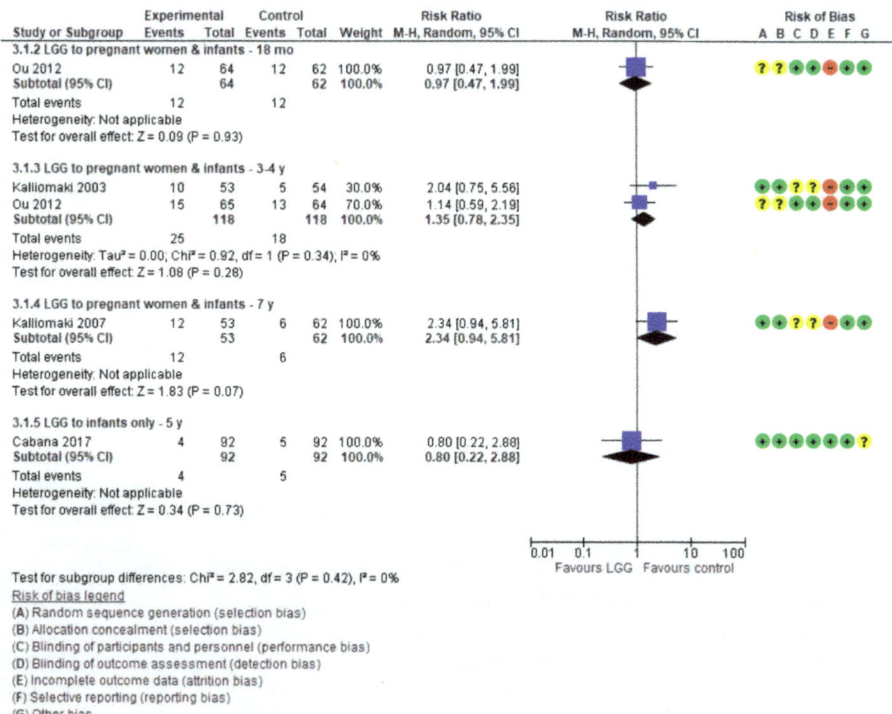

Figure 5. Secondary outcome: Effect of LGG supplementation on allergic rhinitis (data presented based on the timing of LGG administration and the timing of assessment).

LGG Administration during Pregnancy and after Delivery

Three publications [16,19,21] in which LGG was administered during pregnancy and to infants reported data on allergic rhinitis at various time intervals; no significant differences between the study groups were found.

LGG Administration to Infants Only

One RCT [18] in which LGG was administered only to infants reported no significant difference between groups in the risk of allergic rhinitis at 5 years (RR 0.80 (0.22, 2.88)).

3.3. *Food Allergy*

None of the trials reported data on food allergy.

3.4. *Adverse Events*

Only 2 RCTs reported data on adverse events. [17] found a non-significant reduction in the risk of adverse event in the LGG group compared with the placebo group (RR 0.66 (0.4, 1.1)). [20] found no difference between the groups (data were not shown).

4. Discussion

4.1. Summary of Findings

This meta-analysis adds to two recently published meta-analyses [9,10] by focusing on a single, specific probiotic strain. We found no consistent effect of the administration of LGG for reducing the risk of eczema up to 4 years of age, regardless of the timing of LGG administration (during pregnancy and/or during breastfeeding or to infants only). One trial reported a reduced risk of eczema at 7 years of age in the LGG group. However, the 7-year follow-up was completed by only a subset of participants initially randomized into the study (115 of 159, i.e., 72%); hence, this finding had to interpreted with caution. There was no effect of LGG administration on reducing the risk of wheezing/asthma, with the exception of one trial that reported an increased risk of asthma at 7 years in the LGG group compared with the placebo group. However, the high attrition rate in this trial (as mentioned earlier), the borderline statistical significance, and wide confidence intervals around the estimate call for caution in interpreting these findings. There was no effect of LGG administration on allergic rhinitis. Adverse events were similar in both study groups.

4.2. Comparison with Other Reviews

Two previously published meta-analyses pooled data on different probiotics [9,10]. A 2015 systematic review (search date: December 2014) by Cuello-Garcia et al. [9] identified 29 publications in which 12 various probiotics, single or in combinations, were used. The authors concluded that there are significant benefits of probiotic supplementation in reducing the risk of eczema when used by women during the last trimester of pregnancy (RR 0.71, 95% CI 0.60 to 0.84), when used by breastfeeding mothers (RR 0.57, 95% CI 0.47 to 0.69), or when given to infants (RR 0.80, 95% CI 0.68 to 0.94). Based on this systematic review, the WAO guidelines were published [5].

A 2018 systematic review (search date: December 2015) concluded that, overall, probiotic supplementation during pregnancy and breastfeeding reduced the risk of both eczema (19 studies; RR 0.78; 95% CI 0.68 to 0.90; substantial heterogeneity was found (I^2 = 61%)) and "atopic" eczema (11 studies; RR 0.78; 95% CI 0.65 to 0.92; no heterogeneity was found (I^2 = 0%) at age $\leq$ 4 years. However, there was no reduction in the risk of eczema in children aged 5 to 14 years. Subgroup analysis for eczema showed a significant difference between studies that supplemented mothers during the postnatal period (9 interventions; RR 0.64; 95% CI 0.51 to 0.80) and studies that just supplemented infants during the postnatal period (11 interventions; RR 0.93; 95% CI 0.81 to 1.06) [10]. For both meta-analyses, the risk is that pooling data from different genera, species, strains, and doses of probiotics obtained in different settings and/or populations, presumably with variations in their native intestinal microbiota, may result in misleading conclusions. The results could be erroneously extrapolated to other probiotics, including those that have not been adequately studied.

4.3. Strengths and Limitations

Our meta-analysis focused exclusively on one type of a clearly defined, single-organism, probiotic microorganism, specifically LGG. Thus, it provides an answer to the question as to whether current evidence should change practice. Nevertheless, several limitations must be emphasized. First, our search depended on the studies identified via reviewing previously completed systematic reviews. However, as the results were consistent, we decided to rely on these searches. Available data were too limited to allow an examination as to whether the timing of probiotic administration matters (i.e., during pregnancy only, or during pregnancy and to infants, or to infants only), even if each timing was assessed separately. All trials were conducted in high-income countries, thus, the generalizability of these findings to less privileged settings remains unclear. Overall, the quality of studies was sound. Still, some methodological issues should be considered when interpreting the results. For example, the high attrition bias in the trial by Kalliomaki et al. [17] is one methodological limitation. However, this was unavoidable in a trial with a 7-year follow-up. Included trials used different definitions of eczema, and atopic eczema was assessed separately in only one trial [15] As the definitions of wheezing and asthma were often overlapping, these data were presented jointly. However, not all cases of early life wheezing will progress into asthma later on. Most children will eventually grow out of the symptoms and will never develop asthma [23]. Regardless, as some trials have indicated an increased risk of wheezing/asthma, more data are needed to evaluate this potentially harmful effect of using probiotics. This is important as a 2018 systematic review found that of nearly 400 RCT interventions aimed at modifying microbiota, only 6% adequately reported harms [24]. Consequently, the safety and potential harms of using probiotics, particularly very early in life and for a prolonged period, remains questionable. Trials included in our review did not report differences in adverse effects. However, only limited data were available.

5. Conclusions

This meta-analysis does not support the use of LGG for reducing the risk of eczema. Our findings indicate that current guidelines on the use of probiotics for preventing eczema in infants at high risk for this allergic disease should be revised and be more specific with regard to which strain(s) to use.

Supplementary Materials: The following are available online at http://www.mdpi.com/2072-6643/10/9/1319/s1, Figure S1: Identification process for eligible trials, Table S1: Characteristics of the included studies, Table S2: GRADE evidence profile summarizing the effect of *Lactobacillus* GG supplementation vs. placebo or no intervention on eczema.

Author Contributions: Guarantor of the article: H.S. Author contributions: H.S. initially conceptualized this study. Both authors contributed to the initial protocol of the study. Both authors were responsible for data collection, data analysis, data interpretation, and preparation of the report. H.S. assumed the main responsibility for the writing of this manuscript. Both authors approved the final version of the manuscript.

Funding: This research received no external funding from funding agencies in the public, commercial, or not-for-profit sectors.

Conflicts of Interest: Declaration of personal interests: H.S. has served as a speaker for Dicofarm, Vitis Pharma, Bayer, i.e., the manufacturers and/or distributors of LGG. A.H. has served as a speaker for Nutricia, Mead Johnson, Vitis Pharma.

References

1. Asher, M.I.; Montefort, S.; Bjorksten, B.; Lai, C.K.; Strachan, D.P.; Weiland, S.K.; Williams, H.; ISAAC Phase Three Study Group. Worldwide time trends in the prevalence of symptoms of asthma, allergic rhinoconjunctivitis, and eczema in childhood: ISAAC Phases One and Three repeat multicountry cross-sectional surveys. *Lancet* **2006**, *368*, 733–743. [CrossRef]
2. Pascal, M.; Perez-Gordo, M.; Caballero, T.; Escribese, M.M.; Lopez Longo, M.N.; Luengo, O.; Manso, L.; Matheu, V.; Seoane, E.; Zamorano, M. Microbiome and allergic diseases. *Front. Immunol.* **2018**, *17*, 1584. [CrossRef] [PubMed]
3. Hill, C.; Guarner, F.; Reid, G.; Gibson, G.R.; Merenstein, D.J.; Pot, B.; Morelli, L.; Canani, R.B.; Flint, H.J.; Salminen, S.; et al. Expert consensus document. The international scientific association for probiotics and prebiotics consensus statement on the scope and appropriate use of the term probiotic. *Nat. Rev. Gastroenterol. Hepatol.* **2014**, *11*, 506–514. [CrossRef] [PubMed]
4. Szajewska, H.; Nowak-Węgrzyn, A. Allergic and immunologic disorders. In *The Microbiota in Gastrointestinal Pathophysiology Implications for Human Health, Prebiotics, Probiotics, and Dysbiosis*; Floch, M.H., Ringel, Y., Walker, W.A., Eds.; Elsevier Inc.: New York, NY, USA, 2017; pp. 285–298.
5. Fiocchi, A.; Pawankar, R.; Cuello-Garcia, C.; Ahn, K.; Al-Hammadi, S.; Agarwal, A.; Beyer, K.; Burks, W.; Canonica, G.W.; Ebisawa, M.; et al. World allergy organization-mcmaster university guidelines for allergic disease prevention (GLAD-P): Probiotics. *World Allergy Organ. J.* **2015**, *27*, 4. [CrossRef] [PubMed]
6. Ricci, G.; Cipriani, F.; Cuello-Garcia, C.A.; Brożek, J.L.; Fiocchi, A.; Pawankar, R.; Yepes-Nuñes, J.J.; Terraciano, L.; Gandhi, S.; Agarwal, A.; et al. A clinical reading on "World Allergy Organization-McMaster University Guidelines for Allergic Disease Prevention (GLAD-P): Probiotics". *World Allergy Organ. J.* **2016**, *9*, 9. [CrossRef] [PubMed]

7. Szajewska, H.; Shamir, R.; Turck, D.; van Goudoever, J.B.; Mihatsch, W.A.; Fewtrell, M. Recommendations on probiotics in allergy prevention should not be based on pooling data from different strains. *J. Allergy Clin. Immunol.* **2015**, *136*, 1422. [CrossRef] [PubMed]
8. Kalliomäki, M.; Salminen, S.; Arvilommi, H.; Kero, P.; Koskinen, P.; Isolauri, E. Probiotics in primary prevention of atopic disease: A randomized placebo-controlled trial. *Lancet* **2001**, *357*, 1076–1079. [CrossRef]
9. Szajewska, H.; Horvath, A. A partially hydrolyzed 100% whey formula and the risk of eczema and any allergy: An updated meta-analysis. *World Allergy Organ. J.* **2017**, *10*, 27. [CrossRef] [PubMed]
10. Higgins, J.P.T.; Green, S. *Cochrane Handbook for Systematic Reviews of Interventions Version 5.1.0*; Wiley: Hoboken, NJ, USA, 2011.
11. Cuello-Garcia, C.A.; Brożek, J.L.; Fiocchi, A.; Pawankar, R.; Yepes-Nuñez, J.J.; Terracciano, L.; Gandhi, S.; Agarwal, A.; Zhang, Y.; Schünemann, H.J. Probiotics for the prevention of allergy: A systematic review and meta-analysis of randomized controlled trials. *J. Allergy Clin. Immunol.* **2015**, *136*, 952–961. [CrossRef] [PubMed]
12. Garcia-Larsen, V.; Ierodiakonou, D.; Jarrold, K.; Cunha, S.; Chivinge, J.; Robinson, Z.; Geoghegan, N.; Ruparelia, A.; Devani, P.; Trivella, M.; et al. Diet during pregnancy and infancy and risk of allergic or autoimmune disease: A systematic review and meta-analysis. *PLoS Med.* **2018**, *15*, e1002507. [CrossRef] [PubMed]
13. Higgins, J.P.T.; Altman, D.G.; Sterne, J.A.C. On behalf of the cochrane statistical methods group and the cochrane bias methods group. In *Cochrane Handbook for Systematic Reviews of Interventions Version 5.1.0*; Higgins, J.P.T., Green, S., Eds.; Wiley: Hoboken, NJ, USA, 2011.
14. Higgins, J.P.T.; Deeks, J.J. Special topics in statistics. In *Cochrane Handbook for Systematic Reviews of Interventions Version 5.1.0*; Higgins, J.P.T., Green, S., Eds.; Wiley: Hoboken, NJ, USA, 2011.
15. Egger, M.; Smith, G.D.; Schneider, M.; Minder, C. Bias in meta-analysis detected by a simple, graphical test. *Br. Med. J.* **1997**, *315*, 629–634. [CrossRef]
16. Kalliomäki, M.; Salminen, S.; Poussa, T.; Arvilommi, H.; Isolauri, E. Probiotics and prevention of atopic disease: 4-year follow-up of a randomised placebo-controlled trial. *Lancet* **2003**, *361*, 1869–1871. [CrossRef]
17. Boyle, R.J.; Ismail, I.H.; Kivivuori, S.; Licciardi, P.V.; Robins-Browne, R.M.; Mah, L.J.; Axelrad, C.; Moore, S.; Donath, S.; Carlin, J.B.; et al. Lactobacillus GG treatment during pregnancy for the prevention of eczema: A randomized controlled trial. *Allergy* **2011**, *66*, 509–516. [CrossRef] [PubMed]
18. Cabana, M.D.; McKean, M.; Caughey, A.B.; Fong, L.; Lynch, S.; Wong, A.; Leong, R.; Boushey, H.A.; Hilton, J.F. Early probiotic supplementation for eczema and asthma prevention: A randomized controlled trial. *Pediatrics* **2017**, *140*, e20163000. [CrossRef] [PubMed]
19. Kalliomäki, M.; Salminen, S.; Poussa, T.; Isolauri, E. Probiotics during the first 7 years of life: A cumulative risk reduction of eczema in a randomized, placebo-controlled trial. *J. Allergy Clin. Immunol.* **2007**, *119*, 1019–1021. [CrossRef] [PubMed]
20. Kopp, M.V.; Hennemuth, I.; Heinzmann, A.; Urbanek, R. Randomized, double-blind, placebo-controlled trial of probiotics for primary prevention: No clinical effects of Lactobacillus GG supplementation. *Pediatrics* **2008**, *121*, e850–e856. [CrossRef] [PubMed]
21. Ou, C.Y.; Kuo, H.C.; Wang, L.; Hsu, T.Y.; Chuang, H.; Liu, C.A.; Chang, J.C.; Yu, H.R.; Yang, K.D. Prenatal and postnatal probiotics reduces maternal but not childhood allergic diseases: A randomized, double-blind, placebo-controlled trial. *Clin. Exp. Allergy* **2012**, *42*, 1386–1396. [CrossRef] [PubMed]
22. Rautava, S.; Kalliomäki, M.; Isolauri, E. Probiotics during pregnancy and breast-feeding might confer immunomodulatory protection against atopic disease in the infant. *J. Allergy Clin. Immunol.* **2002**, *109*, 119–121. [CrossRef] [PubMed]
23. Van Bever, H.P.; Han, E.; Shek, L.; Yi Chng, S.; Goh, D. An approach to preschool wheezing: To label as asthma? *World Allergy Organ. J.* **2010**, *3*, 253–257. [CrossRef] [PubMed]
24. Bafeta, A.; Koh, M.; Riveros, C.; Ravaud, P. Harms Reporting in Randomized Controlled Trials of Interventions Aimed at Modifying Microbiota: A Systematic Review. *Ann. Intern. Med.* **2018**. [CrossRef] [PubMed]

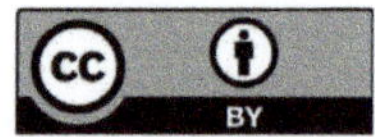

© 2018 by the authors. Licensee MDPI, Basel, Switzerland. This article is an open access article distributed under the terms and conditions of the Creative Commons Attribution (CC BY) license (http://creativecommons.org/licenses/by/4.0/).

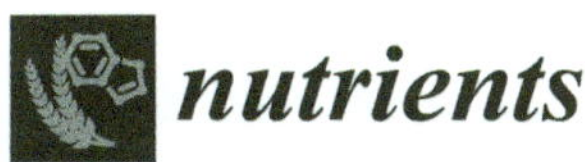

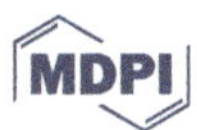

Review

Human Milk Oligosaccharides to Prevent Gut Dysfunction and Necrotizing Enterocolitis in Preterm Neonates

Stine Brandt Bering

Comparative Paediatrics and Nutrition, Department of Veterinary and Animal Sciences, Faculty of Health and Medical Sciences, University of Copenhagen, 1958 Frederiksberg C, Denmark; sbb@sund.ku.dk; Tel.: +45-35-33-10-92

Received: 28 September 2018; Accepted: 5 October 2018; Published: 8 October 2018

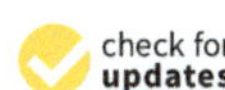

Abstract: This review focuses on the evidence for health benefits of human milk oligosaccharides (HMOs) for preterm infants to stimulate gut adaptation and reduce the incidence of necrotizing enterocolitis (NEC) in early life. The health benefits of breastfeeding are partly explained by the abundant HMOs that serve as prebiotics and immunomodulators. Gut immaturity in preterm infants leads to difficulties in tolerating enteral feeding and bacterial colonization and a high sensitivity to NEC, particularly when breast milk is insufficient. Due to the immaturity of the preterm infants, their response to HMOs could be different from that in term infants. The concentration of HMOs in human milk is highly variable and there is no evidence to support a specifically adapted high concentration in preterm milk. Further, the gut microbiota is not only different but also highly variable after preterm birth. Studies in pigs as models for preterm infants indicate that HMO supplementation to formula does not mature the gut or prevent NEC during the first weeks after preterm birth and the effects may depend on a certain stage of gut maturity. Supplemented HMOs may become more important for gut protection in the preterm infants when the gut has reached a more mature phase.

Keywords: human milk oligosaccharides; human milk; infant formula; necrotizing enterocolitis; preterm infant

---

1. Introduction

Preterm birth (<37 weeks' gestation) is a major health concern and the leading cause of neonatal mortality. Rates of preterm delivery remain high and even increase in some countries but medical advancements have greatly improved survival rates, even for the extremely and very preterm infants (<28 and <32 weeks' gestation, respectively) [1]. Transition to enteral feeding at birth poses a great challenge for the immature gastrointestinal tract of very preterm infants due to their compromised digestive and immune functions. Diet-related neonatal diseases for very preterm infants include sepsis and necrotizing enterocolitis (NEC). The NEC is a devastating intestinal inflammatory disease that leads to necrosis and perforation of the gut epithelium. The NEC complications may relate to morbidities later in life, including compromised neurodevelopment, atopic diseases and retinopathy [2]. Improved long-term survival of preterm infants also reflect improvements in nutritional care and it is now widely recognized that mother's own milk is the optimal diet for preterm new-borns [1]. Mother's own milk reduces morbidity and mortality [3,4], protects against NEC [5–8] and sepsis [9] and is trophic to the gastrointestinal tract [10]. Donor human milk is considered the best alternative to mother's own milk but donor milk is mature-derived milk and pasteurized and the content of bioactive components are therefore reduced [11]. Comparisons of donor human milk with preterm formula, as a supplement to mother's own milk for the first 10 days, did not improve protection against severe infections and mortality in very low-birth-weight infants [12].

Human milk oligosaccharides (HMO) are highly abundant in human milk. With the unique and complex carbohydrate structure, they resist gastrointestinal hydrolysis and digestion by pancreatic and brush-border enzymes and are therefore not absorbed in significant amounts. Instead, they serve as prebiotic substrates for specific commensal bacteria in the gut. Thus, HMOs help to shape the developing microbiome and the innate immune system in the infant gut, as documented from mother-infant cohort studies [13,14]. Several beneficial effects have been associated with HMOs, based on preclinical studies. These HMO effects include antiadhesive properties, modulation of intestinal epithelial cell responses, microbiota and immune modulation, protection against NEC and improved brain development. Reviews on the metabolism and effects of HMOs, mainly in term infants, are available [15–18]. Much less information is available about HMO effects in preterm infants. With the recent industrial capacity to isolate HMOs or synthesize HMO analogues in bulk amounts, the first clinical trials in healthy infants receiving formula have been performed. It is documented that supplementation of 2′-fucosyllactose (2′-FL) and lacto-*N*-neo-tetraose (LNnT) is tolerable and stimulate normal growth within the first 4–6 months of life [19,20]. In general, the number of publications on HMO effects is increasing with the capacity to isolate or produce HMOs in bulk amounts within the recent years, both as regards infant trials and preclinical studies in larger animals. These results now warrant clinical trials to investigate effects of specific HMO interventions for special groups of infants, such as preterm infants.

The prebiotic and immunomodulatory effects of HMOs may be particularly important for the population of very preterm infants to improve their intestinal maturation and protection. On the other hand, it is possible that the physiologically immature intestine in preterm infants hinders or changes the normal HMO-related improvements in gut functions, microbiota composition and immune modulation. This review highlights the current documentation for effects of HMOs to prevent gut dysfunction and NEC in the very preterm infants. The review is based on evidence from clinical trials and cohort studies in infants, preclinical animal models and in vitro studies.

2. Oligosaccharides in Human Milk after Preterm Birth

The HMOs are composed of the monosaccharides glucose (Glc), galactose (Gal), *N*-acetyl glucosamine (GlcNAc), fucose (Fuc) and sialic acid, which in humans is found exclusively as *N*-acetylneuraminic acid (Neu5Ac) [16]. Selected HMOs and their abbreviations are listed in Table 1.

Table 1. Selected human milk oligosaccharide structures and abbreviations [21,22].

Neutral Oligosaccharides		Acidic Oligosaccharides	
2′-Fucosyllactose	2′-FL	Disialyllacto-*N*-tetraose	DSLNT
Lactodifucotetraose	LDFT	Siallylacto-*N*-neo-tetraose b	LST b
Lacto-*N*-tetraose	LNT	Siallylacto-*N*-neo-tetraose c	LST c
Lacto-*N*-neo-tetraose	LNnT	Siallylacto-*N*-tetraose a	LST a
Lacto-*N*-hexaose	LNH	3′-Sialyllactose	3′SL
3-Fucosyllactose	3FL	6′-Sialyllactose	6′SL
Lacto-*N*-fucopentaose I	LNFP I		
Lacto-*N*-fucopentaose II	LNFP II		
Lacto-*N*-fucopentaose III	LNFP III		
Lacto-*N*-fucopentaose V	LNFP V		
Lacto-*N*-difucohexaose I	LNDFH I		
Lacto-*N*-difucohexaose II	LNDFH II		

The HMO composition in human milk is determined by genetic factors and dependent on the mother's Secretor (Se) and Lewis (Le) blood group characteristics. The blood group characteristics determine the expression of the specific α1-2-fucosyltransferase (FUT2) and α1-3/4-fucosyltransferase (FUT3), which gives rise to four different milk groups (Table 2). Group 1 are the Secretor Lewis-positive (Se^+/Le^+) and derives from the most common phenotype. They comprise approximately 70% of the European population and contains the highest concentration of total and fucosylated HMOs, primarily 2′-FL [23]. Group 2 are Nonsecretor Lewis-positive (Se^-/Le^+) and Group 3 are Secretor Lewis-negative (Se^+/Le^-). Group 4 are Nonsecretor Lewis-negative (Se^-/Le^-), which have the lowest levels of total oligosaccharides [24].

Table 2. Milk oligosaccharide groups and the related genotypes.

Milk Group	Genotypes		Phenotypes		Fucosyl-Oligosaccharides [24] *
	Secretor	Lewis	Secretor	Lewis	
1	Se/-	Le/-	Secretor	Lewis positive	2′-FL, LNDFH I + II, LNFP I + II + III, 3FL, LDFT, LNnT, LNT, LNH, MFNLH II
2	se/se	Le/-	Non-secretor	Lewis positive	LNDFH I + II, 3FL, LNFP II + III, LNnT, LNT, LNH, MFNLH II
3	Se/-	le/le	Secretor	Lewis negative	3FL, LNFP I + III, LDFT, 2′-FL, LNnT, LNT, LNH, MFNLH II
4	se/se	le/le	Non-secretor	Lewis negative	3FL, LNFP III, MFLNH II, LNnT, LNT, LNH

* All sialyl-oligosaccharides are present in all the milk groups, including DSLNT, LST, 3′SL, 6′SL.

The different HMOs in the four milk groups have been characterized in preterm milk during the first month of lactation [24]. The total amounts of HMOs were highest in Group 1 milk at day 4 (23.4 g/L) and lowest in Group 4 (11.3 g/L), with important decreases in concentrations in these groups within the first month of lactation (15% and 22%, respectively). Although reduced over time, the levels in Group 1 continued to be highest within the first month, also relative to Groups 2 and 3 (~17 g/L). Therefore, the concentration of total HMOs is not particularly high in colostrum and depends more on the blood characteristics of the mother. LNT and LNnT together constituted >90% of the core oligosaccharides in all 4 groups. Group 1 milk was dominated by 2′-FL, LNDFH and LNFP I, Group 2 by LDFNH, LNFP II and 3′-FL, Group 3 by 2′-FL and LNFP I and Group 4 by MFLNH II and LNFP III. The identified fucosyl-oligosaccharides are listed in Table 2. No differences in the average levels of sialyl-oligosaccharides were observed among the groups but levels were reduced during the first month of lactation in Groups 1, 2 and 4 [24]. Thus, considerable differences in HMO contents were found within the milk groups and were primarily related to the presence or absence of specific fucosyl-oligosaccharides. In another study, LNT was found to be more abundant and with higher variability in preterm milk [25]. Further, 2′-FL was not consistently present across lactation in milk from mothers delivering preterm, which added to the variation in concentrations of fucosylated HMOs. The variation was found both between individuals and during lactation in women delivering preterm compared to women delivering at term. Fucosylation may therefore not be as well-regulated in preterm milk as in term milk [25].

When looking at the total HMO concentration in preterm versus term milk, the total HMO concentration in breast milk from Group 1 mothers delivering preterm [26] was higher than that from mothers delivering at term [27] and decreased during the first month. In another study, the content of neutral HMOs in milk from mothers delivering preterm was not different to milk from mothers delivering at term during the first month of lactation but HMO concentrations varied over time from mother to mother [28]. A recent study found similar levels of HMOs in milk from mothers delivering preterm and term, also with large individual variations [22]. For sialic acid, the content in milk from mothers delivering preterm was higher than in milk from mothers delivering at term and decreased within the first three months of lactation [29]. This may correlate to the total number of acidic HMOs. The varying levels and specificity of HMOs in the milk maintained over time may have significant impact on the biological and clinical effects on preterm infants during the breastfeeding period. The infants of non-secretor, Lewis negative mothers are most likely not compensated by improved gut utility and metabolization and a random factor related to the mother's or the donor blood group genetics may thereby impact gut homeostasis and clinical outcome in the infant.

The difference in total HMO levels between the different studies most likely reflects the lack of standardized methods for obtaining quantitative data on HMO content in milk and the number of subjects included in the studies [22]. From the present studies, there is no clear evidence for a higher total concentration of HMOs in preterm versus term milk. Variation in HMO concentrations among mothers may relate more to high individual differences based on genetic variation. This may or may not influence the susceptibility of preterm infants to NEC, late onset sepsis and related neurodevelopmental impairments.

3. Human Milk Oligosaccharides and Necrotizing Enterocolitis

The high prevalence of NEC in preterm infants is closely related to their immature gut and is affected by the diet and bacterial colonization. With HMOs serving as prebiotics and possibly also as antiadhesive antimicrobials and modulators of intestinal epithelial cell and immune responses, they may have a significant impact on NEC by modulating the immune system and gut microbiota in a more appropriate direction. Currently, no randomized clinical trials in preterm infants have been conducted to document direct effects of supplemented HMOs on NEC outcome. Most indications for HMO effects are based on the lower incidence of NEC in breast-fed infants compared to formula-fed infants [6]. Evidence is also found from mother-infant cohort studies correlating HMO concentration in mother's milk with infant outcomes on NEC related parameters such as microbiota modulation [30].

In a multicentre clinical prospective cohort study, correlation between HMO composition in breast milk and NEC outcome in very low-birth-weight infants showed no differences between NEC cases and total HMO concentration in their milk diet. Only DSLNT-concentrations were lower in almost all milk samples in NEC cases compared with controls [31].

The efficacy of HMOs to prevent NEC has mainly been assessed in preclinical NEC animal models. In neonatal rats, formula supplemented with HMOs (10 mg/mL) showed improved survival (73 to 95%) and reduced pathology scores (1.98 to 0.45). Within the pool of HMOs, DSLNT was identified to exert the NEC protective effect [32]. Both 2′-FL and synthesized DSLNT analogues have been documented to improve NEC protective effects, although not to the same extent as pooled HMOs [33,34]. The neonatal rat studies hereby document beneficial effects of specific HMOs to reduce NEC-related intestinal lesions. The rat NEC models are based on term-delivered pups exposed to various insults (e.g., hypoxia and hypothermia) to induce NEC and not to the prematurity of the organs, which is the main driver of NEC in infants. In rodents, gut development occurs relatively rapidly after birth, while the gut of infants matures gradually from the foetal period and into the neonatal period [35]. After preterm birth, the immature gut has to adapt slowly to cope with the challenges of feeding and bacterial colonization. This situation may differ markedly from the rapid postnatal gut development in rodents. Lipopolysaccharide stimulation of foetal murine intestinal epithelial cells ex vivo results in intracellular cell signalling, transcriptional activation and chemokine secretion, whereas cells from new-born and adult mice are non-responsive [36,37]. This indicates that the intestine acquires immunological tolerance to endotoxin after birth and only in the prenatal state the intestine is hyper-responsive and therefore potentially more NEC-sensitive. The neonatal rats as NEC models are suitable and well-recognized to identify potential dietary effector substrates related to NEC but as common for many models, the effect may be more extreme than what would be observed in infants. This needs to be taken into account when translating the results to infants.

Pigs have the same gastrointestinal structure as humans with similar dietary habits and preterm piglet delivery at 88–95% gestation is associated with clinical complications and degrees of gut immaturity similar to those in infants born at 70–90% gestation, such as impaired respiratory, nutritional, immunological and metabolic responses after preterm birth [35]. The high spontaneous susceptibility to enteral feeding and bacterial colonization closely resemble that in infants. This makes the preterm pig model relevant as a large animal model for studies on clinical complications of preterm birth such as NEC. Novel technologies have now made it possible to generate several of the complex HMOs in larger amounts. This makes it feasible to test single and more complex blends of HMOs as dietary supplements in a clinically relevant NEC model with preterm pigs.

Supplementation with 2′-FL (5 g/L) to formula has only shown minimal short-term effects on NEC and gut maturation in preterm pigs within 5 days. Here, eight 2′-FL pigs (50%) and twelve control pigs (71%) developed NEC with no difference in NEC lesion scores ($p = 0.35$). Further, several intestinal functional parameters were not affected by 2′-FL [38]. Also, blends of 4 and >25 HMOs have been investigated as a supplement to formula at 5–10 g/L for 5 or 11 days after preterm birth in pigs. All HMOs were identified in urine and faeces of the HMO-treated pigs. After 5 days, NEC lesions were similar between HMO supplemented and control pigs. Only after 11 days, supplementation with the 4-HMO blend showed minor tendencies towards reduced NEC relative to control pigs (56 vs. 79%, $p = 0.2$). At the same time dehydration and diarrhoea was increased. The diarrhoea is likely induced by infant formula maldigestion and subsequent high intraluminal osmolarity that may be enhanced by non-digested HMOs in the lumen [39].

4. Human Milk Oligosaccharides and the Preterm Gut Microbiota

The microbiota of preterm infants is different from their healthy term counterparts. This is mainly due to organ immaturity, frequent use of antibiotics and hospital stay in the neonatal intensive care units [40]. The microbiota of healthy term infants is dominated by Bifidobacteria and Bacteroidetes, which are also the primary consumers of HMOs. These bacteria are only present at low abundance in preterm infants. Instead, the preterm infants show low diversity with increased colonization of potentially pathogenic bacteria from the gram-negative family Enterobacteriaceae of the Proteobacteria phylum [30,40–42]. Several Proteobacteria are positively associated with development of NEC, whereas the relative abundances of Firmicutes and Bacteroidetes are decreased [43–45]. In the piglet model, Enterobacteriaceae and Lachnospiraceae were predominant in both preterm and term pigs at 11 days after birth and only in the low abundant genera differences were observed between preterm and term pigs [46]. Proteobacteria and Firmicutes phyla have also been identified as predominant in preterm and term pigs at day 5 but in the preterm pigs, the relative abundance of Proteobacteria decreased and Firmicutes increased at day 26, where also *Lactobacillus* was predominant (Shamrul et al., JPGN in press). As for infants, the Bifidobacteria and Bacteroidetes are found in low numbers in the preterm pigs. Instead the Enterobacteriaceae are dominant. In new-born rats, considerable diversity of bacterial populations has been observed but lactobacilli have often been identified as the most common first colonizers in both formula-fed and breast-fed rats [47,48].

Only few studies have investigated the influence of the different HMOs in mother's milk on the gut microbiota pattern in preterm infants. The HMO composition in milk and stools from mother-preterm infant dyads have shown high variability in the content of HMOs between individuals but similar within mother-infant pairs and secretor status of the mother correlated with specific HMO structures in faecal content of the infant [30]. Further, there was a trend towards higher levels of Proteobacteria and lower levels of Firmicutes in preterm infants of non-secretor mothers. This indicated that HMOs influence the intestinal microbiota in preterm infants. Infants of secretor mothers may be protected by fucosylated HMOs that decrease the levels of pathogens related to NEC and sepsis, for example LDFT and LNFP V and structures that are both fucosylated and sialylated. Other structures, such as LNnH and HMOs that contain neither fucose nor sialic acid, may on the other hand lead to dysbiosis [30,49].

In a new-born pig diarrhoea model, the level of *Enterococcus* was reduced in 2′-FL supplemented pigs within the first eight days after birth. When inoculating the pigs with enterotoxigenic *Escherichia coli* F18, 2′-FL tended to reduce the abundance of *Enterobacteriaceae* and increased the relative abundance of an unclassified *Lachnospiraceae* genus [50]. Also, a mix of HMOs (75% neutral and 25% acidic) have shown to reduce Rotavirus-induced diarrhoea in new-born pigs, with increased number of *Lachnospiraceae* and modulation of the mucosal immunity [51]. In the preterm pig NEC model, only minor microbiota effects were observed in 2′-FL supplemented pigs within 5 days. The pigs tended to have less anaerobic bacteria in caecal contents and only *Enterococcus* differed in proportions between 2′-FL and control pigs [38]. In an 11-day study, the overall bacterial adherence and diversity was not changed after supplementation with a mixture of 4 HMOs in the preterm pig model. The short-chain fatty acids, acetic acid, butyric acid and pentanoic acid, did though tend to be higher in the 4-HMO supplemented pigs [39]. Only *Fusobacterium* were reduced in the 4-HMO supplemented pigs and the number of *Fusobacterium* tended to be related to NEC development. Interestingly, although found in lower amounts, Bifidobacteria correlated with total HMO content and specifically with 2′-FL levels in colon contents in 11-day old preterm pigs fed the 4-HMO blend (Rudloff et al. manuscript in review). In contrary, DSLNT did not correlate with bacterial colonization or NEC, although NEC preventive effects of DSLNT have been observed in rats [34]. The effects of the sialylated oligosaccharide, SL, in a bovine based milk supplement has been investigated in preterm pigs for 19 days (Obelitz-Ryom et al. manuscript in review). Even within this slightly longer study period, supplementation of SL-enriched bovine milk oligosaccharides in amounts similar to what is found in mature human milk (380 mg SL/L) did not change either the overall microbiota density or composition nor the short chain fatty acid levels in the gut. Many of the pigs were clinically compromised with diarrhoea during the study period related to their prematurity and the oligosaccharide supplementation was not able to improve the clinical conditions of the piglets, as also observed earlier [39]. Overall, only minor effects of HMOs on gut microbiota has been observed in preterm pigs, including limited effects of 2′-FL on Bifidobacteria. In contrast to the preterm models, models of undernutrition in new-born infants have shown a relationship between sialylated bovine milk oligosaccharides and growth. Here, gnotobiotic 5-week old mice and 3-day old piglets were inoculated with faecal microbiota from a 6-month old stunted Malawian infant [52].

5. Human Milk Oligosaccharide Effects on Gastrointestinal Maturation

Whereas clinical outcomes such as diarrhoea and NEC are common endpoints in clinical infant trials, gut functional and structural changes are more difficult to investigate. The preclinical animal models and in vitro cell models may give insight into more specific functional gastrointestinal effects, such as gut structure and morphology, epithelial differentiation, mucus production, permeability and digestive and absorptive capacity.

The HMO supplemented formula-fed rat pups have shown normal, healthy microscopic architecture of the ileum, comparable to dam fed pups, whereas some ileal sections from formula-fed and galacto-oligosaccharide supplemented pups showed complete destruction of the tissue [32]. Although tissue architecture was improved with HMO supplementation, no effects were observed on weight gain, where only the dam-fed pups improved weight gain compared to formula-fed pups [32]. No other gut parameters have been documented in the identified rodent HMO studies [32,34].

In the preterm pig NEC studies, no major effects on gut parameters have been observed from HMO supplementation within 5 and 11 days. For 2′-FL supplementation, no effects were found on any of the investigated gut parameters [38]. For 4 and >25 HMO blends, only minor effects on the gut were observed [39]. Overall, no effects were observed on daily weight gain, relative organ weights, mucosa proportion of the small intestine, hexose absorption, gut permeability, or plasma citrulline, reflecting enterocyte mass and function. Minor changes were observed for the brush-border enzyme activities. The activities of lactase, aminopeptidase A, aminopeptidase N and dipeptidyl peptidase IV were higher only in the ileum of piglets supplemented with 25-HMO compared to non-supplemented piglets after 5 days. No changes were observed for maltase and sucrase. The same was observed for the piglets supplemented with 4-HMO, which only showed lower villus heights. Supplementary studies in an intestinal epithelial cell model with IPEC-J2 cells showed reduced proliferation with 25-HMO, 2′FL, LNnT, 6′SL and SA, indicating differentiation towards more mature intestinal cells [39], in line with earlier observations in HT-29, Caco-2 and HIEC cells [53]. Overall, only minor effects have been observed from HMO supplementation to formulas on a wide range of investigated parameters related to gut function and maturation in preterm piglets. In contrast, other diets or dietary components have induced significant improvements in both growth, organ weights and brush-border enzyme activities. For example, porcine or bovine colostrum and donor human milk in comparison to infant formula in preterm pigs [11,54–56]. Also supplements like bioactive whey protein concentrate and lactose [57] and amniotic fluid [58] have documented effects.

6. Immunomodulatory Effects of Human Milk Oligosaccharides

The immature mucosal immune system in the intestine of preterm infants is hyper-inflammatory [59] and the disturbance of the development in controlling inflammatory processes potentially contributes to NEC [60]. The bioactive components in human milk are highly important for the quenching of inflammatory processes after birth, by facilitating appropriate immune responses and antigenic memory [61–63].

So far, randomized controlled trials with HMO interventions have only been conducted in healthy term infants. In a randomized multicentre trial, the effects of supplementation of infant formula with 2′-FL (1.0 g/L) and LNnT (0.5 g/L) on growth, tolerance and morbidity in new-born healthy infants has been investigated during the first 6 months of life. Infants receiving HMOs had lower parent-reported morbidity, particularly bronchitis and fewer medication use, such as antipyretics and antibiotics [20]. A randomized controlled study on growth and tolerance was conducted in healthy new-born infants fed formula supplemented with 2′-FL (0.2 and 1.0 g/L) for 114 days. The 2′-FL supplemented formula was well tolerated and comparable to formula-fed infants for average stool consistency, number of stools per day and percent of feedings associated with spitting up or vomit [19]. In a sub-study nested within this clinical trial, effects on biomarkers of immune function were investigated [64]. Here, infants fed 2′-FL supplemented formula had lower levels of plasma (IL-1ra, IL-1a, IL-1b, IL-6, TNF-α) and ex vivo (TNF-α, IFN-γ) inflammatory cytokines than formula-fed infants. The levels were similar to those of breast-fed infants.

The HMOs from human colostrum have shown to modulate mucosal signalling in the immature human intestine by the use of human foetal intestinal explants. The human foetal intestinal epithelial cells overexpressed innate inflammatory genes, such as *NFkB*, *MyD88*, *TLR2*, *TLR4* and *TRAF*, with inadequate expression of negative feedback regulator genes. Accordingly, the immature intestinal mucosa of foetal tissues is prone to exaggerated responses to pro-inflammatory stimuli, increasing the risk of inflammatory diseases of the intestine in the infant. The HMO stimulation enhanced expression of genes involved in immune cell trafficking, proliferation and recruitment of immune cells to the mucosal surface. This could explain the clinical association between human milk consumption and reduced risk of preterm gut inflammation [65]. The HMOs and particularly 2′-FL, have also been shown to suppress CD14 expression in human intestinal epithelial cells, thereby attenuating lipopolysaccharide-induced inflammation. The inhibition of inflammation supports the role HMOs in the innate immune system to protect the infant through the milk [66].

In vitro studies have associated HMOs to systemic immune functions. In leukocytes isolated from human peripheral blood, sialylated HMOs have shown to reduce selectin-mediated platelet-neutrophil complex formation [67] and inhibit adhesion of monocytes, lymphocytes and neutrophils to endothelial cells [68]. Excessive leukocyte infiltration has been linked to the host's immune system involved in NEC pathogenesis [69] but evidence from preterm infants is lacking. Further, the systemic effects require the presence of HMOs in the circulation, which is minor due to the low absorption of HMOs [70–72].

In the preterm pig studies investigating blends of 4 and >25 HMOs, no changes in the levels of IL-8 and IL-1β in the small intestine and colon were observed from HMO supplementation. Supplementation with 4-HMO for 11 days increased the expression of *IL10*, *IL12*, *TGFβ* and *TLR4* [39]. The upregulation of specific immune genes related to the Th1 and Treg balance may represent an ability of the HMOs to control mucosal immune responses to the diet and the bacterial colonization. This may help to educate the immature immunological pathways in the gut. The systemic immunity has been investigated in preterm pigs supplemented with SL-enriched bovine milk oligosaccharides for 19 days. The levels of blood leukocyte subsets remained unchanged and similar neutrophil phagocytotic capacity of *Staphylococcus aureus* was observed in the SL and control group (Ryom-Obelitz et al. manuscript in review). The lacking effects of HMOs to stimulate mucosal and systemic immune maturation in the preterm pigs may be related to their prematurity. In comparison to term pigs with a well-developed immune system, the preterm pigs may not be able to respond appropriately to bioactive immune-stimulating factors in milk to facilitate an appropriate immune response before their immune system is more mature. Even in pigs with NEC, which should have a significant increase in the activation of innate immune parameters, the immune response of the preterm pigs is moderate [73,74]. The low dietary modulation of the immune system in preterm neonates may be particularly compromising when feeding formula diets that predispose to NEC [6].

7. Human Milk Oligosaccharides for the Preterm Newborns

An overview of HMO effects in the compromised preterm neonates is presented in Figure 1, together with the mechanisms of action in healthy term infants as reviewed earlier [15,17]. Reduced peristalsis, lowered digestive and absorptive function, impaired intestinal epithelial barrier and a dysregulated mucosal immune system leads to the uncontrolled cycle of maldigestion, bacterial invasion, immune activation and inflammation in the preterm neonate. This is particularly evident following formula feeding. As reviewed here, there seem not to be a specifically adapted high concentration of HMOs in preterm versus term milk. Rather, the content is related to high individual differences based on genetic variation. Beneficial effects of individual and pooled HMOs on NEC resistance has been documented in neonatal rat studies. The preterm piglets are highly sensitive to dietary interventions and the pig studies support the beneficial effects of feeding optimal diets such as donor human milk for improved health outcome and NEC prevention [11,55,56]. Nonetheless, it has not been possible to document any significant effects of HMOs supplementation of infant formula on NEC prevention [38,39,50]. This indicates that immune parameters and microbial colonization and fermentation may only to a limited extent be modified by HMOs in a formula base in the early life of the very preterm neonates. Either the effects are minor in the new-born immature gut, or the detrimental effects induced by formula feeding, such as food intolerance and NEC, may override any beneficial effects of HMOs. Other milk components may have a higher impact on gut health in the preterm intestine within the first weeks' of life. Several milk diets with optimized protein bioactivity have proven to be beneficial in the preterm pig intestine by modulating the innate immune defence system and improving gut functional parameters and growth [11,55,57,75–77]. These results indicate that bioactive proteins may be more important than prebiotic oligosaccharides for preterm gut development.

The preterm infants are particularly sensitive with immature organs and although HMOs are thought to stimulate gut and immune maturation and appropriate colonization, the undeveloped gut may not be able to tolerate a high microbial load to the same extent as term infants, regardless the composition [78,79]. Reducing the total load of bacteria, rather than stimulating bacterial colonization, may hinder NEC development more efficiently in the early life of very preterm infants [80,81].

Biological effects of HMOs may likely be more effective to improve the immature gastrointestinal functions in preterm neonates beyond the immediate neonatal period. In a later and more robust period of prenatal development and growth, preterm infants who do not have access to human milk may benefit from HMO supplemented bovine milk-based infant formula. This has though not yet been investigated. At least in healthy new-born term infants, the supplementation of 2′-FL and LNnt to infant formula starting <14 days after birth until 6 months of age has proven to be well tolerated without changing weight gain and associated with lower parent-reported morbidity such as bronchitis [19,20]. In general, the number of publications on HMO effects is increasing with the capacity to isolate or produce HMOs in bulk amounts within the recent years, both as regards infant trials and preclinical studies in larger animals. This will add important information to the generated knowledge from breast-fed infants over the years.

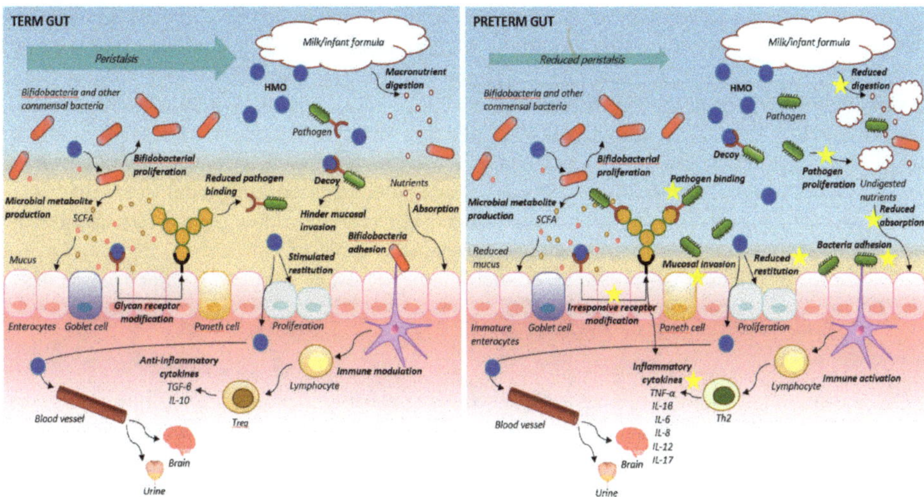

Figure 1. Schematic overview of the suggested mechanisms of action of human milk oligosaccharides (HMOs) in the intestine of term infants (**left panel**) and in the immature intestine of preterm new-born neonates (**right panel**). In the term intestine, appropriate peristalsis, milk digestion and absorption and epithelial barrier protection with well-developed mucus and mature and responsive enterocytes maintain gut and immune homeostasis. Here, HMOs may serve as prebiotics, act as decoy, modify epithelial glycan receptor expression, stimulate epithelial restitution and immune modulation to further secure proper response to feeding. In preterm neonates, gut prematurity may outweigh or hinder the beneficial effects of HMOs. Reduced peristalsis, lowered digestive and absorptive function, a dysregulated mucosal immune system and impaired intestinal epithelial barriers with reduced mucus and epithelial restitution all lead to an imbalance between epithelial cell injury and repair. The HMOs may still serve as a prebiotic substrate for bifidogenic bacteria and support short chain fatty acid (SCFA) production and may also serve as receptor-mediated decoys for specific pathogenic bacteria but the underlying immaturity of the gut with compromised absorptive functions and restitution seem unresponsive to HMOs, with no maturational effects on the basic functions. This is of particularly concern if the HMOs are supplemented to infant formula, where over-fermentation and proliferation of bacteria are inevitable in the preterm gut. Thereby, a vicious cycle of maldigestion, bacterial invasion, immune activation and uncontrolled inflammation appears that does not seem to be hindered by HMO supplementation (indicated with yellow stars).

The preclinical animal studies do not fully represent the NEC pathology of infants and the milk oligosaccharide and gut microbial patterns differ to some extent. Concentrations of oligosaccharides in porcine colostrum is in the range 7.38 to 29.35 g/L and the corresponding value for bovine milk oligosaccharides is about 1 g/L [82]. These data showed big variation among sows, which is similar to observations in humans. The observed range of concentrations is though not very distinct from concentrations in human milk. The highest levels in sows' colostrum correspond to the concentrations found in Group 1 milk and the lowest concentrations similar to the concentrations in Group 4 milk. However, contrary to in humans, the content is significantly reduced (−43%) within the first week after delivery. This may represent the faster ontogeny and shorter time to weaning of the piglet compared to infants. For specific milk oligosaccharides, LNT is highly abundant in human milk and one of the primary drivers of infant colonization with bifidobacteria. In contrary, these bacteria have minor influence in the new-born preterm pig intestine. Human milk is considered unique, as it contains type I oligosaccharides (LNT, LNFP-I, LNFP-II and LNDFH-I), which have not been identified in bovine milk. Unlike bovine milk, LNDFH-I has also been identified in porcine milk and Neu5Gc containing oligosaccharides that are found in bovine milk are absent in porcine milk. Although natural levels of oligosaccharides in porcine milk after the first week is lower than human milk, the higher abundance of fucosylated versus sialylated oligosaccharide structures places porcine milk structurally far closer to human milk than previously assumed [82–84]. From birth, piglets also have endogenous production of fucosylated structures in the gut such as α1,2'-fucose [50]. This may to some extent compensate for the lower levels in the milk. Although the microbial fingerprint in the piglet is different from that of the new-born infants, the presence of fucosylated structures both in the porcine milk and in the gut of the new-born piglets may indicate an impact of these oligosaccharide structures in managing gut homeostasis also in pigs. In both infants and piglets, a balanced milk oligosaccharide composition may be needed to shape the gut microbiome for optimal trophic and protective effects and to keep dysbiosis in check, not only by stimulating bifidobacteria but also by regulating other bacteria such as Enterobacteriaceae that are implicated in NEC.

8. Conclusions

As a major constituent of human milk, HMOs are probably significant contributors to general infant health during breastfeeding. This could be due to their ability to stimulate the immune system and to provide substrates for development of a beneficial gut microbiota. Very preterm infants are born with an immature gut and immune system. Whether the health effects ascribed to HMOs also benefit these neonates in their first difficult weeks of life, when the immature gut needs to adapt to enteral feeding and microbial colonization, is unclear. Reflections on when to introduce HMO supplementation to preterm infants are necessary (e.g., when feeding donor human milk or infant formula). Fortification of donor human milk is often needed to provide enough protein for appropriate growth to the very preterm infant and addition of HMOs in combination with protein supplements may be feasible. Based on the preclinical studies reviewed here, there is limited evidence that addition of HMOs to a milk formula diet of very sensitive preterm neonates in the first weeks of life will reduce NEC sensitivity. Later introduction of HMOs to the preterm neonates, when the gut has adapted to feeding and bacterial colonization may be more beneficial for improved gut health. Larger cohort studies as well as randomized clinical trials with NEC as outcome are needed to validate preclinical findings of HMOs and the discrepancies between preterm and term adaptation and tolerance. Furthermore, the mechanistic actions of HMOs should be tested further in appropriate preclinical animal studies, where specific HMO structures and optimal timing of supplementation should be addressed.

Funding: This research received no external funding.

Conflicts of Interest: The author declares no conflict of interest.

References

1. Cleminson, J.S.; Zalewski, S.P.; Embleton, N.D. Nutrition in the preterm infant: What's new? *Curr. Opin. Clin. Nutr. Metab. Care* **2016**, *19*, 220–225. [CrossRef] [PubMed]
2. Bhatia, J. Human milk and the premature infant. *Ann. Nutr. Metab.* **2013**, *62*, 8–14. [CrossRef] [PubMed]
3. Furman, L.; Taylor, G.; Minich, N.; Hack, M. The effect of maternal milk on neonatal morbidity of very low-birth-weight infants. *Arch. Pediatr. Adolesc. Med.* **2003**, *157*, 66–71. [CrossRef] [PubMed]
4. Abrams, S.A.; Schanler, R.J.; Lee, M.L.; Rechtman, D.J. Greater mortality and morbidity in extremely preterm infants fed a diet containing cow milk protein products. *Breastfeed. Med.* **2014**, *9*, 281–285. [CrossRef] [PubMed]
5. Quigley, M.; McGuire, W. Formula versus donor breast milk for feeding preterm or low birth weight infants. *Cochrane Database Syst. Rev.* **2014**, CD002971. [CrossRef]
6. Lucas, A.; Cole, T.J. Breast milk and neonatal necrotising enterocolitis. *Lancet* **1990**, *336*, 1519–1523. [CrossRef]
7. Meinzen-Derr, J.; Poindexter, B.; Wrage, L.; Morrow, A.L.; Stoll, B.; Donovan, E.F. Role of human milk in extremely low birth weight infants' risk of necrotizing enterocolitis or death. *J. Perinatol.* **2009**, *29*, 57–62. [CrossRef] [PubMed]
8. Corpeleijn, W.E.; Kouwenhoven, S.M.P.; Paap, M.C.; Van Vliet, I.; Scheerder, I.; Muizer, Y.; Helder, O.K.; Van Goudoever, J.B.; Vermeulen, M.J. Intake of own Mother's milk during the first days of life is associated

with decreased morbidity and mortality in very low birth weight infants during the first 60 days of life. *Neonatology* **2012**, *102*, 276–281. [CrossRef] [PubMed]

9. Patel, A.L.; Johnson, T.J.; Engstrom, J.L.; Fogg, L.F.; Jegier, B.J.; Bigger, H.R.; Meier, P.P. Impact of early human milk on sepsis and health-care costs in very low birth weight infants. *J. Perinatol.* **2013**, *33*, 514–519. [CrossRef] [PubMed]
10. Tyson, J.E.; Kennedy, K.A. Trophic feedings for parenterally fed infants. *Cochrane Database Syst. Rev.* **2005**, CD000504. [CrossRef] [PubMed]
11. Li, Y.; Nguyen, D.N.; de Waard, M.; Christensen, L.; Zhou, P.; Jiang, P.; Sun, J.; Bojesen, A.M.; Lauridsen, C.; Lykkesfeldt, J.; et al. Pasteurization Procedures for Donor Human Milk Affect Body Growth, Intestinal Structure and Resistance against Bacterial Infections in Preterm Pigs. *J. Nutr.* **2017**, *147*, 1121–1130. [CrossRef] [PubMed]
12. Corpeleijn, W.E.; De Waard, M.; Christmann, V.; Van Goudoever, J.B.; Jansen-Van Der Weide, M.C.; Kooi, E.M.W.; Koper, J.F.; Kouwenhoven, S.M.P.; Lafeber, H.N.; Mank, E.; et al. Effect of donor milk on severe infections and mortality in very low-birth-weight infants: The early nutrition study randomized clinical trial. *JAMA Pediatr.* **2016**, *170*, 654–661. [CrossRef] [PubMed]
13. Coppa, G.V.; Gabrielli, O.; Zampini, L.; Galeazzi, T.; Ficcadenti, A.; Padella, L.; Santoro, L.; Soldi, S.; Carlucci, A.; Bertino, E.; et al. Oligosaccharides in 4 different milk groups, bifidobacteria and ruminococcus obeum. *J. Pediatr. Gastroenterol. Nutr.* **2011**, *53*, 80–87. [CrossRef] [PubMed]
14. Morrow, A.L.; Ruiz-Palacios, G.M.; Altaye, M.; Jiang, X.; Lourdes Guerrero, M.; Meinzen-Derr, J.K.; Farkas, T.; Chaturvedi, P.; Pickering, L.K.; Newburg, D.S. Human milk oligosaccharides are associated with protection against diarrhea in breast-fed infants. *J. Pediatr.* **2004**, *145*, 297–303. [CrossRef] [PubMed]
15. Bode, L. The functional biology of human milk oligosaccharides. *Early Hum. Dev.* **2015**, *91*, 619–622. [CrossRef] [PubMed]
16. Bode, L. Human milk oligosaccharides: Every baby needs a sugar mama. *Glycobiology* **2012**, *22*, 1147–1162. [CrossRef] [PubMed]
17. Moukarzel, S.; Bode, L. Human Milk Oligosaccharides and the Preterm Infant: A Journey in Sickness and in Health. *Clin. Perinatol.* **2017**, *44*, 193–207. [CrossRef] [PubMed]
18. Musilova, S.; Rada, V.; Vlkova, E.; Bunesova, V. Beneficial effects of human milk oligosaccharides on gut microbiota. *Benef. Microbes* **2014**, *5*, 273–283. [CrossRef] [PubMed]
19. Marriage, B.J.; Buck, R.H.; Goehring, K.C.; Oliver, J.S.; Williams, J.A. Infants Fed a Lower Calorie Formula with 2′FL Show Growth and 2′FL Uptake Like Breast-Fed Infants. *J. Pediatr. Gastroenterol. Nutr.* **2015**, *61*, 649–658. [CrossRef] [PubMed]
20. Puccio, G.; Alliet, P.; Cajozzo, C.; Janssens, E.; Corsello, G.; Sprenger, N.; Wernimont, S.; Egli, D.; Gosoniu, L.; Steenhout, P. Effects of infant formula with human milk oligosaccharides on growth and morbidity: A randomized multicenter trial. *J. Pediatr. Gastroenterol. Nutr.* **2017**, *64*, 624–631. [CrossRef] [PubMed]
21. Kunz, C.; Rudloff, S.; Baier, W.; Klein, N.; Strobel, S. Oligosaccharides in human milk: Structural, functional and metabolic aspects. *Annu. Rev. Nutr.* **2000**, *20*, 699–722. [CrossRef] [PubMed]
22. Kunz, C.; Meyer, C.; Collado, M.C.; Geiger, L.; García-Mantrana, I.; Bertua-Ríos, B.; Martínez-Costa, C.; Borsch, C.; Rudloff, S. Influence of Gestational Age, Secretor and Lewis Blood Group Status on the Oligosaccharide Content of Human Milk. *J. Pediatr. Gastroenterol. Nutr.* **2017**, *64*, 789–798. [CrossRef] [PubMed]
23. Thurl, S.; Henker, J.; Siegel, M.; Tovar, K.; Sawatzki, G. Detection of four human milk groups with respect to Lewis blood group dependent oligosaccharides. *Glycoconj. J.* **1997**, *14*, 795–799. [CrossRef] [PubMed]
24. Gabrielli, O.; Zampini, L.; Galeazzi, T.; Padella, L.; Santoro, L.; Peila, C.; Giuliani, F.; Bertino, E.; Fabris, C.; Coppa, G.V. Preterm Milk Oligosaccharides During the First Month of Lactation. *Pediatrics* **2011**, *128*, e1520–e1531. [CrossRef] [PubMed]
25. De Leoz, M.L.A.; Gaerlan, S.C.; Strum, J.S.; Dimapasoc, L.M.; Mirmiran, M.; Tancredi, D.J.; Smilowitz, J.T.; Kalanetra, K.M.; Mills, D.A.; German, J.B.; et al. Lacto-*N*-tetraose, fucosylation and secretor status are highly variable in human milk oligosaccharides from women delivering preterm. *J. Proteome Res.* **2012**, *11*, 4662–4672. [CrossRef] [PubMed]
26. Coppa, G.V.; Pierani, P.; Zampini, L.; Gabrielli, O.; Carlucci, A.; Catassi, C.; Giorgi, P.L. Lactose, oligosaccharide and monosaccharide content of milk from mothers delivering preterm new-borns over the first month of lactation. *Minerva Pediatr.* **1997**, *49*, 471–475. [PubMed]

27. Coppa, G.V.; Gabrielli, O.; Pierani, P.; Catassi, C.; Carlucci, A.; Giorgi, P.L. Changes in carbohydrate composition in human milk over 4 months of lactation. *Pediatrics* **1993**, *91*, 637–641. [PubMed]
28. Nakhla, T.; Fu, D.; Zopf, D.; Brodsky, N.L.; Hurt, H. Neutral oligosaccharide content of preterm human milk. *Br. J. Nutr.* **1999**, *82*, 361–367. [CrossRef] [PubMed]
29. Wang, B.; Brand-Miller, J.; McVeagh, P.; Petocz, P. Concentration and distribution of sialic acid in human milk and infant formulas. *Am. J. Clin. Nutr.* **2001**, *74*, 510–515. [CrossRef] [PubMed]
30. Underwood, M.A.; Gaerlan, S.; De Leoz, M.L.A.; Dimapasoc, L.; Kalanetra, K.M.; Lemay, D.G.; German, J.B.; Mills, D.A.; Lebrilla, C.B. Human milk oligosaccharides in premature infants: Absorption, excretion and influence on the intestinal microbiota. *Pediatr. Res.* **2015**, *78*, 670–677. [CrossRef] [PubMed]
31. Autran, C.A.; Kellman, B.P.; Kim, J.H.; Asztalos, E.; Blood, A.B.; Spence, E.C.H.; Patel, A.L.; Hou, J.; Lewis, N.E.; Bode, L. Human milk oligosaccharide composition predicts risk of necrotising enterocolitis in preterm infants. *Gut* **2018**, *67*, 1064–1070. [CrossRef] [PubMed]
32. Jantscher-Krenn, E.; Zherebtsov, M.; Nissan, C.; Goth, K.; Guner, Y.S.; Naidu, N.; Choudhury, B.; Grishin, A.V.; Ford, H.R.; Bode, L. The human milk oligosaccharide disialyllacto-N-tetraose prevents necrotising enterocolitis in neonatal rats. *Gut* **2012**, *61*, 1417–1425. [CrossRef] [PubMed]
33. Yu, H.; Yan, X.; Autran, C.A.; Li, Y.; Etzold, S.; Latasiewicz, J.; Robertson, B.M.; Li, J.; Bode, L.; Chen, X. Enzymatic and Chemoenzymatic Syntheses of Disialyl Glycans and Their Necrotizing Enterocolitis Preventing Effects. *J. Org. Chem.* **2017**, *82*, 13152–13160. [CrossRef] [PubMed]
34. Autran, C.A.; Schoterman, M.H.C.; Jantscher-krenn, E.; Kamerling, J.P.; Bode, L. Sialylated galacto-oligosaccharides and 2′-fucosyllactose reduce necrotising enterocolitis in neonatal rats. *Br. J. Nutr.* **2016**, *116*, 294–299. [CrossRef] [PubMed]
35. Sangild, P.T. Gut responses to enteral nutrition in preterm infants and animals. *Exp. Biol. Med.* **2006**, *231*, 1695–1711. [CrossRef]
36. Nanthakumar, N.N.; Fusunyan, R.D.; Sanderson, I.; Walker, W.A. Inflammation in the developing human intestine: A possible pathophysiologic contribution to necrotizing enterocolitis. *Proc. Natl. Acad. Sci. USA* **2000**, *97*, 6043–6048. [CrossRef] [PubMed]
37. Lotz, M.; Gütle, D.; Walther, S.; Ménard, S.; Bogdan, C.; Hornef, M.W. Postnatal acquisition of endotoxin tolerance in intestinal epithelial cells. *J. Cell Biol.* **2006**, *173*, 973–984. [CrossRef]
38. Cilieborg, M.S.; Bering, S.B.; Østergaard, M.V.; Jensen, M.L.; Krych, Ł.; Newburg, D.S.; Sangild, P.T. Minimal short-term effect of dietary 2′-fucosyllactose on bacterial colonisation, intestinal function and necrotising enterocolitis in preterm pigs. *Br. J. Nutr.* **2016**, *116*, 834–841. [CrossRef] [PubMed]
39. Rasmussen, S.O.; Martin, L.; Østergaard, M.V.; Rudloff, S.; Roggenbuck, M.; Nguyen, D.N.; Sangild, P.T.; Bering, S.B. Human milk oligosaccharide effects on intestinal function and inflammation after preterm birth in pigs. *J. Nutr. Biochem.* **2016**, *40*, 141–154. [CrossRef] [PubMed]
40. Arboleya, S.; Binetti, A.; Salazar, N.; Fernández, N.; Solís, G.; Hernández-Barranco, A.; Margolles, A.; de los Reyes-Gavilán, C.G.; Gueimonde, M. Establishment and development of intestinal microbiota in preterm neonates. *FEMS Microbiol. Ecol.* **2012**, *79*, 763–772. [CrossRef] [PubMed]
41. Butel, M.-J.; Suau, A.; Campeotto, F.; Magne, F.; Aires, J.; Ferraris, L.; Kalach, N.; Leroux, B.; Dupont, C. Conditions of bifidobacterial colonization in preterm infants: A prospective analysis. *J. Pediatr. Gastroenterol. Nutr.* **2007**, *44*, 577–582. [CrossRef] [PubMed]
42. Morowitz, M.J.; Denef, V.J.; Costello, E.K.; Thomas, B.C.; Poroyko, V.; Relman, D.A.; Banfield, J.F. Strain-resolved community genomic analysis of gut microbial colonization in a premature infant. *Proc. Natl. Acad. Sci. USA* **2011**, *108*, 1128–1133. [CrossRef] [PubMed]
43. Torrazza, R.M.; Ukhanova, M.; Wang, X.; Sharma, R.; Hudak, M.L.; Neu, J.; Mai, V. Intestinal microbial ecology and environmental factors affecting necrotizing enterocolitis. *PLoS ONE* **2013**, *8*, e83304. [CrossRef] [PubMed]
44. Morrow, A.L.; Lagomarcino, A.J.; Schibler, K.R.; Taft, D.H.; Yu, Z.; Wang, B.; Altaye, M.; Wagner, M.; Gevers, D.; Ward, D.V.; et al. Early microbial and metabolomic signatures predict later onset of necrotizing enterocolitis in preterm infants. *Microbiome* **2013**, *1*, 13. [CrossRef] [PubMed]
45. Pammi, M.; Cope, J.; Tarr, P.I.; Warner, B.B.; Morrow, A.L.; Mai, V.; Gregory, K.E.; Kroll, J.S.; McMurtry, V.; Ferris, M.J.; et al. Intestinal dysbiosis in preterm infants preceding necrotizing enterocolitis: A systematic review and meta-analysis. *Microbiome* **2017**, *5*, 31. [CrossRef] [PubMed]

46. Ren, S.; Hui, Y.; Obelitz-Ryom, K.; Brandt, A.B.; Kot, W.; Nielsen, D.S.; Thymann, T.; Sangild, P.T.; Nguyen, D.N. Neonatal gut and immune maturation is determined more by postnatal age than by post-conceptional age in moderately preterm pigs. *Am. J. Physiol. Gastrointest. Liver Physiol.* **2018**. [CrossRef] [PubMed]
47. Isani, M.; Bell, B.A.; Delaplain, P.T.; Bowling, J.D.; Golden, J.M.; Elizee, M.; Illingworth, L.; Wang, J.; Gayer, C.P.; Grishin, A.V.; et al. Lactobacillus murinus HF12 colonizes neonatal gut and protects rats from necrotizing enterocolitis. *PLoS ONE* **2018**, *13*, e0196710. [CrossRef] [PubMed]
48. Hemme, D.; Raibaud, P.; Ducluzeau, R.; Galpin, J.V.; Sicard, P.; Van Heijenoort, J. "Lactobacillus murinus" n. sp., a new species of the autochtoneous dominant flora of the digestive tract of rat and mouse (author's transl). *Ann. Microbiol. (Paris)* **1980**, *131*, 297–308. [PubMed]
49. Morrow, A.L.; Meinzen-Derr, J.; Huang, P.; Schibler, K.R.; Cahill, T.; Keddache, M.; Kallapur, S.G.; Newburg, D.S.; Tabangin, M.; Warner, B.B.; et al. Fucosyltransferase 2 non-secretor and low secretor status predicts severe outcomes in premature infants. *J. Pediatr.* **2011**, *158*, 745–751. [CrossRef] [PubMed]
50. Cilieborg, M.S.; Sangild, P.T.; Jensen, M.L.; Østergaard, M.V.; Christensen, L.; Rasmussen, S.O.; Mørbak, A.L.; Jørgensen, C.B.; Bering, S.B. α1,2-Fucosyllactose Does Not Improve Intestinal Function or Prevent Escherichia coli F18 Diarrhea in Newborn Pigs. *J. Pediatr. Gastroenterol. Nutr.* **2017**, *64*, 310–318. [CrossRef] [PubMed]
51. Li, M.; Monaco, M.H.; Wang, M.; Comstock, S.S.; Kuhlenschmidt, T.B.; Fahey G.C., Jr.; Miller, M.J.; Kuhlenschmidt, M.S.; Donovan, S.M. Human milk oligosaccharides shorten rotavirus-induced diarrhea and modulate piglet mucosal immunity and colonic microbiota. *ISME J.* **2014**, *8*, 1609–1620. [CrossRef] [PubMed]
52. Charbonneau, M.R.; O'Donnell, D.; Blanton, L.V.; Totten, S.M.; Davis, J.C.C.; Barratt, M.J.; Cheng, J.; Guruge, J.; Talcott, M.; Bain, J.R.; et al. Sialylated Milk Oligosaccharides Promote Microbiota-Dependent Growth in Models of Infant Undernutrition. *Cell.* **2016**, *164*, 859–871. [CrossRef] [PubMed]
53. Kuntz, S.; Rudloff, S.; Kunz, C. Oligosaccharides from human milk influence growth-related characteristics of intestinally transformed and non-transformed intestinal cells. *Br. J. Nutr.* **2008**, *99*, 462–471. [CrossRef] [PubMed]
54. Bjornvad, C.R.; Thymann, T.; Deutz, N.E.; Burrin, D.G.; Jensen, S.K.; Jensen, B.B.; Mølbak, L.; Boye, M.; Larsson, L.-I.; Schmidt, M.; et al. Enteral feeding induces diet-dependent mucosal dysfunction, bacterial proliferation and necrotizing enterocolitis in preterm pigs on parenteral nutrition. *Am. J. Physiol. Gastrointest. Liver Physiol.* **2008**, *295*, G1092–G1103. [CrossRef] [PubMed]
55. Rasmussen, S.O.; Martin, L.; Østergaard, M.V.; Rudloff, S.; Li, Y.; Roggenbuck, M.; Bering, S.B.; Sangild, P.T. Bovine colostrum improves neonatal growth, digestive function and gut immunity relative to donor human milk and infant formula in preterm pigs. *Am. J. Physiol. Gastrointest. Liver Physiol.* **2016**, *311*, G480–G491. [CrossRef] [PubMed]
56. Jensen, M.L.; Sangild, P.T.; Lykke, M.; Schmidt, M.; Boye, M.; Jensen, B.B.; Thymann, T. Similar efficacy of human banked milk and bovine colostrum to decrease incidence of necrotizing enterocolitis in preterm piglets. *Am. J. Physiol. Regul. Integr. Comp. Physiol.* **2013**, *305*, R4–R12. [CrossRef] [PubMed]
57. Li, Y.; Nguyen, D.N.; Obelitz-Ryom, K.; Andersen, A.D.; Thymann, T.; Chatterton, D.E.W.; Purup, S.; Heckmann, A.B.; Bering, S.B.; Sangild, P.T. Bioactive Whey Protein Concentrate and Lactose Stimulate Gut Function in Formula-fed Preterm Pigs. *J. Pediatr. Gastroenterol. Nutr.* **2018**, *66*, 128–134. [CrossRef] [PubMed]
58. Siggers, J.; Ostergaard, M.V.; Siggers, R.H.; Skovgaard, K.; Mølbak, L.; Thymann, T.; Schmidt, M.; Møller, H.K.; Purup, S.; Fink, L.N.; et al. Postnatal amniotic fluid intake reduces gut inflammatory responses and necrotizing enterocolitis in preterm neonates. *Am. J. Physiol. Gastrointest. Liver Physiol.* **2013**, *304*, G864–G875. [CrossRef] [PubMed]
59. Rognum, T.O.; Thrane, S.; Stoltenberg, L.; Vege, A.; Brandtzaeg, P. Development of intestinal mucosal immunity in fetal life and the first postnatal months. *Pediatr. Res.* **1992**, *32*, 145–149. [CrossRef] [PubMed]
60. Lin, P.W.; Stoll, B.J. Necrotising enterocolitis. *Lancet* **2006**, *368*, 1271–1283. [CrossRef]
61. Ballard, O.; Morrow, A.L. Human milk composition: Nutrients and bioactive factors. *Pediatr. Clin. N. Am.* **2013**, *60*, 49–74. [CrossRef] [PubMed]
62. Buescher, E.S. Anti-inflammatory characteristics of human milk: How, where, why. *Adv. Exp. Med. Biol.* **2001**, *501*, 207–222. [PubMed]
63. Chatterton, D.E.W.; Nguyen, D.N.; Bering, S.B.; Sangild, P.T. Anti-inflammatory mechanisms of bioactive milk proteins in the intestine of new-borns. *Int. J. Biochem. Cell. Biol.* **2013**, *45*, 1730–1747. [CrossRef] [PubMed]

64. Goehring, K.C.; Marriage, B.J.; Oliver, J.S.; Wilder, J.A.; Barrett, E.G.; Buck, R.H. Similar to Those Who Are Breastfed, Infants Fed a Formula Containing 2′-Fucosyllactose Have Lower Inflammatory Cytokines in a Randomized Controlled Trial. *J. Nutr.* **2016**, *146*, 2559–2566. [CrossRef] [PubMed]
65. He, Y.; Liu, S.; Leone, S.; Newburg, D.S. Human colostrum oligosaccharides modulate major immunologic pathways of immature human intestine. *Mucosal Immunol.* **2014**, *7*, 1326–1339. [CrossRef] [PubMed]
66. He, Y.; Liu, S.; Kling, D.E.; Leone, S.; Lawlor, N.T.; Huang, Y.; Feinberg, S.B.; Hill, D.R.; Newburg, D.S. The human milk oligosaccharide 2′-fucosyllactose modulates CD14 expression in human enterocytes, thereby attenuating LPS-induced inflammation. *Gut* **2016**, *65*, 33–46. [CrossRef] [PubMed]
67. Bode, L.; Rudloff, S.; Kunz, C.; Strobel, S.; Klein, N. Human milk oligosaccharides reduce platelet-neutrophil complex formation leading to a decrease in neutrophil β 2 integrin expression. *J. Leukoc. Biol.* **2004**, *76*, 820–826. [CrossRef] [PubMed]
68. Bode, L.; Kunz, C.; Muhly-Reinholz, M.; Mayer, K.; Seeger, W.; Rudloff, S. Inhibition of monocyte, lymphocyte and neutrophil adhesion to endothelial cells by human milk oligosaccharides. *Thromb. Haemost.* **2004**, *92*, 1402–1410. [CrossRef] [PubMed]
69. Stefanutti, G.; Lister, P.; Smith, V.V.; Peters, M.J.; Klein, N.J.; Pierro, A.; Eaton, S. P-selectin expression, neutrophil infiltration and histologic injury in neonates with necrotizing enterocolitis. *J. Pediatr. Surg.* **2005**, *40*, 942–948. [CrossRef] [PubMed]
70. Engfer, M.B.; Stahl, B.; Finke, B.; Sawatzki, G.; Daniel, H. Human milk oligosaccharides are resistant to enzymatic hydrolysis in the upper gastrointestinal tract. *Am. J. Clin. Nutr.* **2000**, *71*, 1589–1596. [CrossRef] [PubMed]
71. Rudloff, S.; Pohlentz, G.; Diekmann, L.; Egge, H.; Kunz, C. Urinary excretion of lactose and oligosaccharides in preterm infants fed human milk or infant formula. *Acta Paediatr.* **1996**, *85*, 598–603. [CrossRef] [PubMed]
72. Gnoth, M.J.; Kunz, C.; Kinne-Saffran, E.; Rudloff, S. Human milk oligosaccharides are minimally digested in vitro. *J. Nutr.* **2000**, *130*, 3014–3020. [CrossRef] [PubMed]
73. Østergaard, M.V.; Cilieborg, M.S.; Skovgaard, K.; Schmidt, M.; Sangild, P.T.; Bering, S.B. Preterm Birth Reduces Nutrient Absorption with Limited Effect on Immune Gene Expression and Gut Colonization in Pigs. *J. Pediatr. Gastroenterol. Nutr.* **2015**, *61*, 481–490. [CrossRef] [PubMed]
74. Støy, A.C.F.; Heegaard, P.M.H.; Skovgaard, K.; Bering, S.B.; Bjerre, M.; Sangild, P.T. Increased Intestinal Inflammation and Digestive Dysfunction in Preterm Pigs with Severe Necrotizing Enterocolitis. *Neonatology* **2017**, 289–296. [CrossRef] [PubMed]
75. Støy, A.C.F.; Heegaard, P.M.H.; Thymann, T.; Bjerre, M.; Skovgaard, K.; Boye, M.; Stoll, B.; Schmidt, M.; Jensen, B.B.; Sangild, P.T. Bovine colostrum improves intestinal function following formula-induced gut inflammation in preterm pigs. *Clin. Nutr.* **2014**, *33*, 322–329. [CrossRef] [PubMed]
76. Li, Y.; Jensen, M.L.; Chatterton, D.E.W.; Jensen, B.B.; Thymann, T.; Kvistgaard, A.S.; Sangild, P.T. Raw bovine milk improves gut responses to feeding relative to infant formula in preterm piglets. *Am. J. Physiol. Gastrointest. Liver Physiol.* **2014**, *306*, G81–G90. [CrossRef] [PubMed]
77. Li, Y.; Østergaard, M.V.; Jiang, P.; Chatterton, D.E.W.; Thymann, T.; Kvistgaard, A.S.; Sangild, P.T. Whey protein processing influences formula-induced gut maturation in preterm pigs. *J. Nutr.* **2013**, *143*, 1934–1942. [CrossRef] [PubMed]
78. Cilieborg, M.S.; Thymann, T.; Siggers, R.; Boye, M.; Bering, S.B.; Jensen, B.B.; Sangild, P.T. The incidence of necrotizing enterocolitis is increased following probiotic administration to preterm pigs. *J. Nutr.* **2011**, *141*, 223–230. [CrossRef] [PubMed]
79. Siggers, R.H.; Siggers, J.; Boye, M.; Thymann, T.; Mølbak, L.; Leser, T.; Jensen, B.B.; Sangild, P.T. Early administration of probiotics alters bacterial colonization and limits diet-induced gut dysfunction and severity of necrotizing enterocolitis in preterm pigs. *J. Nutr.* **2008**, *138*, 1437–1444. [CrossRef] [PubMed]
80. Birck, M.M.; Nguyen, D.N.; Cilieborg, M.S.; Kamal, S.S.; Nielsen, D.S.; Damborg, P.; Olsen, J.E.; Lauridsen, C.; Sangild, P.T.; Thymann, T. Enteral but not parenteral antibiotics enhance gut function and prevent necrotizing enterocolitis in formula-fed newborn preterm pigs. *Am. J. Physiol. Gastrointest. Liver Physiol.* **2016**, *310*, G323–G333. [CrossRef] [PubMed]
81. Jensen, M.L.; Thymann, T.; Cilieborg, M.S.; Lykke, M.; Mølbak, L.; Jensen, B.B.; Schmidt, M.; Kelly, D.; Mulder, I.; Burrin, D.G.; et al. Antibiotics modulate intestinal immunity and prevent necrotizing enterocolitis in preterm neonatal piglets. *Am. J. Physiol. Gastrointest. Liver Physiol.* **2014**, *306*, G59–G71. [CrossRef] [PubMed]

82. Difilippo, E.; Pan, F.; Logtenberg, M.; Willems, R.; Braber, S.; Fink-Gremmels, J.; Schols, H.A.; Gruppen, H. Milk Oligosaccharide Variation in Sow Milk and Milk Oligosaccharide Fermentation in Piglet Intestine. *J. Agric. Food Chem.* **2016**, *64*, 2087–2093. [CrossRef] [PubMed]
83. Wei, J.; Wang, Z.A.; Wang, B.; Jahan, M.; Wang, Z.; Wynn, P.C.; Du, Y. Characterization of porcine milk oligosaccharides over lactation between primiparous and multiparous female pigs. *Sci. Rep.* **2018**, *8*, 4688. [CrossRef] [PubMed]
84. Mudd, A.T.; Salcedo, J.; Alexander, L.S.; Johnson, S.K.; Getty, C.M.; Chichlowski, M.; Berg, B.M.; Barile, D.; Dilger, R.N. Porcine Milk Oligosaccharides and Sialic Acid Concentrations Vary Throughout Lactation. *Front. Nutr.* **2016**, *3*. [CrossRef] [PubMed]

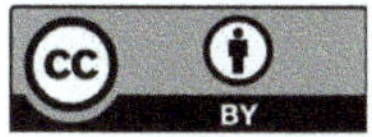

© 2018 by the author. Licensee MDPI, Basel, Switzerland. This article is an open access article distributed under the terms and conditions of the Creative Commons Attribution (CC BY) license (http://creativecommons.org/licenses/by/4.0/).

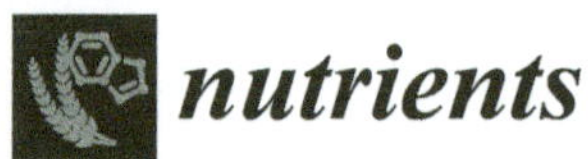

Review

Filling the Gaps: Current Research Directions for a Rational Use of Probiotics in Preterm Infants

Arianna Aceti [1,*,†], Isadora Beghetti [1,†], Luca Maggio [2], Silvia Martini [1], Giacomo Faldella [1] and Luigi Corvaglia [1]

1 Neonatal Intensive Care Unit, AOU Bologna, Department of Medical and Surgical Sciences (DIMEC), University of Bologna, 40138 Bologna, Italy; i.beghetti@gmail.com (I.B.); silvia.martini4@gmail.com (S.M.); giacomo.faldella@unibo.it (G.F.); luigi.corvaglia@unibo.it (L.C.)

2 Department of Woman and Child Health, Obstetric and Neonatology Area, Fondazione Policlinico Universitario A. Gemelli IRCCS, 00168 Rome, Italy; luca.maggio@fastwebnet.it

* Correspondence: arianna.aceti2@unibo.it; Tel.: +39-051-342754

† These authors contributed equally to this work.

Received: 23 September 2018; Accepted: 8 October 2018; Published: 10 October 2018

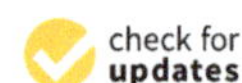

Abstract: The use of probiotics among very low-birth-weight infants is constantly increasing, as probiotics are believed to reduce the incidence of severe diseases such as necrotizing enterocolitis and late-onset sepsis and to improve feeding tolerance. However, despite the enthusiasm towards these products in neonatal medicine, theoretical knowledge and clinical applications still need to be improved. The purpose of this review is to give an overview of the most important gaps in the current literature about potential uses of probiotics in preterm infants, highlighting promising directions for future research. Specifically, further well-designed studies should aim at clarifying the impact of the type of feeding (mother's milk, donor milk, and formula) on the relationship between probiotic supplementation and clinical outcome. Moreover, future research is needed to provide solid evidence about the potential greater efficacy of multi-strain probiotics compared to single-strain products. Safety issues should also be addressed properly, by exploring the potential of paraprobiotics and risks connected to antibiotic resistance in preterm infants. Last, in light of increasing commercial and public interests, the long-term effect of routine consumption of probiotics in such a vulnerable population should be also evaluated.

Keywords: preterm infant; probiotic; human milk; probiotic strain; safety

1. Introduction

Despite continuous improvements in neonatal medicine, prematurity represents the leading cause of both neonatal and childhood mortality through age five years worldwide [1]. Diseases such as necrotizing enterocolitis (NEC) and late-onset sepsis (LOS) pose a serious threat for preterm infants, and are included among the leading causes of morbidity and mortality in this population [2].

There is a growing body of literature directed towards the implementation of preventive measures which could reduce the incidence and severity of these diseases, possibly leading to an improvement in neonatal short- and long-term outcomes [3]. Among these interventions, probiotics appear to be very promising; they have been recently described as living "a golden age" in neonatal medicine [4].

Despite such enthusiasm, it is still difficult to make precise recommendations on the use of probiotics in preterm infants. Recent systematic reviews and meta-analyses of the literature have suggested a beneficial role of probiotics for preventing NEC [5–7] and LOS [8,9], and for improving feeding tolerance by shortening the time to achieve full enteral feeding (FEF) [10,11]; furthermore, it has been suggested that probiotic administration might lead to a global improvement in neonatal health by reducing mortality rates and length of hospital stay [12–14]. However, most of the studies included in these systematic reviews and meta-analyses have not properly addressed all of the potential confounding factors which might interfere in shaping the relationship between probiotic administration and clinical outcomes, thus failing to provide to the clinician a meaningful answer as to which probiotic strain should be used, how long probiotic supplementation should be continued, and which group(s) of infants would likely benefit from the intervention.

Despite concerns about the efficacy and, more importantly, the safety of available probiotic products [15], a recent survey of US Neonatal Intensive Care Units (NICUs) participating to the Vermont Oxford Network has shown that probiotic use among very low-birth-weight (VLBW) infants is increasing, and that there is a wide variability in their indications and in the probiotic products themselves [16].

The purpose of this review is to give an overview of the most important gaps in the current literature about potential uses of probiotics in preterm infants, highlighting promising directions for future research.

2. Defining the Target: Gut Microbiota vs. Clinical Outcomes

In infants, as well as in children and adults, the rationale for using probiotics to treat or prevent any disease relies on their potential ability to restore a healthy gut microbiota. Probiotic action in the gut is mediated through several mechanisms, which include the up- and down-regulation of genes involved in inflammation and cytoprotection, improvement of gut barrier function, production of metabolites such as short-chain fatty acids which modulate the growth of pathogenic bacteria, and competition with other microorganisms [17].

When talking about preterm infants, a clear definition of this probiotic target is challenging, as the characterization of a healthy gut microbiota in these infants is not univocal, being influenced by several factors such as place of birth, mode of delivery, feeding characteristics, antibiotic use, and NICU environment [18]. In addition, despite a generally clear association between dysbiosis and disease, the causality and reversal of disease in response to probiotic-induced changes in gut microbiota have not yet been demonstrated [19]. For this reason, the target for probiotic intervention in preterm infants at present cannot be exclusively microbiological (in other words, a gut microbiota with distinctive "healthy" features), but still needs to be clinical.

Given this premise, a clear definition of clinical outcomes whose improvement might be related to probiotic administration is fundamental. In most clinical trials, sample size calculation is based on single pre-specified outcomes (i.e., mortality, NEC, LOS, feeding tolerance), but other outcomes, for which these studies are probably underpowered, are often analyzed and their results are included among relevant conclusions. This constitutes a limitation of these studies' conclusions, which hopefully should be overcome in the future by calculating the sample size on multiple outcomes.

3. Exploring Feeding Contribution: Human Milk vs. Formula

Infant nutrition in early life has been recognized to play a key role in shaping future health [20]. Specifically, human milk (HM) is known to exert a series of beneficial effects for the infant, including improved neurological, immunological, and metabolic outcomes [21]. In this respect, exclusive HM-feeding appears to be even more important for preterm infants, especially for those born with a VLBW [22]. The beneficial effects of HM are related to its peculiar nutritional and functional components, such as long-chain polyunsaturated fatty acids, immunomodulatory proteins (i.e., lactoferrin, immunoglobulin), and HM oligosaccharides (HMOs) [23]. Some of these HM components have been also related to the decrease in NEC incidence and severity documented in infants receiving exclusive HM [24]. The unique composition of HM possibly confers protection against NEC through several mechanisms implicated in the pathogenesis of the disease, such as reduction in gastric pH, improvement in intestinal motility, and decrease in epithelial permeability. In addition, immunoglobulin A and lactoferrin, contained in HM, might modulate gut inflammation, and HMOs are thought to prevent bacterial adhesion to the intestinal mucosa and exert a prebiotic action on gut microbiota [25]. Furthermore, it is well recognized that HM itself harbors a specific microbiota, which contributes to drive the establishment of the infant gut bacterial community [26]. In this regard, features of gut microbiota in breastfed vs. formula-fed infants are quite different: breastfed infants have a higher abundance of *Bifidobacterium* spp., *Staphylococcus* spp., and *Streptococcus* spp., while *Bacteroides* spp., *Clostridium* spp., *Enterobacteriaceae*, and *Lachnospiraceae* dominate in formula-fed infants [27].

A recent systematic review examined the effect of different enteral feeding strategies, including feeding type and probiotic supplementation, on the establishment of gut microbiota in preterm infants [28], with the aim of identifying feeding factors which would promote gut colonization with beneficial bacteria. Both mother's own milk (MOM) and probiotics were found to promote a healthy gut microbiota, by increasing microbial diversity and promoting colonization with *Bifidobacteria*.

Since the effects of both HM and probiotics on gut microbiota and clinical outcomes such as NEC and LOS have been advocated in so many clinical trials and literature reviews, it is quite surprising that the two interventions have not been examined together. It is plausible that nutrition and supplemental probiotics could act together in the preterm infant's gut, leading to a differential effect of exogenous bacteria depending on type of feeding. Despite the theoretical likeliness of this hypothesis, type of feeding is rarely detailed or considered among confounding factors in trials about probiotics. One might speculate that probiotics would act preferentially in formula-fed infants, as they would counterbalance the negative effect of formula feeding on gut microbiota. However, unexpectedly even for the authors themselves, one clinical trial reported that a combination of probiotic strains (*Lactobacillus acidophilus* and *Bifidobacterium bifidum*) was effective on NEC only in VLBW infants who were exclusively breastfed, but not in those receiving formula [29]. Similarly, two meta-analyses of randomized controlled trials (RCTs) documented a reduction in the incidence of LOS and in the time to achieve FEF only in HM-fed preterm infants [9,11]. More recently, the effect of probiotics on NEC was found to be more pronounced in cohorts where higher proportions of neonates were exclusively breastfed [30].

The available literature does not offer a clear justification for these findings: one hypothesis is that VLBW infants exposed to formula might have a higher baseline risk for diseases such as NEC and feeding intolerance, because intact bovine proteins in infant formula can contribute to intestinal inflammation [25]. Furthermore, it is plausible that the effect of probiotics on clinical outcomes could be mediated by functional HM components such as prebiotic HMOs, immunological factors, and probiotic bacteria [31]. In this respect, recent data suggest that a low abundance of a specific HMO in MOM (disialyllacto-N-tetraose, DSLNT) could represent a marker of the susceptibility of preterm infants to NEC [32], thus highlighting the fundamental role of the crosstalk between HM prebiotic components, gut and HM microbiota, and probiotics in the development of the disease.

While the role of MOM in the prevention of NEC has been established, less is known about donor HM (DHM). In a multicenter clinical trial, the availability of DHM was associated with a 10% increase in MOM availability and a 2.6% decrease in the rate of NEC [33]. Similarly, the introduction of DHM and probiotic supplementation in two clinical settings was linked to a significant reduction in neonatal mortality and to a non-significant decrease in NEC rates [34]. On the contrary, the use of DHM as a supplement to MOM was not associated with any significant benefit in terms in mortality and morbidity indexes, nor in neurodevelopment at 18 months corrected age [35].

The interaction between DHM and probiotic supplementation in shaping neonatal clinical outcomes in far from clear. The manipulation process of DHM, which includes several steps such as freezing, thawing, pooling, and pasteurization, is likely to have a major impact on HM functional components [36]. Whether the changes in DHM composition induced by its manipulation translate into a clinically relevant effect is yet to be demonstrated. Recently, the effect of different feeding types, including MOM, DHM, and formula, on the features of gut microbiota in preterm infants was analyzed: compared to DHM-fed infants, gut microbiota in MOM-fed infants was richer in Bifidobacteriaceae and poorer in Staphylococcaceae, Clostridiaceae, and Pasteurellaceae. Despite these differences, gut microbiota profiles in MOM-fed and DHM-fed infants were more similar than those observed in formula-fed infants [37]. The clinical significance of these observations deserves to be assessed in further trials.

In summary, given the differential effect of MOM, DHM, and formula on both gut microbiota and neonatal clinical outcomes, it is fundamental that further studies exploring probiotic supplementation in preterm infants will plan to describe in greater detail and adjust their data for feeding characteristics of included infants, in order to limit potential confounding factors (i.e., percentage of MOM, duration of exclusive MOM, characteristics of HM fortification, etc.). Even better, it would be ideal to restrict inclusion criteria to infants fed homogeneously (MOM, DHM, or formula), thus overcoming the impracticability of randomizing preterm infants according to type of feeding.

4. Choosing the Probiotic: Is There Strength in (Strain) Numbers?

The strain-specificity of the probiotic effect has been accepted for decades as a pivotal principle of probiotic science and regulation [38]. More than 20 years from the first RCT showing that probiotics could be effective in reducing NEC, several RCTs and cohort studies reporting on NEC, LOS, and/or mortality in preterm infants receiving probiotic supplementation have been conducted. Multiple different probiotic strains or combinations have been used and some of them have been shown to exert beneficial effects. However, it has not been clarified whether a single probiotic or a mixture of probiotics would be more effective in improving preterm infants' outcome, and which probiotic strain or mixture should be better used. Numerous meta-analyses summarizing currently available data have recently been published [4,6,9,11,13,14,30,39–42]: data from these meta-analyses suggest that, beyond the overall benefit, a combination of different strains or species may have advantages over single probiotic organisms [6,9,14,30,39]. Since the same probiotic strain was used in very few studies, strain-specific sub-meta-analyses are difficult to perform, and strain-specific meta-analyses have been conducted only twice [40,41]. In order to provide an overview on the use of probiotics in preterm infants at a strain level and to identify strains with the greatest efficacy, van den Akker et al. carried out a network meta-analysis, combining evidence from direct and indirect comparison across several competing interventions [7]. Single- or multi-strain studies reporting on NEC, LOS, time to FEF, or overall mortality were included. Only a minority of the studied interventions, both single-strain and multi-strain/multi-species, was found to be effective. There was no clear overlap of certain strains which were significantly effective on multiple outcome domains. Most strains or combinations of strains only showed trends towards efficacy, whereas other strains did not demonstrate any. The authors suggested that a lack of effect might be either due to understudied species or to a true lack of effect of certain strains.

The extreme variety of probiotics used in neonatology might lead to conflicting conclusions. The variability of the strains and protocols in the trials included in various meta-analyses is often presented as a weakness. However, given the consistently decreased risk of NEC in RCTs using different probiotic regimens, it could be argued that most of the investigated interventions improve the health of the participants beyond any placebo effect. This evidence might indicate that the concept of strain-specific effects of probiotics may not be relevant to certain outcomes such as NEC [43]. Because of the complexity of the normal gut microbiome and of various cascades involved in the pathogenesis of NEC, different strains may exert their beneficial effect by different pathways. Thus, some authors suggested that commonly used probiotic strains share core benefits providing 'non-specific' or 'generic' protection [44–46]. While some specific mechanisms are rare and present in only a few strains of commonly studied probiotic species, some mechanisms might be frequently observed at a species and even a genus level [45,47]. Shared mechanisms exist among taxonomic groups that include many different strains [48]. On these bases, a multi-strain or multi-species probiotic [49] could be more effective than a single-strain product: more strains give more chances of success for a beneficial effect, provide a greater microbiota diversity and thus more potential niches in combination with individually determined host factors, allow a broader efficacy spectrum, and may exert additive or synergistic effects. However, a combination of probiotic strains does not necessarily ensure, in itself, a greater efficacy than a single-strain probiotic, as different probiotic strains may exert mutual inhibitory properties through the production of antimicrobial substances or differential gene expression [50,51].

Further structured research is needed to address the benefits of single-strain versus multi-strain or multi-species probiotic products in preterm infants. Head-to-head human intervention studies should be performed comparing a multi-strain product with its single-strain components and a placebo. Furthermore, in vitro and animal studies should aim to identify safe probiotic combinations that show additive or synergistic properties, avoiding potential antagonistic effects.

5. Addressing Safety Concerns: Time for Ghost Probiotics?

The routine administration of probiotics to preterm infants is hindered by concerns about the safety of commercially available products. Reasons of concern include fear of probiotic-related sepsis, transmission of antibiotic resistance, and non-availability of high-quality products.

Although none of the meta-analyses on probiotic supplementation in preterm infants reported any serious adverse events in infants receiving probiotics, there are several reports describing the occurrence of probiotic-related infections such as sepsis, pneumonia, and meningitis [31]. In addition, the genome of probiotic bacteria is known to contain genetic elements which confer resistance to several broad-spectrum antibiotics, such as glycopeptides, aminoglycosides, mono-bactams, and fluoroquinolones [52]; these resistant genes are themselves not harmful, but they can be transferred to other gut bacteria and eventually to opportunistic pathogens, leading to an uncontrolled increase in antibiotic-resistance [53], which might lead to longer-term consequences that outweigh the immediate benefits of probiotic supplementation. Furthermore, in many countries probiotics are considered as food supplements, and thus lack the strict quality regulation of other pharmaceuticals [31]. This is linked to a high risk of product contamination which can have serious consequences, especially when probiotics are administered to vulnerable individuals with weak immune systems, enhanced inflammatory responses, and/or compromised gut barrier, such as preterm infants.

To address the safety issues related to currently available probiotics, research is focusing on inactivated products, the so-called "paraprobiotics". The concept of paraprobiotics, or ghost probiotics, was developed by Taverniti et al. [54], who defined them as "non-viable microbial cells or crude cell extracts, which, when administered in adequate amounts, confer a benefit on the human or animal consumer". Inactivation of probiotics has been performed through several methods (i.e., heat, chemical, gamma or ultraviolet rays, sonication), each one having a different effect on cell structure and function [54].

A "probiotic paradox" has been described in relation to paraprobiotics, and is related to the fact that both live and dead microbial cells might exert beneficial responses in the host [55]. Mechanisms of action of paraprobiotics involve the modulation of various steps of the inflammatory and gut immune responses, and theoretical advantages over viable products include enhanced safety and longer shelf-life.

Results of the studies comparing viable vs. non-viable probiotic products on a variety of clinical outcomes have been summarized by Lahtinen et al. The authors concluded that, while it is clear that live bacteria are overall more effective than non-viable ones, there might be some cases where viability is not essential for the health benefit, as suggested by some clinical reports [56]. The evaluation of viable probiotics vs. non-viable ones is further complicated by the fact that, during storage, part of the probiotic population may become "dormant" [57].

At present, few probiotic species, including strains of both *Lactobacillus* and *Bifidobacterium*, have been studied in their inactivated form [58]; current evidence about their potential applications in preterm infants is limited, but it is likely that further research will give new insight into mechanisms of action, most effective and safe probiotic strains to be used in their inactivated form, and most promising clinical applications in preterm infants [59].

6. Choosing the Study Design: The Challenge of Cross-Colonization

Cross-colonization, or cross-contamination, occurs when a microorganism, including a probiotic, is transferred from one individual or environment to another. Early clinical trials on probiotic supplementation to preterm infants reported some cases of cross-colonization with the probiotic organism. Millar et al. documented transient colonization with *Lactobacillus GG* of one infant, whose twin was receiving probiotic supplementation and was being nursed in an adjacent cot [60]. One RCT investigating the colonization with *Bifidobacterium breve* detected the probiotic bacteria in the feces of 44% of the control infants at six weeks [61]. More recently, Hickey et al. [62] assessed the rate of cross-colonization of specific probiotic organisms within a multicenter RCT [63]. The authors reported a low occurrence of probiotic cross-colonization (7.9%) and environmental contamination, suggesting that this phenomenon may be related to physical proximity to infants receiving probiotics, as well as NICU length of stay. In contrast, the Probiotic in Preterm Infants Study (PiPS), the largest multicenter RCT about probiotics in preterm infants, demonstrated that cross-contamination occurred in 49% of the infants in the placebo arm in all study sites. Furthermore, rates of the primary outcomes did not differ significantly between the probiotic and placebo groups [64]. Nonetheless, further analysis based on the colonization status suggested benefits in the colonized infants irrespective of their allocation to the probiotic or placebo treatment groups [65,66].

Mechanisms of cross-contamination in the NICU have not been satisfactorily explored. They likely include transmission through the contamination of NICU surfaces and the body/hands of caregivers [67]. Even if cross-colonization may not result in ingestion of the probiotic bacteria at beneficial doses in the control group, it may be enough to alter the outcomes. The challenges of cross-contamination include both the potential impact on NICU infants and limitations in assessing the true effect of probiotic supplementation in clinical trials. In order to avoid infant-to-infant probiotic dissemination, Totsu et al. [68] performed a cluster RCT involving 19 NICUs, reporting benefits of single-strain *Bifidobacterium bifidum OLB6378* supplementation in preterm infants. Taking these findings together, cross-colonization should be considered when designing further RCTs. Cluster or cross-over cluster randomized trials in which the NICU is randomized rather than the infant should be considered [40,47,64], as well as more standardized hygiene policies and NICU layouts.

7. Conclusions

The interaction between probiotics and the preterm host is extremely complex, due to particular intrinsic and environmental factors. Despite the enthusiasm towards probiotics in neonatal medicine, theoretical knowledge and clinical applications still need to be improved. This review highlights the need for further well-designed studies aimed at clarifying the impact of the type of feeding, as well as related confounding factors, on the relationship between probiotic supplementation and clinical outcome. Furthermore, future research is needed to provide solid evidence about the potential greater efficacy of multi-strain/multi-species probiotics compared to single-strain products. According to recent observations, paraprobiotics could represent an answer to safety concerns related to the routine administration of probiotics in preterm infants, and pre-clinical and clinical studies should be targeted to explore this new frontier. Further RCTs exploring probiotic supplementation in preterm infants should also consider a cluster design to avoid the issue of cross-contamination. Last, in light of increasing commercial and public interests, the long-term effect of the routine consumption of probiotics and the risk connected to antibiotic resistance in this vulnerable population should be explored in ad hoc studies.

Author Contributions: A.A. and I.B. wrote the first draft of the paper. A.A., I.B. and S.M. performed the literature search and review. L.M., G.F. and L.C. made substantial revisions to the first draft. All the authors have approved the submitted version of this work and agree to be personally accountable for their own contributions and for ensuring that questions related to the accuracy or integrity of any part of the work, even ones in which they are not personally involved, are appropriately investigated, resolved, and documented in the literature.

Conflicts of Interest: The authors declare no conflict of interest.

References

1. Harrison, M.S.; Goldenberg, R.L. Global burden of prematurity. *Semin. Fetal Neonatal Med.* **2016**, *21*, 74–79. [CrossRef] [PubMed]
2. Platt, M.J. Outcomes in preterm infants. *Public Health* **2014**, *128*, 399–403. [CrossRef] [PubMed]
3. Schüller, S.S.; Kramer, B.W.; Villamor, E.; Spittler, A.; Berger, A.; Levy, O. Immunomodulation to prevent or treat neonatal sepsis: Past, present, and future. *Front. Pediatr.* **2018**, *6*, 1–17. [CrossRef] [PubMed]
4. Dermyshi, E.; Wang, Y.; Yan, C.; Hong, W.; Qiu, G.; Gong, X.; Zhang, T. The "Golden Age" of probiotics: A systematic review and meta-analysis of randomized and observational studies in preterm infants. *Neonatology* **2017**, *112*, 9–23. [CrossRef] [PubMed]
5. AlFaleh, K.; Anabrees, J. Probiotics for prevention of necrotizing enterocolitis in preterm infants. *Cochrane Database Syst. Rev.* **2014**, *4*, CD005496.
6. Aceti, A.; Gori, D.; Barone, G.; Callegari, M.L.M.L.; Di Mauro, A.; Fantini, M.P.M.P.; Indrio, F.; Maggio, L.; Meneghin, F.; Morelli, L.; et al. Probiotics for prevention of necrotizing enterocolitis in preterm infants: Systematic review and meta-analysis. *Ital. J. Pediatr.* **2015**, *41*, 89. [CrossRef] [PubMed]
7. Van den Akker, C.H.P.; van Goudoever, J.B.; Szajewska, H.; Embleton, N.D.; Hojsak, I.; Reid, D.; Shamir, R. Probiotics for preterm infants: A strain-specific systematic review and network meta-analysis. *J. Pediatr. Gastroenterol. Nutr.* **2018**, *67*, 103–122. [CrossRef] [PubMed]
8. Rao, S.C.; Athalye-jape, G.K.; Deshpande, G.C.; Simmer, K.N.; Patole, S.K. Probiotic supplementation and late-onset sepsis in preterm infants: A meta-analysis. *Pediatrics* **2016**, *137*, 1–16. [CrossRef] [PubMed]
9. Aceti, A.; Maggio, L.; Beghetti, I.; Gori, D.; Barone, G.; Callegari, M.L.; Fantini, M.P.; Indrio, F.; Meneghin, F.; Morelli, L.; et al. Probiotics prevent late-onset sepsis in human milk-fed, very low birth weight preterm infants: Systematic review and meta-analysis. *Nutrients* **2017**, *9*, 904. [CrossRef] [PubMed]
10. Athalye-Jape, G.; Deshpande, G.; Rao, S.; Patole, S. Benefits of probiotics on enteral nutrition in preterm neonates: A systematic review. *Am. J. Clin. Nutr.* **2014**, *100*, 1508–1519. [CrossRef] [PubMed]
11. Aceti, A.; Gori, D.; Barone, G.; Callegari, M.L.; Fantini, M.P.; Indrio, F.; Maggio, L.; Meneghin, F.; Morelli, L.; Zuccotti, G.; et al. Probiotics and time to achieve full enteral feeding in human milk-fed and formula-fed preterm infants: Systematic review and meta-analysis. *Nutrients* **2016**, *8*, 471. [CrossRef] [PubMed]
12. Deshpande, G.; Jape, G.; Rao, S.; Patole, S. Benefits of probiotics in preterm neonates in low-income and medium-income countries: A systematic review of randomised controlled trials. *BMJ Open* **2017**, *7*, e017638. [CrossRef] [PubMed]
13. Sun, J.; Marwah, G.; Westgarth, M.; Buys, N.; Ellwood, D.; Gray, P.H. Effects of probiotics on necrotizing enterocolitis, sepsis, intraventricular hemorrhage, mortality, length of hospital stay, and weight gain in very preterm infants: A meta-analysis. *Adv. Nutr. Int. Rev. J.* **2017**, *8*, 749–763. [CrossRef] [PubMed]
14. Chang, H.Y.; Chen, J.H.; Chang, J.H.; Lin, H.C.; Lin, C.Y.; Peng, C.C. Multiple strains probiotics appear to be the most effective probiotics in the prevention of necrotizing enterocolitis and mortality: An updated meta-analysis. *PLoS ONE* **2017**, *12*, e0171579. [CrossRef] [PubMed]
15. Cohen, P.A. Probiotic safety-No guarantees. *JAMA Intern. Med.* **2018**. [CrossRef] [PubMed]
16. Viswanathan, S.; Lau, C.; Akbari, H.; Hoyen, C.; Walsh, M.C. Survey and evidence based review of probiotics used in very low birth weight preterm infants within the United States. *J. Perinatol.* **2016**, *36*, 1106–1111. [CrossRef] [PubMed]
17. Patel, R.M.; Underwood, M.A. Probiotics and necrotizing enterocolitis. *Semin. Pediatr. Surg.* **2018**, *27*, 39–46. [CrossRef] [PubMed]
18. Iozzo, P.; Sanguinetti, E. Early dietary patterns and microbiota development: Still a way to go from descriptive interactions to health-relevant solutions. *Front. Nutr.* **2018**, *5*, 5. [CrossRef] [PubMed]
19. Sanders, M.E.; Guarner, F.; Guerrant, R.; Holt, P.R.; Quigley, E.M.M.; Sartor, R.B.; Sherman, P.M.; Mayer, E. An update on the use and investigation of probiotics in health and disease. *Gut* **2013**, *62*, 787–796. [CrossRef] [PubMed]
20. Koletzko, B.; Brands, B.; Grote, V.; Kirchberg, F.F.; Prell, C.; Rzehak, P.; Uhl, O.; Weber, M. Long-term health impact of early nutrition: The power of programming. *Ann. Nutr. Metab.* **2017**, *70*, 161–169. [CrossRef] [PubMed]
21. Schneider, N.; Garcia-Rodenas, C.L. Early nutritional interventions for brain and cognitive development in preterm infants: A review of the literature. *Nutrients* **2017**, *9*, 187. [CrossRef] [PubMed]

22. American Academy of Pediatrics. Breastfeeding and the use of human milk. *Pediatrics* **2012**, *129*, e827–e841. [CrossRef] [PubMed]
23. Chong, C.; Bloomfield, F.; O'Sullivan, J. Factors affecting gastrointestinal microbiome development in neonates. *Nutrients* **2018**, *10*, 274. [CrossRef] [PubMed]
24. De la Cruz, D.; Bazacliu, C. Enteral feeding composition and necrotizing enterocolitis. *Semin. Fetal Neonatal Med.* **2018**. [CrossRef]
25. Maffei, D.; Schanler, R.J. Human milk is the feeding strategy to prevent necrotizing enterocolitis! *Semin. Perinatol.* **2017**, *41*, 36–40. [CrossRef] [PubMed]
26. Biagi, E.; Quercia, S.; Aceti, A.; Beghetti, I.; Rampelli, S.; Turroni, S.; Faldella, G.; Candela, M.; Brigidi, P.; Corvaglia, L. The bacterial ecosystem of mother's milk and infant's mouth and gut. *Front. Microbiol.* **2017**, *8*, 1214. [CrossRef] [PubMed]
27. Zimmermann, P.; Curtis, N. Factors Influencing the intestinal microbiome during the first year of life. *Pediatr. Infect. Dis. J.* **2018**. [CrossRef] [PubMed]
28. Xu, W.; Judge, M.; Maas, K.; Hussain, N.; McGrath, J.M.; Henderson, W.A.; Cong, X. Systematic review of the effect of enteral feeding on gut microbiota in preterm infants. *J. Obstet. Gynecol. Neonatal Nurs.* **2017**, *47*, 451–463. [CrossRef] [PubMed]
29. Repa, A.; Thanhaeuser, M.; Endress, D.; Weber, M.; Kreissl, A.; Binder, C.; Berger, A.; Haiden, N. Probiotics (*Lactobacillus acidophilus* and *Bifidobacterium bifidum*) prevent NEC in VLBW infants fed breast milk but not formula. *Pediatr. Res.* **2015**, *77*, 381–388. [CrossRef] [PubMed]
30. Thomas, J.P.; Raine, T.; Reddy, S.; Belteki, G. Probiotics for the prevention of necrotising enterocolitis in very low-birth-weight infants: A meta-analysis and systematic review. *Acta Paediatr.* **2017**, *106*, 1729–1741. [CrossRef] [PubMed]
31. Embleton, N.D.; Zalewski, S.; Berrington, J.E. Probiotics for prevention of necrotizing enterocolitis and sepsis in preterm infants. *Curr. Opin. Infect. Dis.* **2016**, *29*, 256–261. [CrossRef] [PubMed]
32. Autran, C.A.; Kellman, B.P.; Kim, J.H.; Asztalos, E.; Blood, A.B.; Spence, E.C.H.; Patel, A.L.; Hou, J.; Lewis, N.E.; Bode, L. Human milk oligosaccharide composition predicts risk of necrotising enterocolitis in preterm infants. *Gut* **2018**, *67*, 1064–1070. [CrossRef] [PubMed]
33. Kantorowska, A.; Wei, J.C.; Cohen, R.S.; Lawrence, R.A.; Gould, J.B.; Lee, H.C. Impact of Donor Milk Availability on Breast Milk Use and Necrotizing Enterocolitis Rates. *Pediatrics* **2016**, *137*, e20153123. [CrossRef] [PubMed]
34. Sharpe, J.; Way, M.; Koorts, P.J.; Davies, M.W. The availability of probiotics and donor human milk is associated with improved survival in very preterm infants. *World J. Pediatr.* **2018**. [CrossRef] [PubMed]
35. O'Connor, D.L.; Gibbins, S.; Kiss, A.; Bando, N.; Brennan-Donnan, J.; Ng, E.; Campbell, D.M.; Vaz, S.; Fusch, C.; Asztalos, E.; et al. Effect of supplemental donor human milk compared with preterm formula on neurodevelopment of very low-birth-weight infants at 18 months: A randomized clinical trial. *JAMA* **2016**, *316*, 1897–1905. [CrossRef] [PubMed]
36. Peila, C.; Moro, G.E.; Bertino, E.; Cavallarin, L.; Giribaldi, M.; Giuliani, F.; Cresi, F.; Coscia, A. The effect of holder pasteurization on nutrients and biologically-active components in donor human milk: A review. *Nutrients* **2016**, *8*, 477. [CrossRef] [PubMed]
37. Parra-Llorca, A.; Gormaz, M.; Alcántara, C.; Cernada, M.; Nuñez-Ramiro, A.; Vento, M.; Collado, M.C. Preterm gut microbiome depending on feeding type: Significance of donor human milk. *Front. Microbiol.* **2018**, *9*, 1376. [CrossRef] [PubMed]
38. Guarner, F.; Malagelada, J.R. Gut flora in health and disease. *Lancet* **2003**, *361*, 512–519. [CrossRef]
39. Zhang, G.-Q.; Hu, H.-J.; Liu, C.-Y.; Shakya, S.; Li, Z.-Y. Probiotics for preventing late-onset sepsis in preterm neonates: A PRISMA-compliant systematic review and meta-analysis of randomized controlled trials. *Medicine* **2016**, *95*, e2581. [CrossRef] [PubMed]
40. Athalye-Jape, G.; Rao, S.; Simmer, K.; Patole, S. Bifidobacterium breve M-16V as a probiotic for preterm infants: A strain-specific systematic review. *J. Parenter. Enter. Nutr.* **2018**, *42*, 677–688. [CrossRef] [PubMed]
41. Athalye-Jape, G.; Rao, S.; Patole, S. Lactobacillus reuteri DSM 17938 as a probiotic for preterm neonates: A strain-specific systematic review. *J. Parenter. Enter. Nutr.* **2016**, *40*, 783–794. [CrossRef] [PubMed]
42. Hu, H.J.; Zhang, G.Q.; Zhang, Q.; Shakya, S.; Li, Z.Y. Probiotics prevent candida colonization and invasive fungal sepsis in preterm neonates: A systematic review and meta-analysis of randomized controlled trials. *Pediatr. Neonatol.* **2017**, *58*, 103–110. [CrossRef] [PubMed]

43. Ganguli, K.; Walker, W.A. Probiotics in the prevention of necrotizing enterocolitis. *J. Clin. Gastroenterol.* **2011**, *45*, 133–138. [CrossRef] [PubMed]
44. Hill, C.; Sanders, M.E. Rethinking "probiotics". *Gut Microbes* **2013**, *4*, 269–270. [CrossRef] [PubMed]
45. Hill, C.; Guarner, F.; Reid, G.; Gibson, G.R.; Merenstein, D.J.; Pot, B.; Morelli, L.; Canani, R.B.; Flint, H.J.; Salminen, S.; et al. Expert consensus document: The international scientific association for probiotics and prebiotics consensus statement on the scope and appropriate use of the term probiotic. *Nat. Rev. Gastroenterol. Hepatol.* **2014**, 11, 506–514. [CrossRef] [PubMed]
46. Patole, S. Probiotics for preterm infants-The story searching for an end. *Indian Pediatr.* **2017**, *54*, 361–362. [CrossRef] [PubMed]
47. Underwood, M.A. Impact of probiotics on necrotizing enterocolitis. *Semin. Perinatol.* **2017**, *41*, 41–51. [CrossRef] [PubMed]
48. Sanders, M.E.; Benson, A.; Lebeer, S.; Merenstein, D.J.; Klaenhammer, T.R. Shared mechanisms among probiotic taxa: Implications for general probiotic claims. *Curr. Opin. Biotechnol.* **2018**, *49*, 207–216. [CrossRef] [PubMed]
49. Timmerman, H.M.; Koning, C.J.M.; Mulder, L.; Rombouts, F.M.; Beynen, A.C. Monostrain, multistrain and multispecies probiotics-A comparison of functionality and efficacy. *Int. J. Food Microbiol.* **2004**, *96*, 219–233. [CrossRef] [PubMed]
50. Ouwehand, A.C.; Invernici, M.M.; Furlaneto, F.A.C.; Messora, M.R. Effectiveness of multistrain versus single-strain probiotics current status and recommendations for the future. *J. Clin. Gastroenterol.* **2018**. [CrossRef] [PubMed]
51. Deshpande, G.C.; Rao, S.C.; Keil, A.D.; Patole, S.K. Evidence-based guidelines for use of probiotics in preterm neonates. *BMC Med.* **2011**, *9*, 92. [CrossRef] [PubMed]
52. Wong, A.; Saint Ngu, D.Y.; Dan, L.A.; Ooi, A.; Lim, R.L.H. Detection of antibiotic resistance in probiotics of dietary supplements. *Nutr. J.* **2015**, *14*, 95. [CrossRef] [PubMed]
53. Zheng, M.; Zhang, R.; Tian, X.; Zhou, X.; Pan, X.; Wong, A. Assessing the risk of probiotic dietary supplements in the context of antibiotic resistance. *Front. Microbiol.* **2017**, *8*, 1–8. [CrossRef] [PubMed]
54. Taverniti, V.; Guglielmetti, S. The immunomodulatory properties of probiotic microorganisms beyond their viability (ghost probiotics: Proposal of paraprobiotic concept). *Genes Nutr.* **2011**, *6*, 261–274. [CrossRef] [PubMed]
55. Adams, C.A. The probiotic paradox: Live and dead cells are biological response modifiers. *Nutr. Res. Rev.* **2010**, *23*, 37–46. [CrossRef] [PubMed]
56. Lahtinen, S.J. Probiotic viability-does it matter? *Microb. Ecol. Heal. Dis.* **2012**, *23*, 10–14. [CrossRef] [PubMed]
57. Lahtinen, S.J.; Gueimonde, M.; Ouwehand, A.C.; Reinikainen, J.P.; Salminen, S.J. Probiotic bacteria may become dormant during storage. *Appl. Environ. Microbiol.* **2005**, *71*, 1662–1663. [CrossRef] [PubMed]
58. Zorzela, L.; Ardestani, S.K.; McFarland, L.V.; Vohra, S. Is there a role for modified probiotics as beneficial microbes: A systematic review of the literature. *Benef. Microbes* **2017**, *8*, 739–754. [CrossRef] [PubMed]
59. Deshpande, G.; Athalye-Jape, G.; Patole, S. Para-probiotics for preterm neonates-The next frontier. *Nutrients* **2018**, *10*, 871. [CrossRef] [PubMed]
60. Millar, M.R.; Bacon, C.; Smith, S.L.; Walker, V.; Hall, M.A. Enteral feeding of premature infants with *Lactobacillus GG. Arch. Dis. Child.* **1993**, *69*, 483–487. [CrossRef] [PubMed]
61. Kitajima, H.; Sumida, Y.; Tanaka, R.; Yuki, N.; Takayama, H.; Fujimura, M. Early administration of Bifidobacterium breve to preterm infants: Randomised controlled trial. *Arch. Dis. Child. Fetal Neonatal Ed.* **1997**, *76*, F101–F107. [CrossRef] [PubMed]
62. Hickey, L.; Garland, S.M.; Jacobs, S.E.; O'Donnell, C.P.F.; Tabrizi, S.N. Cross-colonization of infants with probiotic organisms in a neonatal unit. *J. Hosp. Infect.* **2014**, *88*, 226–229. [CrossRef] [PubMed]
63. Jacobs, S.E.; Tobin, J.M.; Opie, G.F.; Donath, S.; Tabrizi, S.N.; Pirotta, M.; Morley, C.J.; Garland, S.M. Probiotic Effects on Late-onset Sepsis in Very Preterm Infants: A Randomized Controlled Trial. *Pediatrics* **2013**, *132*, 1055–1062. [CrossRef] [PubMed]
64. Costeloe, K.; Hardy, P.; Juszczak, E.; Wilks, M.; Millar, M.R. *Bifidobacterium breve* BBG-001 in very preterm infants: A randomised controlled phase 3 trial. *Lancet* **2016**, *387*, 649–660. [CrossRef]
65. Deshpande, G.; Rao, S.; Athalye-Jape, G.; Conway, P.; Patole, S. Probiotics in very preterm infants: The PiPS trial. *Lancet* **2016**, *388*, 655. [CrossRef]

66. Karthikeyan, G.; Bhat, B.V. The PiPS (Probiotics in Preterm Infants Study) trial-controlling the confounding factor of crosscontamination unveils significant benefits. *Indian Pediatr.* **2017**, *54*, 162. [PubMed]
67. Meadow, J.F.; Altrichter, A.E.; Bateman, A.C.; Stenson, J.; Brown, G.; Green, J.L.; Bohannan, B.J.M. Humans differ in their personal microbial cloud. *PeerJ* **2015**, *3*, e1258. [CrossRef] [PubMed]
68. Totsu, S.; Yamasaki, C.; Terahara, M.; Uchiyama, A.; Kusuda, S. Bifidobacterium and enteral feeding in preterm infants: Cluster-randomized trial. *Pediatr. Int.* **2014**, *56*, 714–719. [CrossRef] [PubMed]

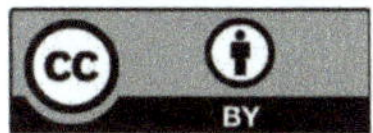
© 2018 by the authors. Licensee MDPI, Basel, Switzerland. This article is an open access article distributed under the terms and conditions of the Creative Commons Attribution (CC BY) license (http://creativecommons.org/licenses/by/4.0/).

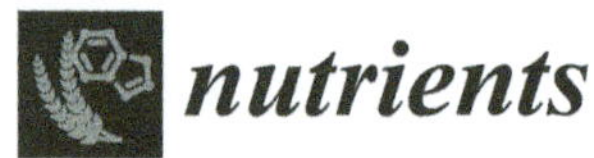

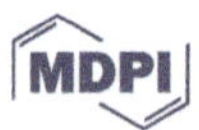

Article

Microbiota and Derived Parameters in Fecal Samples of Infants with Non-IgE Cow's Milk Protein Allergy under a Restricted Diet

María Díaz [1,†], Lucía Guadamuro [1,†], Irene Espinosa-Martos [2], Leonardo Mancabelli [3], Santiago Jiménez [4], Cristina Molinos-Norniella [5], David Pérez-Solis [6], Christian Milani [3], Juan Miguel Rodríguez [2], Marco Ventura [3], Carlos Bousoño [4], Miguel Gueimonde [1], Abelardo Margolles [1], Juan José Díaz [4,*] and Susana Delgado [1,*]

1. Department of Microbiology and Biochemistry of Dairy Products, Instituto de Productos Lácteos de Asturias (IPLA)-Consejo Superior de Investigaciones Científicas (CSIC), 33300 Villaviciosa, Spain; Maria.Diaz@quadram.ac.uk (M.D.); luciagg@ipla.csic.es (L.G.); mgueimonde@ipla.csic.es (M.G.); amargolles@ipla.csic.es (A.M.)
2. Department of Nutrition and Food Science, Universidad Complutense de Madrid (UCM), 28040 Madrid, Spain; irene.espinosa@probisearch.com (I.E.-M.); jmrodrig@ucm.es (J.M.R.)
3. Department of Chemistry, Life Sciences and Environmental Sustainability, University of Parma, 43121 Parma, Italy; leonardo.mancabelli@genprobio.com (L.M.); christian.milani@unipr.it (C.M.); marco.ventura@unipr.it (M.V.)
4. Pediatric Gastroenterology and Nutrition Section, Hospital Universitario Central de Asturias (HUCA), 33011 Oviedo, Spain; principevegeta@hotmail.com (S.J.); ringerbou@yahoo.es (C.B.)
5. Pediatrics, Hospital Universitario de Cabueñes, 33394 Gijón, Spain; cristinamolinos@gmail.com
6. Pediatrics, Hospital Universitario San Agustín, 33401 Avilés, Spain; doctorin@gmail.com

* Correspondence: juanjo.diazmartin@gmail.com (J.J.D.); sdelgado@ipla.csic.es (S.D.)

† These authors contribute equally to this work.

Received: 21 September 2018; Accepted: 6 October 2018; Published: 11 October 2018

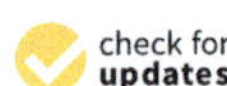

Abstract: Cow's milk protein allergy (CMPA) is the most common food allergy in infancy. Non-IgE mediated (NIM) forms are little studied and the responsible mechanisms of tolerance acquisition remain obscure. Our aim was to study the intestinal microbiota and related parameters in the fecal samples of infants with NIM-CMPA, to establish potential links between type of formula substitutes, microbiota, and desensitization. Seventeen infants between one and two years old, diagnosed with NIM-CMPA, were recruited. They were all on an exclusion diet for six months, consuming different therapeutic protein hydrolysates. After this period, stool samples were obtained and tolerance development was evaluated by oral challenges. A control group of 10 age-matched healthy infants on an unrestricted diet were included in the study. Microbiota composition, short-chain fatty acids, calprotectin, and transforming growth factor (TGF)-β_1 levels were determined in fecal samples from both groups. Infants with NIM-CMPA that consumed vegetable protein-based formulas presented microbiota colonization patterns different from those fed with an extensively hydrolyzed formula. Differences in microbiota composition and fecal parameters between NIM-CMPA and healthy infants were observed. Non-allergic infants showed a significantly higher proportion of Bacteroides compared to infants with NIM-CMPA. The type of protein hydrolysate was found to determine gut microbiota colonization and influence food allergy resolution in NIM-CMPA cases.

Keywords: fecal microbiota; protein hydrolyzed formulas; cow's milk protein; tolerance acquisition; non-IgE mediated allergy

1. Introduction

Cow's milk protein (CMP) is the main cause of food allergy in the first year of life. Based on the involvement of IgE antibodies, CMP allergy (CMPA) is classified as classic IgE-mediated, non-IgE mediated (NIM), and mixed pathophysiology [1]. Typically, clinical presentation is delayed, and digestive symptoms are more frequent, with NIM-CMPA than with IgE-mediated CMPA [2]. In both types, treatment involves the avoidance of cow's milk formula and the use of a therapeutic formula as a substitute. Clinical guidelines recommend the use of an extensively hydrolyzed formula (EHF) as the first choice, while amino acid-based formulas are reserved for those cases not responding to an EHF [3]. Soy formulas represent an option in infants older than six months [4], and rice formulas have been safely used during the last few years [5]. Nowadays, a wide number of articles highlight the importance of the correct establishment/development of gut microbiota in early life and its impact on allergic diseases, including food allergies [6,7]. Although some studies have related intestinal microbiota and allergy resolution in IgE-mediated CMPA [8,9], research on gut microbiota exclusively in NIM-CMPA has been hampered by the difficulty of diagnosis [10]. However, differences in microbial composition between infants with IgE-mediated and non-IgE mediated food allergies have been reported [11]. The present study was designed to evaluate intestinal microbiota and fecal associated parameters in infants with NIM-CMPA, under a milk elimination diet, compared to healthy infants, with an unrestricted conventional diet, with the aim of establishing potential links among microbiota, main feeding sources, and tolerance acquisition.

2. Materials and Methods

2.1. Subjects

Infants 12 to 24 months old diagnosed with NIM-CMPA (n = 17) were prospectively recruited for study participation at three different regional hospitals in Asturias (Northern Spain): *Hospital Universitario Central de Asturias, Hospital Universitario de Cabueñes, and Hospital Universitario San Agustín.* All participants had symptoms suggestive of CMPA, a negative skin prick test, values lower than 0.35 kU/L cow's milk-specific IgE determined in their blood, and a clear positive standardized oral challenge (SOC), performed under medical supervision following the European Society for Pediatric Gastroenterology, Hepatology, and Nutrition (ESPGHAN) guidelines. Infants that were exclusively breastfed at the diagnosis, and those that had used antibiotics or had symptoms of an infectious disease in the four weeks prior to the stool sample collection, were excluded from the study.

The study was approved by the Regional Ethics Committee for Clinical Research of Principality of Asturias (Ref. number 105/15, approved on 22 June 2015). Personal data of the children that provided stool samples conformed to the ethical guidelines outlined in the Declaration of Helsinki and its amendments. Individual signed informed consents were obtained from all the families participating in the study.

2.2. Study Design

This was a prospective cohort study. A detailed medical history, including type of feeding and formula used, were recorded by the clinicians. All infants were on a cow's-milk-free diet for at least six months before a new SOC was performed. Following the elimination diet period, and before the new SOC, stool samples were collected. A control group of 10 age-matched healthy infants (range 12–24 months old), with a normal diet consuming CMP, were included in the study and provided stool samples. Feces from all the participants were collected by their parents in sterile containers and immediately frozen at −20 °C. All samples were thawed on ice once they had been delivered to the laboratory and processed accordingly for different analyses.

2.3. Intestinal Microbial Community Analysis

Extraction of DNA from feces was based on the method of Zoetendal et al. [12] using the QIAamp DNA Stool mini kit (Qiagen, Hilden, Germany), with some modifications as previously described [13]. Partial 16S rRNA gene sequences were amplified from the DNA of the samples according to previous reports [14]. Samples were submitted to 2 × 250 bp paired-end sequencing by an Illumina MiSeq System (Illumina, San Diego, CA, USA). All Illumina quality-approved, trimmed, and filtered sequences were processed using a custom script based on the QIIME software suite [15]. Sequences were classified to the lowest possible taxonomic rank considered (i.e., genus level), using QIIME and the SILVA database as reference. Weighted UniFrac was employed to assess the similarity of the microbial communities between infants. The raw sequences data were deposited in the Sequence Read Archive (SRA) of the NCBI (https://www.ncbi.nlm.nih.gov/sra) under accession numbers SRR6884553 to SRR6884580.

2.4. Analysis of Short-Chain Fatty Acids (SCFAs)

A chromatographic system, composed of 6890N gas chromatography (GC) apparatus (Agilent Technologies, Santa Clara, CA, USA) connected to a flame ionization detector (FID), was used. All samples were analyzed in duplicate and SCFAs were quantified as previously described [16].

2.5. Calprotectin Assays

Calprotectin levels were determined using the commercially available enzyme-linked immunosorbent assay (ELISA) kit CALPROLAB™ (Calpro, Lysaker, Norway) according to the manufacturer's instructions.

2.6. Transforming Growth Factor-β_1 (TGF-β_1) Determination

The concentration of TGF-β_1 in the feces was determined by using a Bio-Plex 200 system instrument and the Bio-Plex Pro™ TGF-β Assay (both from Bio-Rad, Hercules, CA, USA). Analysis of samples was carried out as previously described [17].

2.7. Statistical Analysis

Statistical analysis of microbiological sequences was performed with the Metastats statistical method [18]. Multiple hypothesis tests were adjusted using a false discovery rate (FDR) correction of 0.25. Multivariable statistical analysis was performed by principal coordinates analysis (PCoA) and the plot was visualized in the EMPeror Visualization Program [19]. Differences in the microbial distribution between infants were sought by analysis of molecular variance (AMOVA). Biochemical fecal data were analyzed using IBM SPSS 23 statistic software. Normality was checked by the Shapiro–Wilk test. As the variables were not normally distributed, medians and interquartile ranges (Q1 and Q3) were calculated, and comparisons were performed, by using the non-parametric Mann–Whitney test. The level of significance was set at p values of <0.05. Finally, the Spearman correlation method was conducted to elucidate the relationship between the variables of the study.

3. Results

Seventeen infants (nine male and eight female) were recruited into the NIM-CMPA group and 10 infants into the control group. No statistically significant differences were found with respect to sex and age between the two groups: median of 17 (13–23) months in the NIM-CMPA group vs. 18 (14.3–24) months in the control group. Infants in the NIM-CMPA group were fed with EHFs (12 patients, 70.6%), soy protein-based formulas (two patients, 11.8%), and hydrolyzed rice formulas (three patients, 17.6%). All of them developed tolerance to CMP by the end of the study with the exception of the three infants fed a rice formula.

3.1. Microbiota Analysis in NIM-CMPA in Relation to Tolerance and Diet

The three infants who did not develop tolerance to CMP, after the exclusion diet for six months, presented a clear distinct microbiota colonization pattern characterized by a low abundancy of sequences of Actinobacteria, in particular the genus *Bifidobacteria* (Table 1). Distinctively, the infant that reported the quickest and severest gastrointestinal (GI) symptoms after the SOC presented a clear dysbiotic pattern, with a marked presence of sequences belonging to the phylas Verrucomicrobia and Proteobacteria (infant code 12; Figure S1). The PCoA plot showed that the samples from the three non-tolerant infants did not clearly cluster and were separated from the infants who acquired desensitization to CMP (Figure 1). However, when AMOVA was used to assess the statistical significance of the spatial separation, significant differences in the microbial clustering between tolerant and non-tolerant infants (the latter ones consuming rice formula) were revealed (p value = 0.02).

Table 1. Significant differences (at different taxonomic ranks) in fecal microbial abundances (%) between tolerant and non-tolerant infants with non-IgE mediated cow's milk protein allergy (NIM-CMPA) after a period with a diet free of cow's milk protein (CMP).

Phylum	p Value [a]	Relative Abundance [b]	
		Non-Tolerant CMPA Infants (n = 3)	Tolerant CMPA Infants (n = 14)
Actinobacteria	0.002	0.428 ± 0.200	21.775 ± 15.731
Family			
Bifidobacteriaceae	0.002	0.087 ± 0.141	17.705 ± 15.513
Coriobacteriaceae	0.009	0.266 ± 0.224	3.990 ± 4.087
Genus			
Bifidobacterium	0.002	0.087 ± 0.141	17.680 ± 15.506

[a] Significance was considered below a p value of 0.05, multiple hypothesis test correction of Benjamini and Hochberg was applied with a false discovery rate (FDR) of 0.25. [b] Mean relative abundance ± standard deviation.

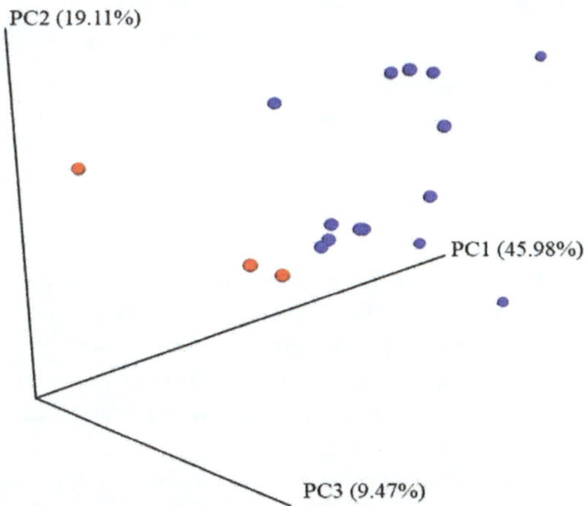

Figure 1. Principal coordinates analysis (PCoA) plot. For its construction, the weighted Unifrac method was used to compare the bacterial communities among samples from non-tolerant (n = 3) and tolerant (n = 14) infants with non-IgE mediated cow's milk protein allergy (NIM-CMPA), based on their phylogenetic relationship. Percentages shown in the axes represent the explained variance. Blue circles illustrate samples from tolerant infants whereas red circles illustrate those that maintain active hypersensitivity after the standardized oral challenge (SOC). Analysis of molecular variance (AMOVA) was used to assess the statistical significance of the spatial separation between both groups (p = 0.02).

Other members of the Actinobacteria phylum, in particular the family *Coriobacteriaceae*, was significantly diminished in the infants with NIM-CMPA that consumed vegetable protein-based formulas ($n = 5$; mean of 0.64% of total assigned reads; range 0.02–2.38%), both rice and soy, compared to those infants fed with an EHF (mean of 4.45%; range 0.08–13.44%).

3.2. Microbiota Analysis Comparison between the NIM-CMPA and Control Groups

Differences in the composition of the gut microbial communities between the infants with NIM-CMPA and the infants in the control group were observed. The non-allergic group, following an unrestricted diet, showed a significantly higher proportion of sequences of the phylum Bacteroidetes, the family *Bacteroidaceae*, and the genus *Bacteroides* compared to the NIM-CMPA group (Figure 2). In contrast, some members of the Clostridiales order, such as the *Eubacterium fissicatena* group (of the family *Lachnospiraceae*), were significantly higher in allergic infants, which also included the aforementioned *Coriobacteriaceae* family (mean of 3.33% of assigned reads, ranging from 0.02% to 13.44%, in the NIM-CMPA group versus 0.86% of assigned reads, ranging from 0.01% to 4.12%, in the control group).

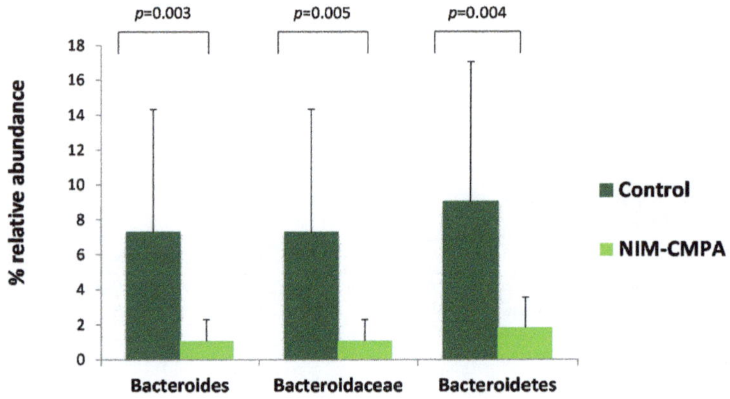

Figure 2. Differences in relative abundances (%) of sequences belonging to the phylum Bacteriodetes, the family *Bacteroidaceae*, and the genus *Bacteroides* in fecal samples of infants with non-IgE mediated cow's milk protein allergy (NIM-CMPA) ($n = 17$) and non-allergic control infants ($n = 10$). Comparisons were corrected with a false discovery rate (FDR) of 0.25.

3.3. Fecal Excreted SCFAs

Regarding the quantification of the SCFAs in the feces, there were no statistically significant differences in the acetic, butyric, and propionic levels between the NIM-CMPA and control groups (Table 2). For butyric acid, levels were higher in the infants with NIM-CMPA; however, the difference was borderline and not statistically significant ($p = 0.06$). There was a positive correlation (Spearman correlation coefficient $r = 0.48$, $p = 0.01$) between butyric acid levels and fecal *Coriobacteriaceae*, both of which were higher in the allergic group (see Figure S2).

Conversely, the branched chain fatty acids (BCFAs), isobutyric and isovaleric acids, presented significantly higher levels in the infants with NIM-CMPA than in the control group ($p = 0.03$).

Table 2. Levels of main short-chain fatty acids (SCFAs), branched chain fatty acids (BCFAs), transforming growth factor-β$_1$ (TGF-β$_1$), and calprotectin excreted in feces of infants with non-IgE mediated cow's milk protein allergy (NIM-CMPA) and infants in the control group.

Median (IQR) [a]	Infants		p Value [b]
	NIM-CMPA (n = 17)	Control (n = 10)	
BCFAs (μmol/g)	5.13 (3.08–6.52)	2.59 (1.94–3.37)	0.03
Acetic (μmol/g)	54.88 (48.05–89.63)	68.61 (50.49–69.96)	0.90
Propionic (μmol/g)	16.19 (13.09–21.48)	15.64 (11.66–24.06)	0.94
Butyric (μmol/g)	17.59 (12.74–21.41)	12.88 (6.14–14.3)	0.06
TGF-β$_1$ (pg/mL)	1774.79 (1153.10–3810.88)	1496.29 (382.23–5820.20)	0.73
Calprotectin (μg/g)	47.25 (28.80–106.10)	68.40 (30.38–76.73)	1.00

[a] Concentrations represent median and interquartile ranges (IQR). [b] Mann–Whitney U test. Significance was set at p = 0.05.

3.4. *Inflammatory Parameters*

The levels of the TGF-β$_1$ in feces of infants with NIM-CMPA were quite similar compared with values obtained in the control group, and statistical differences between both groups were not found (Table 2). In one infant of the control group and in three of the NIM-CMPA group, the levels of TGF-β$_1$ were below the lower limit of quantification (0.62 pg/mL). A significant negative correlation between fecal levels of butyric acid and excretion of TGF-β$_1$ was observed (r = 0.53, p = 0.04), but only in the group of infants with NIM-CMPA (Figure S3).

Fecal calprotectin concentrations in allergic infants did not show statistical differences with those found in control infants (Table 2). Calprotectin levels in the samples from the three infants that did not acquire tolerance, after the elimination diet, were no different from the levels found in the remaining NIM-CMPA patients, nor in the infants in the control group.

4. Discussion

NIM-CMPA is difficult to diagnose because clinical symptoms appear with a delayed onset and no specific diagnostic tests are available [20]. For this reason, there are only a few studies focusing on non-IgE mediated cases [10], and almost none of them consider the description of gut microbiota. The development of the intestinal microbiota and immune system could be playing a critical role in this condition, which affects children during their first two years of life. The important association between GI microbiota and food allergies in early infancy has been clearly pointed to in recent years [6,7,21], although the precise mechanisms of desensitization and interaction with the host remains poorly understood in most cases.

Our study was designed to evaluate intestinal microbiota and fecal associated parameters in infants with NIM-CMPA, under a milk elimination diet, compared to healthy infants, on an unrestricted diet, in an effort to establish potential links among microbiota and its metabolites, main feeding sources, and tolerance acquisition. The importance of formula selection for the management of infants with CMPA (both IgE and non-IgE mediated) and the acquisition of tolerance has been previously stated in studies by Berni Canani and colleagues, who demonstrated that an EHF supplemented with a probiotic (*Lactobacillus rhamnosus* GG) was able to accelerate tolerance acquisition in infants with CMPA [22,23]. However, the microbiota was not analyzed in these works. In our study, we observed that only those infants who were consuming rice hydrolyzed formulas did not develop clinical tolerance after six months of an exclusion diet, and presented significant differences in their microbiota with respect to those who outgrew their CMPA. To the best of our knowledge, this is the first study focusing exclusively on NIM-CMPA. A recent work has also been published in NIM-CMPA patients, but in that case, in suspected not challenge-proven cases [10]. In that interventional study, only a few groups of fecal microorganisms (bifidobacteria and *Clostridium coccoides* group (reclassified now as *Blautia coccoides*, belonging to the clostridial cluster XIVa)) were evaluated by fluorescence in situ hybridization. In our study, we obtain detailed insights into the microbiota composition using next-generation sequencing (NGS) techniques. We found that infants with NIM-CMPA that consumed vegetable protein-based formulas had less *Coriobacteriaceae*. Specifically, those fed with rice formulas presented low abundances of representatives of *Coriobacteriaceae* and *Bifidobacteriaceae* in their fecal samples. Members of *Bifidobacteriaceae* (in particular *Bifidobacterium*) and *Coriobacteriaceae* (mainly *Collinsella*) have been reported to be highly prevalent from the early years of life [21,24]. *Coriobacteriaceae*, and certainly the genus *Collinsella*, were present in higher rates in infants with NIM-CMPA that consumed an EHF in our study. Although the biology of these bacteria is still largely ignored [21], experiments in vitro in human models showed that both *Collinsella* spp. and *Bifidobacterium* spp. are the major lactose utilizers in the human gut [24]. In fact, lactose is present is some of the commercial EHFs, but not in vegetable ones. In our work, a positive correlation was found between *Coriobacteriaceae* and butyrate levels. This may be explained by the stimulation of certain butyrate producers, such as members of the *C. coccoides* group, through cross-feeding mechanisms [25] that are triggered by end fermentation metabolites, which are produced by *Coriobacteriaceae*.

We also observed statistically higher levels of BCFAs (isobutyric and isovaleric acids) in infants with NIM-CMPA as compared with infants in the control group. These minor SCFAs have often been associated with protein breakdown [26]. Previous studies of IgE-mediated CMPA revealed fecal concentrations and percentages of butyric acid and BCFAs higher in infants with CMPA than in healthy infants [27].

The most outstanding difference between allergic and healthy infants, in terms of fecal microbiota composition, in our study was the reduction in the relative proportions of the phylum Bacteroidetes, especially the family *Bacteroideaceae* and the genus *Bacteroides*, in the infants with NIM-CMPA (both tolerant and non-tolerant) after the restricted diet period. Bacteroidetes perform metabolic conversions that are essential for the host, often related to the degradation of proteins [24]. Some species may play an important role in protein metabolism since they have proteolytic activity. The association of *Bacteroides* with a high consumption of fat and proteins of animal origin has been previously mentioned [28,29]. It has been described that in the mature intestine of the child, by two to three years of age, the microbiota composition mainly consists of *Bacteroideaceae*, as well as *Lachnospiraceae* and *Ruminococcaceae* members [30]. Other conditions during infancy, such as antibiotic exposure, preterm birth, or cesarean section delivery, have been related with reduced abundance of Bacteroidetes [31–33]. Furthermore, in adults, this group of microorganisms has been reported to be affected in some digestive pathologies, such as irritable bowel syndrome [34].

The precise mechanisms leading to tolerance in NIM-CMPA cases are not yet elucidated. Several immunological mechanisms may be responsible for the non-IgE reactions. Th1/Th2 imbalances are assumed to have an impact, but both humoral and/or cell-mediated mechanisms may be implicated and induce symptoms [35]. The regulatory cytokine TGF-β_1 is known to induce T-cell suppression, contributing to the downregulation of inflammatory processes. The expression of this growth factor in the intestinal mucosa increases with age during infancy [35]. In the present study, significant differences in the fecal levels of TGF-β_1 between infants diagnosed with NIM-CMPA and healthy infants were not found. Additionally, the three infants with persistent CMPA after the second SOC showed values in the same range as those that acquired tolerance. In a previous study of patients with NIM-CMPA, a higher frequency of circulating regulatory T (Treg) cells were found in children who, after a milk-free period, outgrew their allergy compared to those who maintained clinically active hypersensitivity [36]. The authors suggested that the suppressive action of cow's milk-specific Treg cells was exerted partly by direct cell–cell contact, and partly by production of TGF-β. In our study, it should be taken into consideration that fecal samples were taken after a period of six months of a dairy-free diet, during which most of the participants became tolerant, indicating that the underlying inflammatory condition of the gut may have normalized. Contrary to what we expected, we found a moderate, but significant, negative correlation between butyric acid and TGF-β_1 fecal levels in the group of infants with NIM-CMPA. Although we do not have a clear explanation at this stage, we postulate that the relationship between butyric acid levels and TGF-β_1 might be related to the role of the TGF-β receptor. Although this needs to be explored further in future studies, the activity of the type 1 receptor for TGF-β, rather than the cytokine itself, has already been suggested as being related with the pathogenesis of NIM-CMPA [37]. Furusawa and colleagues demonstrated, for the first time in 2013, that butyrate induce differentiation of colonic Treg cells, which have a central role in the suppression of inflammatory and allergic responses [38]. Butyrate exerts anti-inflammatory effects, through epigenetic mechanisms, influencing immune system development and function. The positive role of butyrate epigenetic effects on children's health has been previously highlighted [39].

Calprotectin levels vary with age, and therefore different studies on children have used diverse cut-off values [40]. As observed previously by others [41], differences in calprotectin concentrations between healthy and allergic infants after a CMP elimination diet were not found in our study, probably due to most of the patients outgrowing their allergy after the therapeutic diet restriction stabilization period.

Patterns of formula selection in infants with CMPA are changing with an increased use of soy and rice hydrolyzed formulas [23,42]. Actually, more information is needed for the choice of formula substitutes for children with CMPA [5]. Our findings support the recommendations of the GI Committee of ESPGHAN [3], and show that the use of a vegetable dietary regimen may not be conducive to achieving oral tolerance, due to the absence of exposure to immunomodulatory peptides and the shaping of the gut microbial communities. We realize the limitations of the study, namely the small number of patients included in each group. Therefore, the data found in this pilot study need to be confirmed in a larger population, especially since some studies in the past did not find differences in tolerance acquisition rates between the choice of different vegetable (rice, soy, and protein) formulas with respect to EHFs [43,44].

Our results indicate that the type of formula consumed in early life can determine the composition and diversity of the microbiota established. These preliminary data on NIM-CMPA still have to be taken with caution due to the high inter-individual variability in the microbiota among infants in this age period [21]. Although, with the present data, we hypothesize that differences in a child's main diet may influence the intestinal microbiota and its metabolic products, and, ultimately, influence tolerance acquisition, which has an important impact on clinical practice in NIM-CMPA.

Supplementary Materials: The following are available online at http://www.mdpi.com/2072-6643/10/10/1481/s1, Figure S1: Microbial composition at the phylum level in fecal samples of infants with non-IgE mediated (NIM) cow's milk protein allergy (CMPA) and non-allergic control infants. Figure S2: Regression of butyric acid levels on *Coriobacteriaceaea* abundances in all infants of the study (allergic and control; $n = 27$). Figure S3: Correlation between transforming growth factor (TGF)-β_1 and butyric acid levels in feces of infants with non-IgE mediated (NIM) cow's milk protein allergy (CMPA) ($n = 17$).

Author Contributions: S.D. and J.J.D. contributed with the conception of the study. M.D. and L.G. contributed equally to this work, performing both the laboratory determinations and the statistics. I.E.-M. and J.M.R. were involved in the cytokine analysis. L.M., C.M., and M.V. performed the DNA sequencing and analysis. S.J., C.M.-N., D.P.-S., C.B., and J.J.D. carried out the recruitment and diagnoses of the infants. J.J.D. was in charge of the SOCs and the recovery of information from the participant families. S.D., M.G., and A.M. planned the experimental design of the study and contributed to the interpretation of the data. S.D. provided material and human resources and drafted the manuscript. All authors corrected and approved the final version.

Funding: This research was funded by Instituto Danone through Ayudas a Proyectos de Investigación Científica 2015 and by Fundación Nutrición y Crecimiento.

Acknowledgments: The technical assistance of Jorge Rodríguez Álvarez-Buylla for the chromatographic determinations is greatly acknowledged, as well as the help of Lee Kellingray in the language revision.

Conflicts of Interest: The authors declare no conflicts of interest. The funders had no role in the design of the study; in the collection, analyses, or interpretation of data; in the writing of the manuscript; or in the decision to publish the results.

References

1. Nowak-Wegrzyn, A.; Szajewska, H.; Lack, G. Food allergy and the gut. *Nat. Rev. Gastroenterol. Hepatol.* **2017**, *14*, 241–257. [CrossRef] [PubMed]
2. Venter, C.; Brown, T.; Shah, N.; Fox, A.T. Diagnosis and management of non-IgE-mediated cow's milk allergy in infancy—A UK primary care practical guide. *Clin. Transl. Allergy* **2013**, *3*, 23. [CrossRef] [PubMed]
3. Koletzko, S.; Niggemann, B.; Arato, A.; Dias, J.A.; Heuschkel, R.; Husby, S.; Mearin, M.L.; Papadopoulou, A.; Ruemmele, F.M.; Staiano, A.; et al. Diagnostic approach and management of cow's-milk protein allergy in infants and children: ESPGHAN GI Committee practical guidelines. *J. Pediatr. Gastroenterol. Nutr.* **2012**, *55*, 221–229. [CrossRef] [PubMed]
4. Bhatia, J.; Greer, F. American Academy of Pediatrics Committee on Nutrition. Use of soy protein-based formulas in infant feeding. *Pediatrics* **2008**, *121*, 1062–1068. [CrossRef] [PubMed]
5. Fiocchi, A.; Dahda, L.; Dupont, C.; Campoy, C.; Fierro, V.; Nieto, A. Cow's milk allergy: Towards an update of DRACMA guidelines. *World Allergy Organ. J.* **2016**, *9*, 35. [CrossRef] [PubMed]
6. Simonyte Sjodin, K.; Vidman, L.; Ryden, P.; West, C.E. Emerging evidence of the role of gut microbiota in the development of allergic diseases. *Curr. Opin. Allergy Clin. Immunol.* **2016**, *16*, 390–395. [CrossRef] [PubMed]
7. Rachid, R.; Chatila, T.A. The role of the gut microbiota in food allergy. *Curr. Opin. Pediatr.* **2016**, *28*, 748–753. [CrossRef] [PubMed]
8. Thompson-Chagoyan, O.C.; Vieites, J.M.; Maldonado, J.; Edwards, C.; Gil, A. Changes in faecal microbiota of infants with cow's milk protein allergy—A Spanish prospective case-control 6-month follow-up study. *Pediatr. Allergy Immunol.* **2010**, *21*, e394–e400. [CrossRef] [PubMed]
9. Bunyavanich, S.; Shen, N.; Grishin, A.; Wood, R.; Burks, W.; Dawson, P.; Jones, S.M.; Leung, D.; Sampson, H.; Sicherer, S.; et al. Early-life gut microbiome composition and milk allergy resolution. *J. Allergy Clin. Immunol.* **2016**, *138*, 1122–1130. [CrossRef] [PubMed]
10. Candy, D.C.A.; Van Ampting, M.T.J.; Oude Nijhuis, M.M.; Wopereis, H.; Butt, A.M.; Peroni, D.G.; Vandenplas, Y.; Fox, A.T.; Shah, N.; West, C.E.; et al. A synbiotic-containing amino-acid-based formula improves gut microbiota in non-IgE-mediated allergic infants. *Pediatr. Res.* **2018**, *83*, 677–686. [CrossRef] [PubMed]
11. Ling, Z.; Li, Z.; Liu, X.; Cheng, Y.; Luo, Y.; Tong, X.; Yuan, L.; Wang, Y.; Sun, J.; Li, L.; et al. Altered fecal microbiota composition associated with food allergy in infants. *Appl. Environ. Microbiol.* **2014**, *80*, 2546–2554. [CrossRef] [PubMed]
12. Zoetendal, E.G.; Heilig, H.G.; Klaassens, E.S.; Booijink, C.C.; Kleerebezem, M.; Smidt, H.; De Vos, W.M. Isolation of DNA from bacterial samples of the human gastrointestinal tract. *Nat. Protoc.* **2006**, *1*, 870–873. [CrossRef] [PubMed]
13. Guadamuro, L.; Delgado, S.; Redruello, B.; Flórez, A.B.; Suárez, A.; Martínez-Camblor, P.; Mayo, B. Equol status and changes in fecal microbiota in menopausal women receiving long-term treatment for menopause symptoms with a soy-isoflavone concentrate. *Front. Microbiol.* **2015**, *6*, 777. [CrossRef] [PubMed]
14. Milani, C.; Hevia, A.; Foroni, E.; Duranti, S.; Turroni, F.; Lugli, G.A.; Sánchez, B.; Martín, R.; Gueimonde, M.; van Sinderen, D.; et al. Assessing the fecal microbiota: An optimized ion torrent 16S rRNA gene-based analysis protocol. *PLoS ONE* **2013**, *8*, e68739. [CrossRef] [PubMed]
15. Caporaso, J.G.; Kuczynski, J.; Stombaugh, J.; Bittinger, K.; Bushman, F.D.; Costello, E.K.; Fierer, N.; Gonzalez Peña, A.; Goodrich, J.K.; Gordon, J.I.; et al. QIIME allows analysis of high-throughput community sequencing data. *Nat. Methods* **2010**, *7*, 335–336. [CrossRef] [PubMed]
16. Salazar, N.; Gueimonde, M.; Hernandez-Barranco, A.M.; Ruas-Madiedo, P.; de los Reyes-Gavilán, C.G. Exopolysaccharides produced by intestinal Bifidobacterium strains act as fermentable substrates for human intestinal bacteria. *Appl. Environ. Microbiol.* **2008**, *74*, 4737–4745. [CrossRef] [PubMed]
17. Gómez, M.; Moles, L.; Espinosa-Martos, I.; Bustos, G.; de Vos, W.M.; Fernández, L.; Rodríguez, J.M.; Fuentes, S.; Jiménez, E. Bacteriological and immunological profiling of meconium and fecal samples from preterm infants: A two-year follow-up study. *Nutrients* **2017**, *9*, 1293. [CrossRef] [PubMed]
18. White, J.R.; Nagarajan, N.; Pop, M. Statistical methods for detecting differentially abundant features in clinical metagenomic samples. *PLoS Comput. Biol.* **2009**, *5*, e1000352. [CrossRef] [PubMed]
19. Vazquez-Baeza, Y.; Pirrung, M.; Gonzalez, A.; Knight, R. EMPeror: A tool for visualizing high-throughput microbial community data. *GigaScience* **2013**, *2*, 16. [CrossRef] [PubMed]

20. Hochwallner, H.; Schulmeister, U.; Swoboda, I.; Spitzauer, S.; Valenta, R. Cow's milk allergy: From allergens to new forms of diagnosis, therapy and prevention. *Methods* **2014**, *66*, 22–33. [CrossRef] [PubMed]
21. Milani, C.; Duranti, S.; Bottacini, F.; Casey, E.; Turroni, F.; Mahony, J.; Belzer, C.; Delgado Palacio, S.; Arboleya Montes, S.; Mancabelli, L.; et al. The first microbial colonizers of the human gut: Composition, activities, and health implications of the infant gut microbiota. *Microbiol. Mol. Biol. Rev.* **2017**, *81*, e00036-17. [CrossRef] [PubMed]
22. Berni Canani, R.; Nocerino, R.; Terrin, G.; Coruzzo, A.; Cosenza, L.; Leone, L.; Troncone, R. Effect of Lactobacillus GG on tolerance acquisition in infants with cow's milk allergy: A randomized trial. *J. Allergy Clin. Immunol.* **2012**, *129*, 580–582. [CrossRef] [PubMed]
23. Berni Canani, R.; Nocerino, R.; Terrin, G.; Frediani, T.; Lucarelli, S.; Cosenza, L.; Passariello, A.; Leone, L.; Granata, V.; Di Costanzo, M.; et al. Formula selection for management of children with cow's milk allergy influences the rate of acquisition of tolerance: A prospective multicenter study. *J. Pediatr.* **2013**, *163*, 771–777. [CrossRef] [PubMed]
24. Rajilic-Stojanovic, M.; de Vos, W.M. The first 1000 cultured species of the human gastrointestinal microbiota. *FEMS Microbiol. Rev.* **2014**, *38*, 996–1047. [CrossRef] [PubMed]
25. Flint, H.J.; Duncan, S.H.; Scott, K.P.; Louis, P. Links between diet, gut microbiota composition and gut metabolism. *Proc. Nutr. Soc.* **2015**, *74*, 13–22. [CrossRef] [PubMed]
26. Rios-Covian, D.; Ruas-Madiedo, P.; Margolles, A.; Gueimonde, M.; de los Reyes-Gavilán, C.G.; Salazar, N. Intestinal short chain fatty acids and their link with diet and human health. *Front. Microbiol.* **2016**, *7*, 185. [CrossRef] [PubMed]
27. Thompson-Chagoyan, O.C.; Fallani, M.; Maldonado, J.; Vieites, J.M.; Khanna, S.; Edwards, C.; Doré, J.; Gil, A. Faecal microbiota and short-chain fatty acid levels in faeces from infants with cow's milk protein allergy. *Int. Arch. Allergy Immunol.* **2011**, *156*, 325–332. [CrossRef] [PubMed]
28. Wu, G.D.; Chen, J.; Hoffmann, C.; Bittinger, K.; Chen, Y.-Y.; Keilbaugh, S.A.; Bewtra, M.; Knights, D.; Walters, W.A.; Knight, R.; et al. Linking long-term dietary patterns with gut microbial enterotypes. *Science* **2011**, *334*, 105–108. [CrossRef] [PubMed]
29. David, L.A.; Maurice, C.F.; Carmody, R.N.; Gootenberg, D.B.; Button, J.E.; Wolfe, B.E.; Ling, A.V.; Devlin, A.S.; Varma, Y.; Fischbach, M.A.; et al. Diet rapidly and reproducibly alters the human gut microbiome. *Nature* **2014**, *505*, 559–563. [CrossRef] [PubMed]
30. Arrieta, M.C.; Stiemsma, L.T.; Amenyogbe, N.; Brown, E.M.; Finlay, B. The intestinal microbiome in early life: Health and disease. *Front. Immunol.* **2014**, *5*, 427. [CrossRef] [PubMed]
31. Azad, M.B.; Konya, T.; Persaud, R.R.; Guttman, D.S.; Chari, R.S.; Field, C.J.; Sears, M.R.; Mandhane, P.J.; Turvey, S.E.; Subbarao, P.; et al. Impact of maternal intrapartum antibiotics, method of birth and breastfeeding on gut microbiota during the first year of life: A prospective cohort study. *BJOG* **2016**, *123*, 983–993. [CrossRef] [PubMed]
32. Jakobsson, H.E.; Abrahamsson, T.R.; Jenmalm, M.C.; Harris, K.; Quince, C.; Jernberg, C.; Björkstén, B.; Engstrand, L.; Andersson, A.F. Decreased gut microbiota diversity, delayed Bacteroidetes colonisation and reduced Th1 responses in infants delivered by caesarean section. *Gut* **2014**, *63*, 559–566. [CrossRef] [PubMed]
33. Arboleya, S.; Sanchez, B.; Milani, C.; Duranti, S.; Solís, G.; Fernández, N.; de los Reyes-Gavilán, C.; Ventura, M.; Margolles, A.; Gueimonde, M. Intestinal microbiota development in preterm neonates and effect of perinatal antibiotics. *J. Pediatr.* **2015**, *166*, 538–544. [CrossRef] [PubMed]
34. Rajilic-Stojanovic, M.; Biagi, E.; Heilig, H.G.; Kajander, K.; Kekkonen, R.A.; Tims, S.; de Vos, W.M. Global and deep molecular analysis of microbiota signatures in fecal samples from patients with irritable bowel syndrome. *Gastroenterology* **2011**, *141*, 1792–1801. [CrossRef] [PubMed]
35. Caubet, J.C.; Nowak-Wegrzyn, A. Current understanding of the immune mechanisms of food protein-induced enterocolitis syndrome. *Expert Rev. Clin. Immunol.* **2011**, *7*, 317–327. [CrossRef] [PubMed]
36. Karlsson, M.R.; Rugtveit, J.; Brandtzaeg, P. Allergen-responsive CD4+CD25+ regulatory T cells in children who have outgrown cow's milk allergy. *J. Exp. Med.* **2004**, *199*, 1679–1688. [CrossRef] [PubMed]
37. Chung, H.L.; Hwang, J.B.; Park, J.J.; Kim, S.G. Expression of transforming growth factor beta1, transforming growth factor type I and II receptors, and TNF-alpha in the mucosa of the small intestine in infants with food protein-induced enterocolitis syndrome. *J. Allergy Clin. Immunol.* **2002**, *109*, 150–154. [CrossRef] [PubMed]

38. Furusawa, Y.; Obata, Y.; Fukuda, S.; Endo, T.A.; Nakato, G.; Takahashi, D.; Nakanishi, Y.; Uetake, C.; Kato, K.; Kato, T.; et al. Commensal microbe-derived butyrate induces the differentiation of colonic regulatory T cells. *Nature* **2013**, *504*, 446–450. [CrossRef] [PubMed]
39. Paparo, L.; di Costanzo, M.; di Scala, C.; Cosenza, L.; Leone, L.; Nocerino, R.; Canani, R.B. The influence of early life nutrition on epigenetic regulatory mechanisms of the immune system. *Nutrients* **2014**, *6*, 4706–4719. [CrossRef] [PubMed]
40. Olafsdottir, E.; Aksnes, L.; Fluge, G.; Berstad, A. Faecal calprotectin levels in infants with infantile colic, healthy infants, children with inflammatory bowel disease, children with recurrent abdominal pain and healthy children. *Acta Paediatr.* **2002**, *91*, 45–50. [CrossRef] [PubMed]
41. Beser, O.F.; Sancak, S.; Erkan, T.; Kutlu, T.; Çokuğraş, H.; Çokuğraş, F.Ç. Can fecal calprotectin level be used as a markers of inflammation in the diagnosis and follow-up of cow's milk protein allergy? *Allergy Asthma Immunol. Res.* **2014**, *6*, 33–38. [CrossRef] [PubMed]
42. Vandenplas, Y.; De Greef, E.; Hauser, B. Paradice Study Group. Safety and tolerance of a new extensively hydrolyzed rice protein-based formula in the management of infants with cow's milk protein allergy. *Eur. J. Pediatr.* **2014**, *173*, 1209–1216. [CrossRef] [PubMed]
43. Reche, M.; Pascual, C.; Fiandor, A.; Polanco, I.; Rivero-Urgell, M.; Chifre, R.; Johnston, S.; Martín-Esteban, M. The effect of a partially hydrolysed formula based on rice protein in the treatment of infants with cow's milk protein allergy. *Pediatr. Allergy Immunol.* **2010**, *21*, 577–585. [CrossRef] [PubMed]
44. Terracciano, L.; Bouygue, G.R.; Sarratud, T.; Veglia, F.; Martelli, A.; Fiocchi, A. Impact of dietary regimen on the duration of cow's milk allergy: A random allocation study. *Clin. Exp. Allergy* **2010**, *40*, 637–642. [CrossRef] [PubMed]

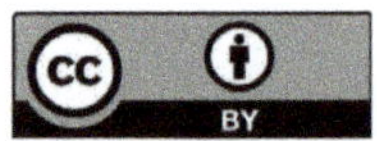

© 2018 by the authors. Licensee MDPI, Basel, Switzerland. This article is an open access article distributed under the terms and conditions of the Creative Commons Attribution (CC BY) license (http://creativecommons.org/licenses/by/4.0/).

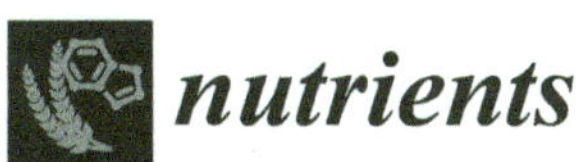

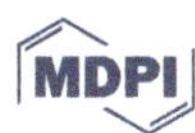

Review

Microbial and Nutritional Programming—The Importance of the Microbiome and Early Exposure to Potential Food Allergens in the Development of Allergies

Bożena Cukrowska

Immunology Laboratory, Department of Pathology, The Children's Memorial Health Institute, Aleja Dzieci Polskich 20, 04-730 Warsaw, Poland; b.cukrowska@ipczd.pl; Tel. +48-22-815-10-91

Received: 30 September 2018; Accepted: 16 October 2018; Published: 18 October 2018

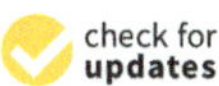

Abstract: The "microbiota hypothesis" ties the increase in allergy rates observed in highly developed countries over the last decades to disturbances in the gut microbiota. Gut microbiota formation depends on a number of factors and occurs over approximately 1000 days of life, including the prenatal period. During this period the microbiota helps establish the functional immune phenotype, including immune tolerance. The development of immune tolerance depends also on early exposure to potential food allergens, a process referred to as nutritional programming. This article elaborates on the concepts of microbial and nutritional programming and their role in the primary prevention of allergy.

Keywords: microbiome; intestinal microbiota; microbial programming; nutritional programming; allergy; prevention

1. Introduction

Allergies are one of the key medical problems in highly developed countries, where the proportion of those affected exceeds 30% and continues to grow [1]. The observed increase in allergy rates is associated with the type of lifestyle and involves excessive cleanliness and antibiotic use, small families, increased Cesarean section (CS) rates, altered dietary habits (increased use of processed foods, ready meals), rapid urbanization, and increasingly limited contact with nature [2,3]. These factors immensely affect the composition of the gut microbiota, which is currently believed to be essential for immune system functioning and the development of immune tolerance. The gut microbiota establishes itself over approximately 1000 initial days of life. During this time, the microbiota programs the baby's immature immune system [4]. Another key factor determining the composition of gut microbiota is nutrition. The baby's diet affects the composition of microbiota (e.g., in the breastfed infants, predominantly bifidobacteria occur) and is a source of exposure to potential allergens. Studies show that the diet of both the mother (during pregnancy and lactation) and the baby influence the development of allergies later in life [5].

This article presents the role of the gut microbiota and controlled exposure to food allergens in allergy development as well as the possible preventive measures intended to stem the rise in allergy rates.

2. Gut Microbiota and Allergic Conditions

The gut microbiota is a complex of microorganisms colonizing the mucous membranes (mainly the intestinal mucosa) and constitutes an integral part of the human body. The number of bacteria colonizing the gastrointestinal tract (10^{14} cells) is comparable to that of all the cells in the body and, as demonstrated by recent calculations, exceeds the number of nucleated human cells 10-fold [6]. However, the microbiome (all the genetic material within the microbiota, i.e., the microbiota genome) is over a hundred-fold bigger than that of the human genome [7]. Modern molecular methods show the intestinal microbiome to be very diverse and individually specific [8,9]. In addition, the composition of the intestinal microbiome undergoes short- and long-term changes throughout life, which are induced by numerous factors such as diet, antibiotic therapy, stress, infections etc. However, the largest modifications of the microbiome, which seem to be permanent, occur during the period of intestinal biocenosis formation [9]. Studies by Lozupone et al. comparing the microbiomes of the citizens of the Republic of Malawi and the United States showed considerable differences in microbiota composition between developing and highly developed countries [10]. By comparing the microbiome of Malavians (Malawi-born individuals who emigrated to the US) and citizens of United States, the study demonstrated that the "Westernized" diet had limited effects on the microbiome established in early childhood. This confirms the theory that the window of opportunity for changing the intestinal microbiome extends over no more than the first two years of a child's life and any microbiome disturbances (dysbiosis) occurring in this period may result in an abnormal immune system activation and development of pathological conditions such as allergy [3,4].

Studies show that the microbiota in children with allergies are less diversified, with the observed bacterial colonization (predominantly with *Bacteoidetes*, and *Bifidobacterium* and *Lactobacillus* species) reportedly delayed and less numerous in this age group [11,12]. One important fact in microbial programming is that the differences in microbiota composition between children with allergies and healthy children occur during early infancy, even before the first signs of allergy. Assessing 3-week-old neonates who developed allergic symptoms during their first year of life, Kalliomaki et al. demonstrated an increased number of *Clostridium* species, with a concurrent decrease in *Bifidobacterium* genera, compared with healthy children [13]. Moreover, a reduced biodiversity of gut-colonizing bacteria at the age of 1 year was associated with increased allergy rates at age 6 years and the development of asthma at age 7 years [14,15]. Furthermore, a reduced colonization with *Bifidobacterium* and *Lactobacillus* species at the age of 1–2 months induced the development of allergy by the age of 5 years [16].

3. The Impact of Gut Microbiota on Immune System Development

Despite developed lymphatic organs, the immune system of neonates is immature. Neonatal lymphocytes are referred to as naïve, i.e., never before exposed to external antigens [17]. Gut-colonizing bacteria are among the first antigens to activate the body's defense mechanisms, and help seal the intestinal barrier, establish immune tolerance, and modify the body's response to potential allergens [18]. The gut microbiota forms the first line of defense against pathogens, activates the synthesis of secretory immunoglobulins A (IgA), and increases the expression of the proteins (e.g., zonulin, occludin) that form intraepithelial junctions.

Studies carried out on gnotobiotic experimental models demonstrated that in contrast to conventionally raised mice, germ-free (GF) mice have hypoplastic Peyer's patches and decreased number of both IgA-secreting plasma cells and lymphocytes located in the lamina propria [19,20]. Colonization of GF animals with components of the gut microbiota induced production of secretory IgA, which are natural antibodies reacting with a wide spectrum of microorganisms and food molecules including allergens. Recently, using transmission electron microscopy we have presented that the gut microbiota improves the immature intestinal epithelium of GF mice [20]. Brush borders of GF-mouse enterocytes were irregularly arranged with decreased numbers of cytoskeletal microfilaments and a lack of elongation into the terminal web. Colonization of GF mice with *Lactobacillus* species obtained from the stool of healthy infants significantly improved this condition. In addition, the adherens junctions of *Lactobacillus* colonized mice were significantly elongated and narrow compared with those in the GF mice and resembled those found in mice colonized with physiological microbiota.

This fortification of the intestinal barrier was further evident from the increased levels of the zonulin and occludin proteins in *Lactobacillus*-colonized animals [20].

Gut-colonizing bacteria, which react with Toll-like receptors located on the intestinal epithelium and dendritic cells, stimulate also signaling pathways that activate a number of immune effector cells, such as macrophages, B cells, NK cells, helper T cells (Th1 and Th2), cytotoxic T cells, and regulatory T (Treg) cells [18]. Treg cells regulate the immune response and are characterized by a specific cytokine profile. They produce interleukin (IL)-10 and transforming growth factor (TGF)-beta 1. Treg cells are responsible for maintaining Th1/Th2 cytokine equilibrium and the development of immune tolerance [21]. Our results obtained in gnotobiotic animals showed that stimulation of the immune system by defined components of the intestinal microbiota in early ontogeny is followed by the induction of regulatory mechanisms that maintain the stability of both the local mucosal and systemic immunity [19,20]. This is especially important during the infancy period, as the T cell cytokine profile during early life is pro-allergenic (Th2-like), while Th1 capacity to produce cytokines (IL-12, IFN-gamma) is impaired during this period [17].

4. Factors Affecting Gut Microbiota Formation

Despite reports demonstrating the presence of bacteria in the amniotic fluid and placenta, which could indicate the formation of the gut microbiota already in the prenatal period [22,23], in 2017 a study contradicting this theory was published [24]. The assertion that the fetal gastrointestinal tract is sterile and the first gut-colonizing bacteria appear during delivery is believed to be true, and the delivery is the time when the newborn is in direct contact with the microorganisms of the mother or environment [24]. However, the child's intestinal ecosystem may be affected by the mother's microbiota as early as during the prenatal period, e.g., via low-molecular-weight metabolites, such as butyric acid. During the prenatal period, butyric acid can induce colonocyte proliferation and growth as well as activate adhesion receptors (on the intestinal epithelium) for the bacteria constituting the newborn's microbiome [25].

In newborns 98% of intestinal bacteria belong to one of these four phyla: *Firmicutes*, *Bacteroidetes*, *Proteobacteria*, and *Actinobacteria* [9]. From the second week of life, the gastrointestinal tracts of breastfed infants contain predominantly bifidobacteria. As the child develops and solids are introduced into its diet, the microbiota composition becomes more diversified [26]. At the age of approximately 2 years, the gut microbiota stabilizes and the proportion of individual types of bacteria is similar to that observed in adults (i.e., predominantly *Bacteroidetes*). There are a number of factors that shape the infant gut microbiota: the mother's microbiome, gestational age, mode of delivery, hospital environment, diet (both of the mother and the child), hospitalization period, medication, e.g., antibiotics [26–28]. The optimal microbiota composition that may reduce the risk of developing an allergy is observed in infants whose mothers are healthy, did not take antibiotics during pregnancy or lactation, as well as infants who were delivered vaginally, breastfed, living in contact with nature, animals, peers, and siblings, with no antibiotics or excessively sanitized living conditions [27].

The 1000-day pre- and postnatal period of gut ecosystem formation marks the formation of the microbiome—a new organ, which programs mainly the function of the immature immune system but also metabolism and the gut–brain axis [29].

5. The Impact of the Mode of Delivery on the Gut Microbiome and Allergy Development

During vaginal delivery, the baby is in contact with the microbiota of the mother's gastrointestinal tract and birth canal and this microbiota is the main source of microorganisms colonizing the newborn [9]. During the first day of life, neonatal intestines are colonized predominantly by facultative anaerobic bacteria (*Escherichia coli* and enterococci), which proliferate in an oxygen-rich infant gut and prepare the conditions for further colonization with bacteria of the genera: *Bifidibacterium*, *Lactobacillus*, *Bacteroides*, and *Clostridium* [26]. One beneficial effect observed in vaginally delivered newborns is a decrease in the number of *Clostridium* bacteria in favor of *Bifidobacterium* bacteria as early as on day 3 of life [30]. Newborns delivered via a CS are deprived of any contact with the mother's intestinal microbiota, which results in dysbiosis (an imbalance in the composition of the gut microbiota) observed as early as in the first few hours after birth and over the next days. One-day-old CS-born neonates were shown to be colonized predominantly by the microorganisms colonizing the mother's skin [31]. These 1-day-old neonates had also a smaller number of *Escherichia coli* and *Bacteroides fragilis*, with higher rates of *Clostridium difficile* isolates and hospital-derived bacteria (including antibiotic-resistant strains) [30]. Despite being breastfed, 3-day-old CS-born neonates exhibited no bifidobacteria [31]. It seems that neonatal period dysbiosis observed after CS delivery may lead to disturbances in microbiotic homeostasis in the subsequent months and years of life. Children delivered via CS demonstrated microbiotic abnormalities such as reduced microbiotic biodiversity, delayed and reduced colonization with *Bacteroidetes* also at the age of 3, 6, 12, and even 24 months [32]. Our studies confirmed an absence of *Bacteroidetes* in the gut of preterm, CS-born neonates one week after birth, with this absence persisting for a period of at least 8 weeks independently on supplementation with *Saccharomyces boulardii* [33].

Disturbances of gut microbiota resulting from CS may affect the development of allergies in the future, which is suggested by epidemiological studies. These studies show that CS deliveries correlate with higher incidence of food allergy and asthma [34–37]. American cohort studies conducted in 136,098 children indicated that the risk of developing asthma by children aged 4.5–6 years was over seven-fold higher (odds ratio (OR) = 7.77, 95% confidence interval (CI): 6.25–9.65) in the presence of additional factors (besides CS), which negatively affect the gut microbiome. These additional factors included antibiotic therapy during pregnancy and infancy as well as a lack of siblings [38].

6. The Effect of Gut Microbiome and Breastfeeding on Allergy Development

Breast milk is the best food for infants, providing the child with all essential nutrients (except vitamins D and K), supporting the function of immature gastrointestinal and immune systems and optimally shaping the development of the gut microbiota [39]. The gut of breastfed infants is colonized predominantly by bifidobacteria [26]. The microbiota of formula-fed children is more diversified and includes *Enterobacteriaceae*, *Enterococcus* species, and *Bacteroides* species [9,26].

The most important component of breast milk (absent from cow's milk) responsible for the formation of the microbiome are human milk oligosaccharides (HMOs) [40]. There are more than 200 currently known HMOs (resistant to digestive enzymes) which become a selective medium for *Bifidobacteria*, inducing their proliferation in the gut, increasing short-chain fatty acid (e.g., butyric acid) levels, and lowering stool pH. HMOs can also bind to specific intestinal epithelial receptors, which prevents the adhesion of pathogenic bacteria.

Recent studies demonstrated that apart from natural prebiotics (HMOs), breast milk also contains live probiotic bacteria from the genera *Lactobacillus* and *Bifidobacterium* [41,42]. The most commonly isolated *Bifidobacterium* species found in breast milk was *Bifidobacterium breve*, and the most commonly isolated *Lactobacilli* were *Lactobacillus salivarius* and *Lactobacillus fermentum*. Therefore, breast milk is a natural synbiotic containing both probiotics and prebiotics. However, not all mothers' breastmilk contains probiotic bacteria. The breastmilk of over 50% of women yields no bifidobacterial isolates; moreover, the breastmilk of approximately 30% of women contains no *Lactobacillus* species. The microbiotic profile of breastmilk depends on a number of factors, including the composition of the woman's gut and skin microbiota, the woman's health, medication (mainly antibiotics), and the type of delivery [43–45]. Antibiotic therapy during pregnancy and lactation dramatically lowers the number of *Lactobacillum* and *Bifidobacterium* genera in breastmilk [43]. The breastmilk of women who delivered via CS contains a lower number of bifidobacteria compared with that of women after a vaginal delivery [44]. The breastmilk of obese mothers was shown to contain a lower number of bifidobacteria and higher number of *Staphylococcus* species as well as to exhibit an altered immunomodulatory capacity, which was associated with lowered levels of such immunostimulating factors as TGF-beta2 and soluble CD14 [45].

Despite the observed differences in the composition of breast milk, studies demonstrate that breast-feeding has a beneficial effect on the occurrence of many diseases associated with the improper functioning of the immune system. Reduced immunity, immaturity of the intestinal barrier and intestinal dysbiosis is primarily associated with premature births. Thus, preterm infants are particularly vulnerable to severe infections such as necrotizing enterocolitis and sepsis. It is now believed that mother's milk is the optimal diet for such newborns. Human milk has been shown to reduce morbidity and mortality in preterm newborns [46] and protects against necrotizing enterocolitis in early life [47].

In studies on the impact of breast feeding on occurrence of allergies exclusive breastfeeding for 3 months was proven to reduce the risk of atopic dermatitis in genetically predisposed children as well as in those without genetic predisposition [48]. The CHILD (Canadian Healthy Infant Longitudinal Development Birth Cohort) study involving 3296 children showed that, compared with exclusive breastfeeding for the first three months, other diets (such as formula feeding (OR = 2.14; 95% CI 1.37–3.35) or mixed feeding (OR = 1.73; 95% CI 1.17–2.57)) increase the risk of developing asthma at the age of 3 years [49]. Moreover, studies by Chu et al. indicated that breastfeeding for the first 6 months may lower the elevated risk of asthma in children born via CS [50].

7. Infant Formulas Supplemented with Prebiotics and Probiotics in Allergy Prevention

Formula-fed or mixed-fed children are more prone to developing allergy. Infant formulas are based on cow's milk, whose composition is fundamentally different from that of human breast milk. This is why, manufacturers supplement infant formulas with bioactive ingredients present in human breast milk, including substances directly affecting the baby's microbiome, such as oligosaccharides with prebiotic properties or probiotic bacteria derived from human breast milk (e.g., *Bifidobacterium breve*). There are also synbiotic formulas containing both oligosaccharides and probiotic bacteria.

The most thoroughly studied oligosaccharides are a mixture of short-chain galacto-oligosaccharides (scGOS) and long-chain fructo-oligosaccharides (lcFOS) in a 9:1 ratio, at a dose of 8 g per liter. It was demonstrated that supplementation of infant formulas with a scGOS/lcFOS mixture shifts the microbiotic profile in formula-fed infants towards the profile observed in breastfed infants [51,52]. Consequently, these infants were shown to bear an increased number of bacteria from the genera *Bifidobacterium* and *Lactobacillus*. In addition, formula supplementation with scGOS/lcFOS helped resolve post-antibiotic-therapy dysbiosis, lowered stool pH (the pH reached the values similar to those observed in breastfed infants), and made the short-chain fatty acid profile similar to that present in breastfed infants. The use of a synbiotic formula supplemented with scGOS/lcFOS and the probiotic bacteria *Bifidobacterium breve* M-16V in infants born via CS induced elimination of dysbiosis by increasing the number of bifidobacteria [53]. In older, healthy children aged 1–3 years, a 3-month-long diet of synbiotic formula also resulted in an increase in bacteria of the genus *Bifidobacterium* [54].

Moro et al. are the authors of the first randomized placebo-controlled clinical study on the use of scGOS/lcFOS-supplemented infant formulas conducted in infants at risk of developing allergy [55]. The study group was fed with a partially hydrolyzed whey formula supplemented with scGOS/lcFOS at 8 g/L for 6 months. After this period, the risk of developing atopic dermatitis was halved in the group fed a scGOS/lcFOS-supplemented formula. This beneficial effect persisted for at least 2 years. A 2-year-long prospective study by Arslanoglu et al. demonstrated that feeding infants formulas containing extensively hydrolyzed whey and supplemented with scGOS/lcFOS for 6 months not only lowers the rates of atopic dermatitis, but also significantly reduces the number of children with wheezing and urticaria in comparison with those rates in the group receiving formula without prebiotic supplementation [56]. A 5-year follow-up confirmed persistent, long-term benefits of the evaluated dietary intervention [57].

In 2016, World Allergy Organization (WAO) experts issued their guidelines on the use of prebiotics in allergy prevention [58]. These guidelines suggest that all formula-fed infants should receive formulas supplemented with prebiotics. This WAO guideline was based on an analysis of 18 randomized placebo-controlled trials, which demonstrated that supplementing the diet of healthy formula-fed infants with prebiotics during the first year of life lowers the risk of asthma and recurrent wheezing (relative risk (RR): 0.37; 95% CI 0.17–0.80) as well as the risk of food allergy (RR 0.28; 95% CI 0.08–1.00). The published guidelines emphasized that there is no need to provide prebiotic supplementation either to breastfed infants or to lactating mothers.

One year earlier, by analyzing randomized placebo-controlled studies, WAO experts issued a statement suggesting the potential use of probiotics in primary prevention of allergy in high-risk families (in pregnant women, breastfeeding women, and infants) [59]. A 2013 meta-analysis of 25 randomized placebo-controlled clinical studies involving 4031 children showed probiotics administered both pre- and postnatally to be the most effective [60]. Probiotic supplementation was demonstrated to reduce total IgE levels over a long-term (at least 2-year) follow-up and to lower the risk of allergy, but they had no effect on reducing the incidence of asthma. The WAO guideline does not recommend specific strains for primary prevention of allergy. The authors emphasize that the recommendations are conditional and depend on the results of the further research. Recently, Szajewska and Horvath published a meta-analysis of randomized double blind placebo controlled studies, which presented that pre- and/or postnatal supplementation with *Lactobacillus rhamnosus* GG strain does not affect the occurrence of atopic dermatitis, and this strain should not be recommended in allergy prevention [61]. However, it is necessary to remember that probiotic effects are both strain- and population-specific. Thus, the clinical efficacy may be dependent on the strain, but also on a mode of birth (CS or vaginal delivery) or geographical place of birth (northern or southern countries), and these determinants were not taken into account in the meta-analysis. On the other hand, it should be emphasized that the *Lactobacillus rhamnosus* GG strain does not originate from breast milk, only from the intestine. How much it can affect the specific action of probiotics we do not know, and further research is necessary.

8. The Effect of Nutritional Programming on Allergy Development

A baby's diet affects the development of allergies by acting at least bi-directionally (Figure 1). On the one hand food influences the composition of the gut microbiota influencing the development and functioning of the immune system. On the other hand an induction of immune tolerance can be achieved by direct exposure to potential allergens during pregnancy, lactation, and weaning. The contact of the immune system with small doses of allergens activates the formation of Treg lymphocytes [21]. The 20th century was an era of eliminating potential allergens from the diet of both the mother (during pregnancy and lactation) and child (late—often over the age of 1 year—introduction of allergenic foods). The advent of the 21st century completely altered our attitudes toward exposure to potential allergens. The PASTURE study (Protection against Allergy: Study in Rural Environments) of 2014 demonstrated that the less varied the diet during the first year, the higher the risk of developing food allergy at the age of 4, 5, and 6 years [62]. This study also showed a significant reduction of 26% for the development of asthma, with each additional food item introduced in the first year of life. Likewise, a study called LEAP (Learning Early about Peanut Allergy) demonstrated that introducing a potential allergen (in this case: peanuts) at small doses into the diet early (at the age of 4–6 months) reduced the incidence of allergy to this allergen by 80% [63]. Recent studies confirmed that allergen introduction reduced peanut allergy incidence most effectively when peanuts were introduced into the mother's diet during pregnancy and lactation and then into the infant's diet [64]. Thus, dietary interventions during gestation and lactation period include a balanced diet without elimination of potential allergens (Table 1). In the postnatal period breastfeeding for a minimum of 4–6 months, the introduction of solid foods according to the recent recommendation of the European Society for Paediatric Gastroenterology Hepatology and Nutrition from week 17 and no later than at week 26 including potential allergens may also have a positive impact on allergy development [65].

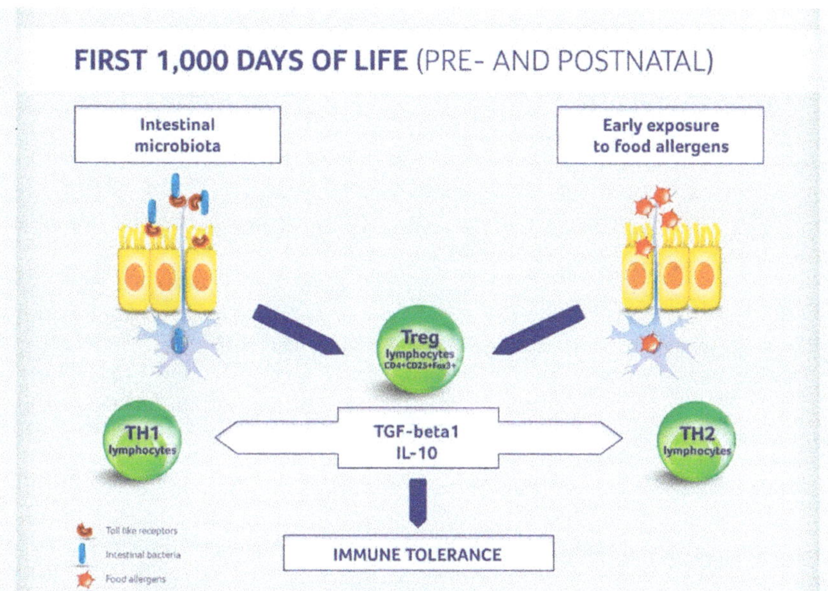

Figure 1. Immune tolerance development in children. Regulatory (Treg) T lymphocytes are activated by the gut microbiota and contact with potential food allergens.

Table 1. Dietary intervention in pre- and postnatal period which could play role in induction of immune tolerance.

Prenatal Period	Postnatal Period
• Balanced and varied diet • No elimination of potential allergens • The use of probiotics may be considered in families at risk of allergy	• Breastfeeding for a minimum 4–6 months • Introduction of solid foods starting from week 17; no later than at week 26 • No elimination of potential allergens • Formulas supplemented with prebiotic oligosaccharides may be considered in formula-fed and non-exclusively fed infants • Partially hydrolyzed formulas, optionally supplemented with prebiotics and/or probiotics may be considered in formula-fed and non-exclusively fed infants in families at risk of allergy

The development of cow's milk (CM) allergy in formula-fed infants may depend on the degree of CM protein hydrolysis [66,67]. Formulas with extensively hydrolyzed proteins and amino acid-based elemental formulas are not intended for healthy infants. Instead, they are for infants with symptomatic allergy to CM proteins. In contrast, partially hydrolyzed formulas (pHF), also called hypoallergenic formulas, which contain partially broken down proteins are especially recommended for children from families at risk of allergy (i.e., when the parents and/or siblings have allergies). It seems that partially hydrolyzed CM proteins can be more effective in induction of specific Treg cells. Gouw et al. identified specific peptides with tolerogenic potential in a whey-based pHF [68]. They presented that partial hydrolysis induced the occurrence of peptides overlapping the specific regions of beta-lactoglobulin, which were found to contain T-cell epitopes with tolerogenic potential. In experimental mice studies partially hydrolyzed whey proteins increased the percentage of Treg cells in the mesenteric lymph nodes leading to a significantly reduced acute allergic skin response to whey [69]. Also, in a clinical trial performed by Boyle et al. the effect of whey-based pHF on Treg cells was investigated. In this randomized, placebo-controlled study after 6 months of intervention, increased percentages of $CD4^{+}CD25^{high}Foxp3^{high}$ Treg lymphocytes were detected in infants who received pHF compared to the ones who received a standard infant formula. In spite of positive effects on T reg cells, pHF did not prevent eczema in the first year in high-risk infants [70]. In contrast, an update meta-analysis performed by Szajewska and Horvath in 2017 showed that 100% whey-based pHF (manufactured by a single manufacturer), given to infants at risk of allergy development decreased the occurrence of eczema, and reduced the risk of eczema and all allergic diseases among children at high risk of allergy at different time points [66]. Although the certainty of the evidence is low, as the authors underline, such intervention could have beneficial effects in primary prevention of allergies. In a review article by Vandeplas, it is suggested that pHF may be used for all infants, irrespective of family history of allergy [67]; however, at this time, there are no studies confirming the effectiveness of such action.

9. Conclusions and Recommendations

Current preventive measures intended to stem the development of allergies focus on inducing immune tolerance via microbial and nutritional programing. Primary prevention of allergies is focused on dietary intervention during both pre- and postnatal periods, and includes a balanced diet without elimination of potential allergens in pregnant and lactating mothers as well as promoting breast feeding for a minimum of 4–6 months, with early introduction of solid foods in the infant diet. To prevent dysbiosis in infants, CS should be only performed when medically indicated, and antibiotic therapy should be limited in both pregnant/lactating women and in infants. In formula- or non-exclusively fed infants, the introduction of synbiotic formulas or those supplemented with prebiotic oligosaccharides can have positive effects on allergy development; however, additional research in this field would be still needed.

Funding: The study was support by the grant of the Children's Memorial Health Institute S156/2017 and S163/2018.

Conflicts of Interest: B.C. has served as a speaker for Nutritia, Mead Johnson, Bayer, Apotex, and Polpharma.

Abbreviations

CI	Confidence interval
CM	Cow milk
CS	Cesarean section
GF	Germ-free
HMOs	Human milk oligosaccharides
IgA (E)	immunoglobulins A (E)
IL	interleukin
lcFOS	long chain fructo-oligosaccharides
OR	Odds ratio
pHF	partially hydrolyzed formula
RR	Relative risk
scGOS	short chain galacto-oligosaccharides
TGF	transforming growth factor
Th	T helper
Treg	regulatory T cells
WAO	World Allergy Organization

References

1. Von Mutius, E. The Rising Trends in Asthma and Allergic Diseases. *Clin. Exp. Allergy* **1998**, *28* (Suppl. 5), 45–49. [CrossRef] [PubMed]
2. Holt, P.G.; Inouye, M.; Logan, A.C.; Prescott, S.L.; Sly, P.D. An Exposome Perspective: Early-Life Events and Immune Development in a Changing World. *J. Allergy Clin. Immunol.* **2017**, *140*, 24–40. [CrossRef]
3. Shreiner, A.; Huffnagle, G.B.; Noverr, M.C. The "Microflora Hypothesis" of Allergic Diseases. *Adv. Exp. Med. Biol.* **2008**, *635*, 113–134. [CrossRef] [PubMed]

4. Wopereis, H.; Oozeer, R.; Knipping, K.; Belzer, C.; Knol, J. The First Thousand Days—Intestinal Microbiology of Early Life: Establishing a Symbiosis. *Pediatr. Allergy Immunol.* **2014**, *25*, 428–438. [CrossRef] [PubMed]
5. Greer, F.R.; Sicherer, S.H.; Burks, A.W. Effects of Early Nutrition Interventions on the Development of Atopic Disease in Infants and Children: The Role of Maternal Dietary Restriction, Breastfeeding, Timing of Introduction of Complementary Foods, and Hydrolyzed Formulas. *Pediatrics* **2008**, *121*, 183–191. [CrossRef] [PubMed]
6. Sender, R.; Fuchs, S.; Milo, R. Revised Estimates for the Number of Human and Bacteria Cells in the Body. *PLoS Biol.* **2016**, *14*, e1002533. [CrossRef] [PubMed]
7. Human Microbiome Project Consortium, Structure, Function and Diversity of the Healthy Human Microbiome. *Nature* **2012**, *486*, 207–214. [CrossRef] [PubMed]
8. Eckburg, P.B.; Bik, E.M.; Bernstein, C.N.; Purdom, E.; Dethlefsen, L.; Sargent, M.; Gill, S.R.; Relman, D.A. Diversity of the Human Intestinal Microbial Flora. *Science* **2005**, *308*, 11635–11638. [CrossRef] [PubMed]
9. Collado, M.C.; Cernada, M.; Baüerl, C.; Vento, M.; Pérez-Martínez, G. Microbial Ecology and Host-Microbiota Interactions During Early Life Stages. *Gut Microbes* **2012**, *3*, 352–365. [CrossRef] [PubMed]
10. Lozupone, C.A.; Stombaugh, J.I.; Gordon, J.I.; Jansson, J.K.; Knight, R. Diversity, Stability and Resilience of the Human Gut Microbiota. *Nature* **2012**, *489*, 220. [CrossRef] [PubMed]
11. Björksten, B.; Naaber, P.; Sepp, E.; Mikelsaar, M. The Intestinal Microflora in Allergic Estonian and Swedish 2-year-old Children. *Clin. Exp. Allergy* **1999**, *29*, 342–346. [CrossRef] [PubMed]
12. Abrahamsson, T.R.; Jakobsson, H.E.; Andersson, A.F.; Björkstén, B.; Engstrand, L.; Jenmalm, M.C. Low Diversity of the Gut Microbiota in Infants with Atopic Eczema. *J. Allergy Clin. Immunol.* **2012**, *129*, 434–440. [CrossRef] [PubMed]
13. Kalliomäki, M.; Kirjavainen, P.; Kero, P.; Salminen, S.; Isolauri, E. Distinct Patterns of Neonatal Gut Microflora in Infants in Whom Atopy Was Not Developing. *J. Allergy Clin. Immunol.* **2001**, *107*, 129–134. [CrossRef] [PubMed]
14. Bisgaard, H.; Li, N.; Bonnelykke, K.; Chawes, B.L.; Skov, T.; Paudan-Müller, G.; Stokholm, J.; Smith, B.; Krogfelt, K.A. Reduced Diversity of the Intestinal Microbiota During Infancy Is Associated With Increased Risk of Allergic Disease at School Age. *J. Allergy Clin. Immunol.* **2011**, *128*, 646–652. [CrossRef] [PubMed]
15. Abrahamsson, T.R.; Jakobsson, H.E.; Andersson, A.F.; Björkstén, B.; Engstrand, L.; Jenmalm, M.C. Low Gut Microbiota Diversity in Early Infancy Precedes Asthma at School Age. *Clin. Exp. Allergy* **2014**, *44*, 842–850. [CrossRef] [PubMed]
16. Sjögren, Y.M.; Jenmalm, M.C.; Böttcher, M.F.; Björkstén, B.; Sverremark-Ekström, E. Altered Early Infant Gut Microbiota in Children Developing Allergy up to 5 Years of Age. *Clin. Exp. Allergy* **2009**, *39*, 518–526. [CrossRef]
17. Brugman, S.; Perdijk, O.; van Neerven, R.J.; Savelkoul, H.F. Mucosal Immune Development in Early Life: Setting the Stage. *Arch. Immunol. Ther. Exp.* **2015**, *63*, 251–268. [CrossRef] [PubMed]
18. Tlaskalová-Hogenová, H.; Stepánková, R.; Hudcovic, T.; Tucková, L.; Cukrowska, B.; Lodinová-Zádníková, R.; Kozáková, H.; Rossmann, P.; Bártová, J.; Sokol, D.; et al. Commensal Bacteria (Normal Microflora), Mucosal Immunity and Chronic Inflammatory and Autoimmune Diseases. *Immunol. Lett.* **2004**, *93*, 97–108. [CrossRef] [PubMed]
19. Cukrowska, B.; Kozakova, H.; Rehakova, Z.; Sinkora, J.; Tlaskalova-Hogenova, H. Specific Antibody and Immunoglobulin Responses after Intestinal Colonization of Germ-Free Piglets with Non-Pathogenic Escherichia coli O86. *Immunobiology* **2001**, *204*, 425–433. [CrossRef] [PubMed]
20. Kozakova, H.; Schwarzer, M.; Tuckova, L.; Srutkova, D.; Czarnowska, E.; Rosiak, I.; Hudcovic, T.; Schabussova, I.; Hermanova, P.; Zakostelska, Z.; et al. Colonization of Germ-Free Mice with a Mixture of Three Lactobacillus Strains Enhances the Integrity of Gut Mucosa and Ameliorates Allergic Sensitization. *Cell. Mol. Immunol.* **2016**, *13*, 251–262. [CrossRef] [PubMed]
21. Akdis, C.A.; Akdis, M. Mechanisms of Immune Tolerance to Allergens: Role of IL-10 and Tregs. *J. Clin. Investig.* **2014**, *124*, 4678–4680. [CrossRef] [PubMed]
22. Aagaard, K.; Ma, J.; Antony, K.M.; Ganu, R.; Petrosino, J.; Versalovic, J. The Placenta Harbors a Unique Microbiome. *Sci. Transl. Med.* **2014**, *6*, 237ra65. [CrossRef] [PubMed]
23. Collado, M.C.; Rautava, S.; Aakko, J.; Isolauri, E.; Salminen, S. Human Gut Colonisation May be Initiated in Utero by Distinct Microbial Communities in the Placenta and Amniotic Fluid. *Sci. Rep.* **2016**, *22*, 23129. [CrossRef] [PubMed]

24. Perez-Muñoz, M.E.; Arrieta, M.C.; Ramer-Tait, A.E.; Walter, J. A Critical Assessment of the "Sterile Womb" and "in Utero Colonization" Hypotheses: Implications for Research on the Pioneer Infant Microbiome. *Microbiome* **2017**, *28*, 48. [CrossRef] [PubMed]
25. Tan, J.; McKenzie, C.; Potamitis, M.; Thorburn, A.N.; Mackay, C.R.; Macia, L. The Role of Short-Chain Fatty Acids in Health and Disease. *Adv. Immunol.* **2014**, *121*, 91–119. [CrossRef] [PubMed]
26. Penders, J.; Thijs, C.; Vink, C.; Stelma, F.F.; Snijders, B.; Kummeling, I.; van den Brandt, P.A.; Stobberingh, E.E. Factors Influencing the Composition of the Intestinal Microbiota in Early Infancy. *Pediatrics* **2006**, *118*, 511–521. [CrossRef] [PubMed]
27. Prescott, S.L.; Larcombe, D.L.; Logan, A.C.; West, C.; Burks, W.; Caraballo, L.; Levin, M.; Etten, E.V.; Horwitz, P.; Kozyrskyj, A.; et al. The Skin Microbiome: Impact of Modern Environments on Skin Ecology, barrier Integrity, and Systemic Immune Programming. *World Allergy Organ. J.* **2017**, *10*, 29. [CrossRef] [PubMed]
28. Martin, R.; Makino, H.; Cetinyurek Yavuz, A.; Ben-Amor, K.; Roelofs, M.; Ishikawa, E.; Kubota, H.; Swinkels, S.; Sakai, T.; Oishi, K.; et al. Early-Life Events, Including Mode of Delivery and Type of feeding, Siblings and Gender, Shape the Developing Gut Microbiota. *PLoS ONE* **2016**, *11*, e0158498. [CrossRef] [PubMed]
29. Holzer, P.; Farzi, A. Neuropeptides and the Microbiota-Gut-Brain Axis. *Adv. Exp. Med. Biol.* **2014**, *817*, 195–219. [CrossRef] [PubMed]
30. Dominguez-Bello, M.G.; Costello, E.K.; Contreras, M.; Magris, M.; Hidalgo, G.; Fierer, N.; Knight, R. Delivery Mode Shapes the Acquisition and Structure of the Initial Microbiota Across Multiple Body Habitats in Newborns. *Proc. Natl. Acad. Sci. USA* **2010**, *107*, 11971–11975. [CrossRef] [PubMed]
31. Biasucci, G.; Benenati, B.; Morelli, L.; Bessi, E.; Boehm, G. Cesarean Delivery May Affect the Early Biodiversity of Intestinal Bacteria. *J. Nutr.* **2008**, *138*, 1796S–1800S. [CrossRef] [PubMed]
32. Jakobsson, H.E.; Abrahamsson, T.R.; Jenmalm, M.C.; Harris, K.; Quince, C.; Jernberg, C.; Björkstén, B.; Engstrand, L.; Andersson, A.F. Decreased Gut Microbiota Diversity, Delayed Bacteroidetes Colonisation and Reduced Th1 Responses in Infants Delivered by Caesarean Section. *Gut* **2014**, *63*, 559–566. [CrossRef] [PubMed]
33. Zeber-Lubecka, N.; Kulecka, M.; Ambrozkiewicz, F.; Paziewska, A.; Lechowicz, M.; Konopka, E.; Majewska, U.; Borszewska-Kornacka, M.; Mikula, M.; Cukrowska, B.; et al. Effect of Saccharomyces boulardii and Mode of Delivery on the Early Development of the Gut Microbial Community in Preterm Infants. *PLoS ONE* **2016**, *11*, e0150306. [CrossRef] [PubMed]
34. Papathoma, E.; Triga, M.; Fouzas, S.; Dimitriou, G. Cesarean Section Delivery and Development of Food Allergy and Atopic Dermatitis in Early Childhood. *Pediatr. Allergy Immunol.* **2016**, *27*, 419–424. [CrossRef] [PubMed]
35. Magnus, M.C.; Håberg, S.E.; Stigum, H.; Nafstad, P.; London, S.J.; Vangen, S.; Nystad, W. Delivery by Cesarean Section and Early Childhood Respiratory Symptoms and Disorders the Norwegian Mother and Child Cohort Study. *Am. J. Epidemiol.* **2011**, *174*, 1275–1285. [CrossRef] [PubMed]
36. Guibas, G.V.; Moschonis, G.; Xepapadaki, P.; Roumpedaki, E.; Androutsos, O.; Manios, Y.; Papadopoulos, N.G. Conception via in vitro Fertilization and Delivery by Caesarean Section Are Associated with Paediatric Asthma Incidence. *Clin. Exp. Allergy* **2013**, *43*, 1058–1066. [CrossRef] [PubMed]
37. Tollånes, M.C.; Moster, D.; Daltveit, A.K.; Irgens, L.M. Cesarean Section and Risk of Severe Childhood Asthma: A Population-Based Cohort Study. *J. Pediatrics* **2008**, *153*, 112–116. [CrossRef] [PubMed]
38. Wu, P.; Feldman, A.S.; Rosas-Salazar, C.; James, K.; Escobar, G.; Gebretsadik, T.; Li, S.X.; Carroll, K.N.; Walsh, E.; Mitchel, E.; et al. Relative Importance and Additive Effects of Maternal and Infant Risk Factors on Childhood Asthma. *PLoS ONE* **2016**, *11*, e0151705. [CrossRef] [PubMed]
39. Musilova, S.; Rada, V.; Vlkova, E.; Bunesova, V. Beneficial Effects of Human Milk Oligosaccharides on Gut Microbiota. *Benef. Microbes* **2014**, *5*, 273–283. [CrossRef] [PubMed]
40. Chen, X. Human Milk Oligosaccharides (HMOS): Structure, Function, and Enzyme-Catalyzed Synthesis. *Adv. Carbohydr. Chem. Biochem.* **2015**, *72*, 113–190. [CrossRef] [PubMed]
41. Fernández, L.; Langa, S.; Martín, V.; Jiménez, E.; Martín, R.; Rodríguez, J.M. The Microbiota of Human Milk in Healthy Women. *Cell. Mol. Biol.* **2013**, *59*, 31–42. [PubMed]

42. Martín, R.; Jiménez, E.; Heilig, H.; Fernández, L.; Marín, M.L.; Zoetendal, E.G.; Rodríguez, J.M. Isolation of Bifidobacteria from Breast Milk and Assessment of the Bifidobacterial Population by PCR-Denaturing Gradient Gel Electrophoresis and Quantitative Real-Time PCR. *Appl. Environ. Microbiol.* **2009**, *75*, 965–969. [CrossRef] [PubMed]
43. Soto, A.; Martín, V.; Jiménez, E.; Mader, I.; Rodríguez, J.M.; Fernández, L. Lactobacilli and Bifidobacteria in Human Breast Milk: Influence of Antibiotherapy and Other Host and Clinical factors. *J. Pediatr. Gastroenterol. Nutr.* **2014**, *59*, 78–88. [CrossRef] [PubMed]
44. Khodayar-Pardo, P.; Mira-Pascual, L.; Collado, M.C.; Martínez-Costa, C. Impact of Lactation Stage, Gestational age and Mode of Delivery on Breast Milk Microbiota. *J. Perinatol.* **2014**, *34*, 599–605. [CrossRef] [PubMed]
45. Collado, M.C.; Laitinen, K.; Salminen, S.; Isolauri, E. Maternal Weight and Excessive Weight Gain During Pregnancy Modify the Immunomodulatory Potential of Breast Milk. *Pediatr. Res.* **2012**, *72*, 77–85. [CrossRef] [PubMed]
46. Abrams, S.A.; Schanler, R.J.; Lee, M.L.; Rechtman, D.J. Greater Mortality and Morbidity in Extremely Preterm Infants Fed a Diet Containing Cow Milk Protein Products. *Breastfeed. Med.* **2014**, *9*, 281–285. [CrossRef] [PubMed]
47. Quigley, M.; McGuire, W. Formula versus Donor Breast Milk for Feeding Preterm or Low Birth Weight Infants. *Cochrane Database Syst. Rev.* **2018**, *20*, CD002971. [CrossRef] [PubMed]
48. Kramer, M.S. Breastfeeding and Allergy: The Evidence. *Ann. Nutr. Metab.* **2011**, *59* (Suppl. 1), 20–26. [CrossRef] [PubMed]
49. Klopp, A.; Vehling, L.; Becker, A.B.; Subbarao, P.; Mandhane, P.J.; Turvey, S.E.; Lefebvre, D.L.; Sears, M.R.; CHILD Study Investigators; Azad, M.B. Modes of Infant Feeding and the Risk of Childhood Asthma: A Prospective Birth Cohort Study. *J. Pediatr.* **2017**, *190*, 192–199. [CrossRef] [PubMed]
50. Chu, S.; Chen, Q.; Chen, Y.; Bao, Y.; Wu, M.; Zhang, J. Cesarean Section Without Medical Indication and Risk of Childhood Asthma, and Attenuation by Breastfeeding. *PLoS ONE* **2017**, *18*, e0184920. [CrossRef] [PubMed]
51. Moro, G.E.; Mosca, F.; Miniello, V.; Fanaro, S.; Jelinek, J.; Stahl, B.; Boehm, G. Effects of a New Mixture of Prebiotics on Faecal Flora and Stools in Term Infants. *Acta Paediatr.* **2003**, *91*, 77–79. [CrossRef]
52. Knol, J.; Scholtens, P.; Kafka, C.; Steenbakkers, J.; Gro, S.; Helm, K.; Klarczyk, M.; Schöpfer, H.; Böckler, H.M.; Wells, J. Colon Microflora in Infants Fed Formula with Galacto- and Fructo-Oligosaccharides: More Like Breast-Fed Infants. *J. Pediatr. Gastroenterol. Nutr.* **2005**, *40*, 36–42. [CrossRef] [PubMed]
53. Chua, M.C.; Ben-Amor, K.; Lay, C.; Neo, A.G.E.; Chiang, W.C.; Rao, R.; Chew, C.; Chaithongwongwatthana, S.; Khemapech, N.; Knol, J.; et al. Effect of Synbiotic on the Gut Microbiota of Cesarean Delivered Infants: A Randomized, Double-Blind, Multicenter Study. *J. Pediatr. Gastroenterol. Nutr.* **2017**, *65*, 102–106. [CrossRef] [PubMed]
54. Kosuwon, P.; Lao-Araya, M.; Uthaisangsook, S.; Lay, C.; Bindels, J.; Knol, J.; Chatchatee, P. A Synbiotic Mixture of scGOS/lcFOS and Bifidobacterium breve M-16V Increases Faecal Bifidobacterium in Healthy Young Children. *Benef. Microbes* **2018**, *9*, 541–552. [CrossRef] [PubMed]
55. Moro, G.; Arslanoglu, S.; Stahl, B.; Jelinek, J.; Wahn, U.; Boehm, G. A Mixture of Prebiotic Oligosaccharides Reduces the Incidence of Atopic Dermatitis During the First Six Months of Age. *Arch. Dis. Child.* **2006**, *91*, 814–819. [CrossRef] [PubMed]
56. Arslanoglu, S.; Moro, G.E.; Schmitt, J.; Tandoi, L.; Rizzardi, S.; Boehm, G. Early Dietary Intervention with a Mixture of Prebiotic Oligosaccharides Reduces the Incidence of Allergic Manifestations and Infections During the First Two Years of Life. *J. Nutr.* **2008**, *138*, 1091–1095. [CrossRef] [PubMed]
57. Arslanoglu, S.; Moro, G.E.; Boehm, G.; Wienz, F.; Stahl, B.; Bertino, E. Early Neutral Prebiotic Oligosaccharide Supplementation Reduces the Incidence of Some Allergic Manifestations in the First 5 Years of Life. *J. Biol. Regul. Homeost. Agents* **2012**, *26* (Suppl. 3), 49–59. [PubMed]
58. Cuello-Garcia, C.A.; Fiocchi, A.; Pawankar, R.; Yepes-Nuñez, J.J.; Morgano, G.P.; Zhang, Y.; Ahn, K.; Al-Hammadi, S.; Agarwal, A.; Gandhi, S.; et al. World Allergy Organization-McMaster University Guidelines for Allergic Disease Prevention (GLAD-P.): Prebiotics. *World Allergy Organ J.* **2016**, *9*, 10. [CrossRef] [PubMed]
59. Fiocchi, A.; Pawankar, R.; Cuello-Garcia, C.; Ahn, K.; Al-Hammadi, S.; Agarwal, A.; Beyer, K.; Burks, W.; Canonica, G.W.; Ebisawa, M.; et al. World Allergy Organization-McMaster University Guidelines for Allergic Disease Prevention (GLAD-P.): Probiotics. *World Allergy Organ J.* **2015**, *27*, 4. [CrossRef] [PubMed]

60. Elazab, N.; Mendy, A.; Gasana, J.; Vieira, E.R.; Quizon, A.; Forno, E. Probiotic Administration in Early Life, Atopy, and Asthma: A Meta-analysis of Clinical Trials. *Pediatrics* **2013**, *132*, e666–e676. [CrossRef] [PubMed]
61. Szajewska, H.; Horvath, A. Lactobacillus rhamnosus GG in the Primary Prevention of Eczema in Children: A Systematic Review and Meta-Analysis. *Nutrients* **2018**, *10*. [CrossRef] [PubMed]
62. Roduit, C.; Frei, R.; Depner, M.; Schaub, B.; Loss, G.; Genuneit, J.; Pfefferle, P.; Hyvärinen, A.; Karvonen, A.M.; Riedler, J.; et al. Increased Food Diversity in the First Year of Life is Inversely Associated with Allergic Diseases. *J. Allergy Clin. Immunol.* **2014**, *133*, 1056–1064. [CrossRef] [PubMed]
63. Du Toit, G.; Roberts, G.; Sayre, P.H.; Bahnson, H.T.; Radulovic, S.; Santos, A.F.; Brough, H.A.; Phippard, D.; Basting, M.; Feeney, M.; et al. Randomized Trial of Peanut Consumption in Infants at Risk for Peanut Allergy. *N. Engl. J. Med.* **2015**, *372*, 803–813. [CrossRef] [PubMed]
64. Pitt, T.J.; Becker, A.B.; Chan-Yeung, M.; Chan, E.S.; Watson, W.T.A.; Chooniedass, R.; Azad, M.B. Reduced Risk of Peanut Sensitization Following Exposure through Breast-Feeding and Early Peanut Introduction. *J. Allergy Clin. Immunol.* **2018**, *141*, 620–625. [CrossRef] [PubMed]
65. Fewtrell, M.; Bronsky, J.; Campoy, C.; Domellöf, M.; Embleton, N.; Fidler Mis, N.; Hojsak, I.; Hulst, J.M.; Indrio, F.; Lapillonne, A.; Molgaard, C. Complementary Feeding: A Position Paper by the European Society for Paediatric Gastroenterology, Hepatology, and Nutrition (ESPGHAN) Committee on Nutrition. *J. Pediatr. Gastroenterol. Nutr.* **2017**, *64*, 119–132. [CrossRef] [PubMed]
66. Szajewska, H.; Horvath, A. A Partially Hydrolyzed 100% Whey Formula and the Risk of Eczema and Any Allergy: An Updated Meta-analysis. *World Allergy Organ J.* **2017**, *10*, 27. [CrossRef] [PubMed]
67. Vandenplas, Y. Prevention and Management of Cow's Milk Allergy in Non-Exclusively Breastfed Infants. *Nutrients* **2017**, *9*, 731. [CrossRef] [PubMed]
68. Gouw, J.W.; Jo, J.; Meulenbroek, L.A.P.M.; Heijjer, S.; Kremer, E.; Sandalova, E.; Knulst, A.C.; Jeurink, P.; Garssen, J.; Rijnierse, A.; Knippels, L.M.J. Identification of Peptides with Tolerogenic Potential in a Hydrolyzed Whey-Based Infant Formula. *Clin. Exp. Allergy* **2018**. [CrossRef] [PubMed]
69. Van Esch, B.C.; Schouten, B.; de Kivit, S.; Hofman, G.A.; Knippels, L.M.; Willemsen, L.E.; Garssen, J. Oral Tolerance Induction by Partially Hydrolyzed Whey Protein in Mice is Associated with Enhanced Numbers of Foxp3+ Regulatory T-Cells in the Mesenteric Lymph Nodes. *Pediatr. Allergy Immunol.* **2011**, *22*, 820–826. [CrossRef] [PubMed]
70. Boyle, R.J.; Tang, M.L.; Chiang, W.C.; Chua, M.C.; Ismail, I.; Nauta, A.; Hourihane, J.O.B.; Smith, P.; Gold, M.; Ziegler, J.; et al. Prebiotic-Supplemented Partially Hydrolysed Cow's Milk Formula for the Prevention of Eczema in High-Risk Infants: A Randomized Controlled Trial. *Allergy* **2016**, *71*, 701–710. [CrossRef] [PubMed]

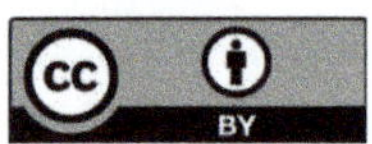

© 2018 by the author. Licensee MDPI, Basel, Switzerland. This article is an open access article distributed under the terms and conditions of the Creative Commons Attribution (CC BY) license (http://creativecommons.org/licenses/by/4.0/).

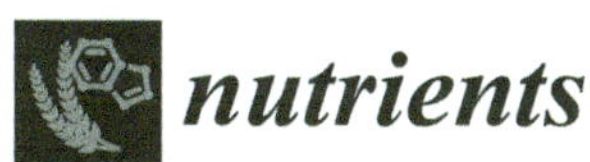

MDPI

Article

Low Diversity of Human Milk Oligosaccharides is Associated with Necrotising Enterocolitis in Extremely Low Birth Weight Infants

Erik Wejryd [1], Magalí Martí [1], Giovanna Marchini [2,3], Anna Werme [1], Baldvin Jonsson [2,3], Eva Landberg [1,4] and Thomas R. Abrahamsson [1,5,*]

1 Department of Clinical and Experimental Medicine, Linköping University, 58183 Linköping, Sweden; erik.wejryd@liu.se (E.W.); magali.marti.genero@liu.se (M.M.); anna.werme@gmail.com (A.W.); eva.landberg@regionostergotland.se (E.L.)
2 Department of Neonatology, Karolinska University Hospital, 17176 Stockholm, Sweden; giovanna.marchini@sll.se (G.M.); baldvin.jonsson@sll.se (B.J.)
3 Department of Women´s and Children´s Health, Karolinska Insitute, 17177 Stockholm, Sweden
4 Department of Clinical Chemistry, Linköping University, 58185 Linköping, Sweden
5 Department of Pediatrics, Linköping University, 58183 Linköping, Sweden
* Correspondence: thomas.abrahamsson@liu.se; Tel.: +46-010-103-0000

Received: 25 September 2018; Accepted: 12 October 2018; Published: 20 October 2018

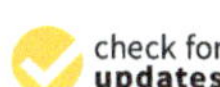

Abstract: Difference in human milk oligosaccharides (HMO) composition in breast milk may be one explanation why some preterm infants develop necrotizing enterocolitis (NEC) despite being fed exclusively with breast milk. The aim of this study was to measure the concentration of 15 dominant HMOs in breast milk during the neonatal period and investigate how their levels correlated to NEC, sepsis, and growth in extremely low birth weight (ELBW; <1000 g) infants who were exclusively fed with breast milk. Milk was collected from 91 mothers to 106 infants at 14 and 28 days and at postmenstrual week 36. The HMOs were analysed with high-performance anion-exchange chromatography with pulsed amperometric detection. The HMOs diversity and the levels of Lacto-N-difucohexaose I were lower in samples from mothers to NEC cases, as compared to non-NEC cases at all sampling time points. Lacto-N-difucohexaose I is only produced by secretor and Lewis positive mothers. There were also significant but inconsistent associations between 3′-sialyllactose and 6′-sialyllactose and culture-proven sepsis and significant, but weak correlations between several HMOs and growth rate. Our results suggest that the variation in HMO composition in breast milk may be an important factor explaining why exclusively breast milk fed ELBW infants develop NEC.

Keywords: neonatal; preterm; breast milk; oligosaccharides; diversity; necrotizing enterocolitis; sepsis; growth

1. Introduction

While the care of premature infants has improved dramatically during the last decades, still about 30% of the extremely low birth weight (ELBW, birth weight < 1000 g) infants die [1]. Severe infections and necrotizing enterocolitis (NEC) are common causes of death in this population, and there are clear links between nutrition and the risk of NEC, infection, and mortality [2]. Definite NEC (Bell's stage II-III [3]) remains among the most devastating diseases encountered in premature infants. It is associated with an excessive inflammatory process in the intestinal mucosa that presents clinically with feeding intolerance, abdominal distension, and bloody stools [4]. The incidence among ELBW infants is approximately 10% [5], but varies in different neonatal settings between 4 to 15% depending on factors such as breastfeeding rates and use of milk banks [6]. The surgical intervention rate is as high as 50% [4], and the mortality rate in affected infants is 15–30%. It is increasingly recognized that NEC is a major adverse factor for subsequent lower intelligence quotient (IQ), motor impairment, visual impairment, and cerebral palsy [7]. Finding new measures to identify and treat infants at-risk is urgently needed.

Exclusive enteral feeding with human breast milk remains the most important prevention strategy for NEC [2]. However, in Scandinavian countries, despite exclusive feeding with breast milk being employed routinely for at least 20 years, the incidence of NEC in ELBW infants is still as high as 10% according to the most recent data available in the Swedish Neonatal Quality Register (www.snq.se). Breast milk not only provides the necessary nutrients for growth and development, it also contains numerous immunological components that compensate the immature and inexperienced mucosal immune system [8]. Such components include immune cells, IGA antibodies, and pro and anti-inflammatory cytokines such as TNF and IL-10 [8,9].

Difference in the composition of bioactive components in breast milk may explain why some preterm infants still develop NEC despite being fed exclusively with breast milk. Among these, non-digestible human milk oligosaccharides (HMOs) are highly abundant (5–15 g/L) as constituents. Besides stimulating beneficial microbes, such as bifidobacteria, in the infant intestinal tract [10], HMOs mimic carbohydrate-binding motifs of certain enteric pathogens, such as enteropathogenic *E. coli*, by acting as a receptor decoy, and thereby prevent adhesion of these pathogens to the apical surface of enterocytes [11]. Certain HMOs also stimulate anti-inflammatory responses in the intestinal epithelium [12,13]. A growing body of evidence suggests that the HMO composition in breast milk influences the risk of developing NEC in preterm infants [14–16]. Supplementation with the HMOs disialyllacto-N-tetraose (DSLNT) [14] and 2′-fucosyllactose (2FL) were identified to be protective against NEC in an experimental murine model. Low DSLNT levels preceded NEC development in very low birth weight preterm infants (VLBW; <1500 g) in a human trial [16]. Interestingly, there was a high variation of DSLNT in different countries in a world-wide study in which Swedish mothers had the lowest levels [17]. HMO levels have also been associated with growth [18] and the risk of infections in infants [19,20].

The aim of this study was to investigate the composition of 15 dominant HMOs in breast milk during the neonatal period and examine how this correlated to NEC, sepsis, and growth in ELBW infants who were exclusively fed with breast milk. The analyses revealed low HMO diversity and low levels of the HMO Lacto-N-difucohexaose (LNDH I) in infants that developed NEC.

2. Materials and Methods

2.1. Study Design and Participants

The present study was a part of the prospective, randomized-controlled, multi-centre trial "Prophylactic Probiotics to Extremely Low Birth Weight Premature Infants" (PROPEL) evaluating the effect of probiotic *Lactobacillus reuteri* DSM 17938 on feeding tolerance, growth, severe morbidities, and mortality in ELBW premature infants (ClinicalTrials.gov ID NCT01603368). A detailed study design and the clinical outcomes have been published elsewhere [21]. Briefly, in total 134 infants born between gestational week (gw) 23 + 0 and 27 + 6 with a birth weight below 1000 g were enrolled between 2012 and 2015 at two level III neonatal intensive care units (Astrid Lindgren Children's Hospital, Stockholm, and Linköping University Hospital, Linköping, Sweden). Exclusion criteria were major congenital or chromosomal anomalies, no realistic hope of survival, the infant could not be fed and thus not receive the study product within three days, or the infant was included in another intervention trial on growth, feeding intolerance, or severe morbidity. Participating infants received daily oral administration of 1.25×10^8 *L. reuteri* DSM 17938 or placebo from birth to postmenstrual week 36 + 0. Written informed consent was obtained from both parents and the study was approved by the Ethics Committee for Human Research at Linköping University (Dnr 2012/28-31, Dnr 2012/433-32).

Due to the 100% coverage of breast milk donor banks, all infants were fed exclusively with breast milk until they had reached a weight of at least 2000 g. Protein and lipid fortification was based individually on analyses of the macronutrient and energy content of the breast milk given to each infant. Oral feeding started during the first day of life and increased gradually at a rate specified in clinical guidelines. Breast milk fortification with bovine protein fortifier started when the enteral feeds had reached 100 mL/kg/day. Breast milk samples were collected from 91 mothers to 106 infants at 14 (n = 78) and 28 (n = 71) days after delivery and at postmenstrual week (PMW) 36 + 0 (n = 51). The milk was frozen in sterile tubes at −20 °C (short-term) and subsequently at −70 °C. The median time until the analysed breast milk was given to the infant was five days (inter-quartile range [IQR] 1–7). Samples were only obtained if the infant was exclusively fed mother´s own milk. All infants to mothers from whom samples were available were included in the present study. Mother´s own milk was not pasteurised before feeding at the neonatal intensive care units (NICUs) at the time of the trial. Analytic staff was blinded to the clinical metadata until the laboratory analyses were concluded.

2.2. Clinical Outcomes

The infants were characterized using comprehensive clinical data including perinatal data, growth, antibiotics, and mild to severe morbidities collected daily in a study specific case report form until gestational week 36 + 0. Necrotizing enterocolitis (NEC) was staged according to Bell's criteria [3], and all cases of stage II or greater were recorded. A diagnosis of culture-proven sepsis required a positive blood culture, clinical deterioration, and a laboratory inflammatory response. Weight, length and head circumference were recorded at birth, at 14 and 28 days, and at PMW 36 + 0. In order to adjust for gestational age, the standard deviation score (z-score) for each measurement was calculated using Niklasson's growth chart, which is based on information of normal deliveries from gestational week 24 to full term in the Swedish medical birth registry, 1990–1999 [22]. The growth rate was calculated using the difference in z-score between the later measurements and birth.

2.3. Purification of Human Milk Oligosaccharides

HMOs were purified from each milk sample by the following method. To remove lipids, 1 mL of the milk sample was centrifuged at 20,000 g for 30 min. Thereafter, 0.5 mL of the infranatant fluid was transferred to another tube and 50 µL of the internal standard was added. The internal standard consisted of 2.4 mg/mL galacturonic acid (Sigma-Aldrich, St Louis, MO, USA) and 12 mg/mL stachyose (Sigma-Aldrich). To precipitate proteins, 1 mL of refrigerated 99.5 % ethanol was added, and the mixture was kept at 4 °C for one hour and subsequently centrifuged at 20,000 g for 10 min at 4 °C. The sample was further purified by applying 1 mL of the supernatant fluid to an Isolute C18 column (Biotage, Uppsala, Sweden), preconditioned with 2 mL of ethanol followed by 2 mL of water. The eluate was collected and then ultra-filtrated using Amicon Ultra-4 (Merck Millipore, Cork, Ireland) with a 3 kDa molecular cut off. The tube was centrifuged at 4000 g for 40 min and the filtered sample was collected. To remove ethanol, the filtrate was evaporated with compressed air for one hour at 40 °C. Neutral oligosaccharides were further purified by applying 50 µL of the sample to an anion exchange bonded silica cartridge (LC-SAX, Supelco, Bellefonte, PA, USA), preconditioned according to instructions. Thereafter, 500 µL of Milli-Q water was added to the column and the eluate was collected.

2.4. Analysis of Human Milk Oligosaccharides

High-performance anion-exchange chromatography (HPAEC) with pulsed amperometric detection (PAD) was used to separate and quantify the major 15 oligosaccharides in human milk (Table 1). The analysis was based on previous published methods [23–25], but adopted to the following system to achieve optimal separation of the measured oligosaccharides.

Table 1. Median human milk oligosaccharides (HMO) levels (μmol/L) in breast milk from mothers to extremely low birth weight (ELBW) infants during the neonatal period.

Name	Type	Secreted by	Day 14 $n = 78$ Median (IQR)	Day 28 $n = 71$ Median (IQR)	36th PMW $N = 56$ Median (IQR)
3′-sialyllactose (3SL)	Sialylated	All	328 (255–395)	292 (226–336)	207 (161–280)
6′-sialyllactose (6SL)	Sialylated	All	1197 (935–1587)	821 (602–1019)	291 (191–488)
Sialyl-lacto-N-tetraose a (LSTa)	Sialylated	All	9 (5–14)	4 (3–8)	3 (2–5)
Sialyl-lacto-N-tetraose b (LSTb)	Sialylated	All	69 (42–127)	102 (45–142)	75 (33–108)
Sialyl-lacto-N-neotetraosec (LSTc)	Sialylated	All	130 (86–197)	79 (48–107)	20 (12–34)
Disialyl-lacto-N-tetraose (DSLNT)	Sialylated	All	657 (475–1049)	669 (394–910)	389 (206–516)
2′-fucosyllactose (2FL)	Neutral	Se+	5390 (0–7383)	4720 (0–7072)	4379 (1964–5840)
3′-fucosyllactose (3FL)	Neutral	All	1241 (569–2005)	1486 (795–2680)	1803 (1061–3003)
Lacto-difucotetraose (LDFT)	Neutral	Se+	394 (0–685)	388 (0–717)	466 (38–645)
Lacto-N-tetraose (LNT)	Neutral	All	2294 (1708–3138)	2205 (1640–2897)	1529 (1112–2189)
Lacto-N-neotetraose (LNnT)	Neutral	All	180 (96–263)	151 (86–220)	155 (90–271)
Lacto-N-fucopentaose I (LNFP I)	Neutral	Se+	1163 (0–1852)	819 (0–1714)	536 (95–1126)
Lacto-N-fucopentaose II (LNFP II)	Neutral	Le+	401 (147–948)	384 (152–826)	324 (177–685)
Lacto-N-fucopentaose III (LNFP III)	Neutral	All	362 (261–496)	402 (301–503)	423 (320–518)
Lacto-N-difucohexaose I (LNDH I)	Neutral	Se+ Le+	652 (0–1176)	726 (0–1173)	454 (0–968)
Σ analyzed HMO			15770 (12694–17393)	14992 (12803–17655)	11676 (10157–13703)

PMW = Postmenstrual week. IQR = Interquartile range. HMO = human milk oligosaccharides.

The high-performance anion-exchange chromatography with pulsed amperometric detection (HPAEC-PAD) system ICS-3000 (Dionex, Sunnyvale, CA, USA) was equipped with a thermostated CarboPac PA-200 column (3 × 50 mm guard column and 3 × 250 mm analytical column), an electrochemical Au detector and an Ag/AgCl reference electrode. The flow rate was 0.5 mL/min and the injection volume 20 μL. Separation was achieved using different gradient programs. For neutral oligosaccharides a constant concentration of 20 mM NaOH and a gradient with sodium acetate (NaOAc) from 0 to 25 mM at 5 to 30 min (30 °C) or 6 to 37 min (25 °C) were used. For acidic (sialylated) oligosaccharides a constant concentration of 0.1 M NaOH and a two-step gradient of NaOAc from 20 mM to 80 mM at 5 to 30 min and from 80 mM to 150 mM at 30 to 40 min were used. HPAEC was performed at both 30 and 40 °C for acidic oligosaccharides, to achieve optimal separation [26]. The different HMOs were identified by comparing their retention times to those of known milk oligosaccharide standards that were analysed in each run. All oligosaccharide standards were from Dextra Laboratories (Reading, UK), except for DSLNT, 3SL and 6SL, which were from Sigma-Aldrich. The oligosaccharide concentrations were calculated from the individual HMOs peak areas in relation to the area of the internal standard (galacturonic acid for acidic and stachyose for neutral oligosaccharides). The results were further corrected for the response factor of each individual oligosaccharide, as determined by the analysis of standards with known concentrations.

2.5. Statistical Analyses

The primary outcome and other continuous variables with skewed distributions were analysed with Mann-Whitney U test, while *t*-test for independent samples were employed for continuous variables with normal distributions. Fisher's exact test was used for categorical outcome variables. Baseline characteristics were summarized by means and standard deviations (SDs) for continuous data and counts and percentages for categorical data. Primary and secondary outcome variables were summarized by means and SD or medians with IQR for continuous data and counts and percentages for categorical data. The analysis of similarity (ANOSIM) was applied to test if HMOs composition was more similar within the same mother over time than between mothers [27]. ANOSIM provides an R-value where R close to 1 indicates dissimilarity and R close to 0 indicates even distribution (of high and low ranks) within and between groups. As a complement to ANOSIM, permutation analysis of variance (PERMANOVA) was also applied to test if HMO composition differed among the mothers and over time. The distribution of HMOs composition across mothers and sampling times were observed by Non-metric Multi-dimensional Scaling (NMDS) plots. NMDS maps the pair-wise (dis)similarity of ranked distances to a k-dimensional ordination space, where the distance between objects corresponds to their (dis)similarity [28]. The statistical discrimination was at a significance level of 0.05. No adjustments for multiple comparisons were made for those outcomes, for which there were separate hypotheses, such as NEC, sepsis, and growth rate parameters. All statistical analyses were performed using IBM SPSS Statistics software, version 25 (IBM Corp, Armonk, NY, USA), except for Shannon diversity index, ANOSIM, PERMANOVA, and NMDS that were performed in R version 3.3.0 [29].

3. Results

3.1. Description of the Study Population

Breast milk samples were collected from 91 mothers to 106 infants at 14 (78 mothers to 89 infants) and 28 (71 mothers to 83 infants) days after delivery and at PMW 36 + 0 (56 mothers to 65 infants). Baseline characteristics of the ELBW infants are displayed in Table 2.

Table 2. Background characteristics in extremely low birth weight (ELBW) infants with and without necrotising enterocolitis (NEC) during the neonatal period.

	No NEC (n = 96)	NEC (n = 10)	p *
Gestational age, weeks + days, mean (SD)	25 + 4 (9 days)	25 + 1 (9 days)	0.3
Birth weight, g, mean (SD)	749 (136)	681 (123)	0.1
Birth weight zscore, mean (SD)	−1.1 (1.2)	−1.4 (1.6)	0.6
Birth length, cm, mean (SD)	32.7 (2.5)	32.0 (2.2)	0.4
Birth length z-score, mean (SD)	−1.5 (1.8)	−1.4 (2.0)	0.9
Birth head circumference, cm, mean (SD)	23.0 (1.5)	22.8 (1.2)	0.5
Birth head circumference z-score, mean (SD)	−0.8 (0.8)	−0.6 (0.7)	0.4
Small for gestational age, n (%)	22 (23)	2 (20)	0.8
Caesarean section, n (%)	62 (65)	6 (60)	0.8
Apgar score 5 min, mean (SD)	6.2 (2.6)	7.0 (2.4)	0.3
Apgar score 10 min, mean (SD)	7.8 (1.9)	8.4 (1.6)	0.3
Male, n (%)	49 (51)	9 (90)	<0.01
Infants from multiple pregnancy, n (%)	35 (36)	4 (40)	0.8
Maternal smoking, n (%)	2 (2)	1 (10)	0.5
Maternal preeclampsia, n (%)	10 (10)	1 (10)	1.0
Preterm premature rupture of membranes, n (%)	30 (30)	4 (40)	0.6
Maternal chorioamnionitis, n (%)	20 (21)	3 (30)	0.6
Maternal prepartal antibiotics, n (%)	51 (53)	5 (50)	0.9
Prenatal steroids, n (%)	94 (81)	10 (100)	0.2
Received surfactant, n (%)	78 (81)	9 (90)	0.4
Antibiotics during first week, n (%)	95 (99)	10 (100)	1.0
Antibiotics during second week, n (%)	76 (79)	10 (100)	0.2
Probiotic supplementation, n (%)	50 (52)	5 (50)	1.0
Patent ductus arteriosus treated, n (%)	70 (73)	7 (70)	1.0

* t-test for independent samples to compare means. Fisher's exact test to compare proportions.

3.2. Development of the HMOs Over Time

Concentrations of the 15 HMOs in breast milk samples from 14 and 28 days after delivery and at PMW 36 + 0 are displayed in Table 1. ANOSIM analyses including the 41 cases with samples from all three time points indicated a higher variability in HMOs composition between mothers (R-value = 0.04; $p = 0.01$) than within the same mother over time (R-value = 0.7; $p = 0.001$). The HMO composition was clearly separated by the secretor status (R-value = 0.9; $p = 0.001$), which was also revealed in the NMDS plot (Figure 1). The PERMANOVA analyses showed that the secretor status explained 63% ($p = 0.001$) of the variance in HMO composition, the mother explained 26% ($p = 0.001$) and sampling time point only 0.07% ($p = 0.001$). When adjusting for secretor status, the mother explained 70% ($p = 0.001$), while the sampling time point explained 17% ($p = 0.001$) of the variance for both, secretor-positive, and secretor-negative cases.

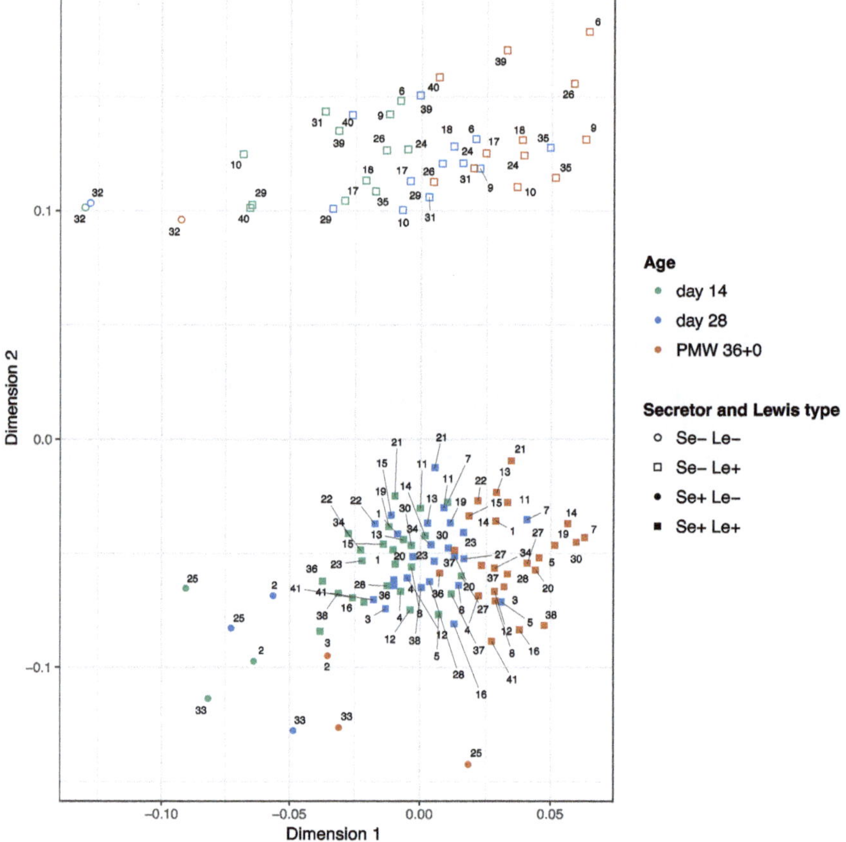

Figure 1. Non-metric multidemension scaling (NMDS) plot of the HMO composition among the 41 mothers with samples from all three time points. Each mother is indicated by a number from 1 to 41. PMW 36 + 0: postmenstrual week 36 + 0. Stress level: 0.08

3.3. Clinical Outcomes in Relation to the HMO Levels

The HMO composition at day 14 in each NEC case is shown in Figure 2, and the levels of the 15 HMOs in samples from mothers to infants who did and did not developed NEC and culture-proven sepsis, respectively, are displayed in Table 3 and 4 (day 14), S1 and S2 (day 28), and S3 and S4 (PMW 36 + 0). NEC development was associated with low levels of the neutral oligosaccharide LNDH

I at all three sampling time points. This HMO is only produced by mothers that are both secretor and Lewis-positive (Table 1). NEC development was also associated with low levels of LSTa and LNnT at 28 days. The diversity of all 15 HMOs was lower in all three samples from mothers to NEC cases as compared to non-NEC cases (Figure 3a), while there was no difference between NEC and non-NEC cases in the total content of HMO in the samples (Table 3, Tables S1 and S3). There was also a trend towards less NEC among infants to secretor and Lewis-positive mothers (Figure S1). The HMO diversity in NEC and non-NEC cases stratified by the different secretor groups is displayed in Figure S2. Male gender was significantly more common among the NEC-cases (Table 2), but there were no differences in HMO diversity in breast milk from mothers of singleton boys and girls ($p = 0.43$ at 14 days, $p = 0.76$ at 28 days, and $p = 0.84$ at postmenstrual week 36 + 0). The incidence of NEC was not associated with probiotic supplementation (Table 2).

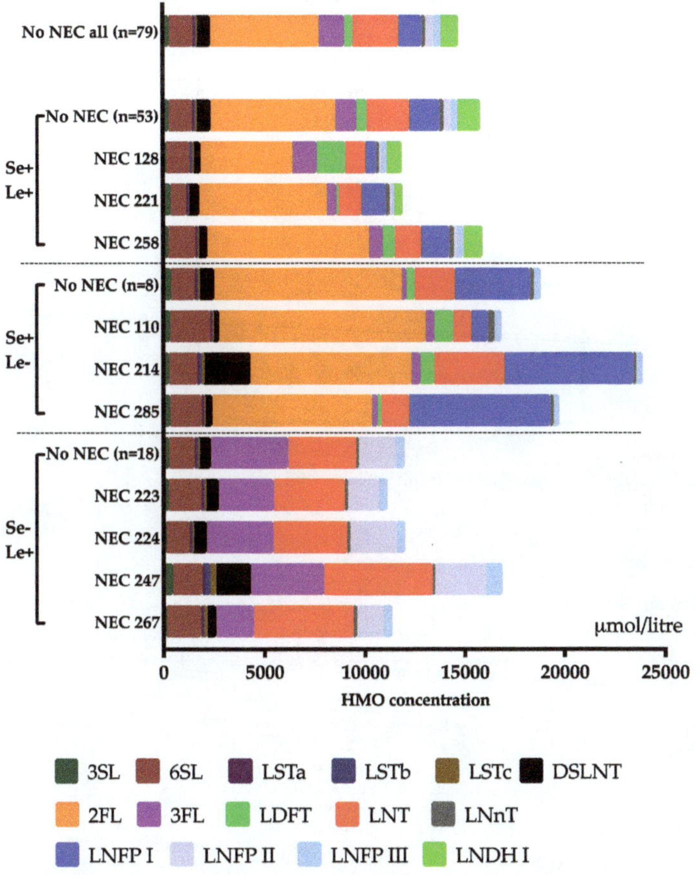

Figure 2. Human milk oligosaccharide (HMO) content in the first breast milk sample from mothers of all NEC-cases, stratified according to secretor (Se) and Lewis (Le) status, and median HMO levels in milk samples from day 14 from the non-NEC cases of the respective Se/Le groups

a) HMO diversity and NEC

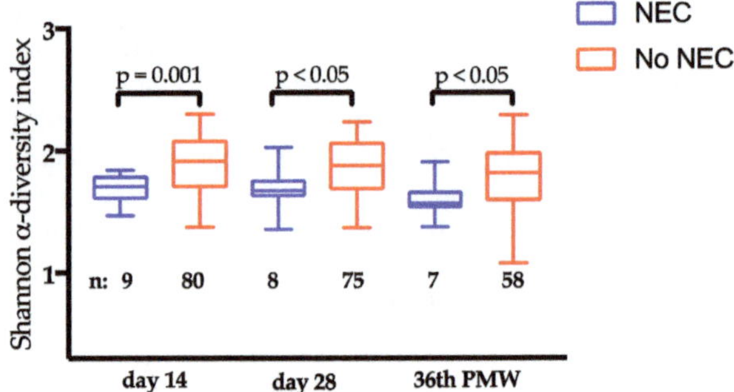

b) HMO diversity and culture proven sepsis

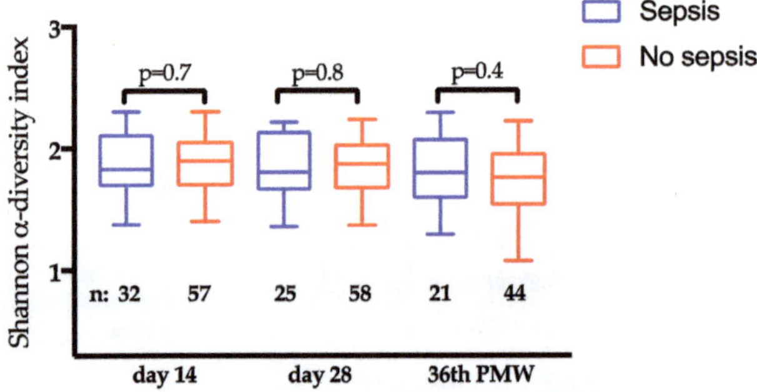

Figure 3. Human milk oligosaccharide (HMO) diversity in breast milk samples and the incidence of NEC (**a**) and culture proven sepsis (**b**). Boxes indicate 25th, 50th and 75th percentiles; whiskers indicate min and max values. *t*-test for independent samples was used to compare means. N indicates the number of patients in each group. PMW=postmenstrual week.

Table 3. Comparison of human milk oligosaccharide (HMO) concentrations (µmol/L) in milk samples from day 14 to infants who developed or did not develop necrotising enterocolitis (NEC).

	Secreted by	NEC (n = 9) Median (IQR)		No NEC (n = 80) Median (IQR)		p *
3SL	All	318	(231–376)	321	(254–395)	0.8
6SL	All	1437	(1220–1635)	1159	(919–1585)	0.2
LSTa	All	9	(7–17)	10	(5–14)	0.6
LSTb	All	49	(29–144)	68	(42–128)	0.4
LSTc	All	138	(103–196)	130	(85–198)	0.7
DSLNT	All	572	(401–1193)	674	(498–1038)	0.4
2FL	Se+	6331	(0–8026)	5390	(3374–7223)	0.9
3FL	All	675	(436–3004)	1255	(575–1841)	0.6
LDFT	Se+	45	(0–651)	410	(28–686)	0.2
LNT	All	3507	(1277–4320)	2294	(1710–2990)	0.7
LNnT	All	129	(90–208)	187	(111–273)	0.2
LNFP I	Se+	797	(0–3903)	1165	(441–1789)	0.5
LNFP II	Le+	124	(0–1996)	413	(191–880)	0.6
LNFP III	All	363	(332–437)	351	(267–526)	0.8
LNDH I	Se+ Le+	0	(0–213)	882	(0–1279)	<0.01
Σ analyzed HMO		15889	(11623–18311)	15770	(13405–17274)	0.8

* Mann Whitney *U*-test for independent samples used to compare distributions.

High levels of 6SL at 14 days (Table 4) and low levels of 3SL and at 28 days of life (Table S2) were significantly associated with the development of culture-proven sepsis, although HMO diversity was not (Figure 3b).

Table 4. Comparison of human milk oligosaccharide (HMO) concentrations (μmol/L) in milk samples from day 14 to infants who developed or did not develop culture-proven sepsis.

	Secretedby	Sepsis (n = 32) Median (IQR)		No Sepsis (n = 57) Median (IQR)		p *
3-SL	All	283	(236–336)	331	(268–399)	0.2
6-SL	All	1313	(1088–1647)	1142	(876–1503)	<0.05
LSTa	All	7	(4–12)	11	(7–14)	0.1
LSTb	All	62	(34–154)	72	(42–114)	0.5
LSTc	All	134	(102–174)	127	(79–199)	0.8
DSLNT	All	622	(426–941)	644	(502–1093)	0.2
2FL	Se+	4829	(0–7674)	5944	(3429–7467)	0.3
3FL	All	1367	(595–2983)	1227	(524–1833)	0.4
LDFT	Se+	386	(0–664)	404	(22–690)	0.7
LNT	All	2459	(1481–3630)	2194	(1768–2710)	0.5
LNnT	All	202	(100–273)	177	(110–257)	0.9
LNFP I	Se+	957	(0–1625)	1490	(475–2042)	0.2
LNFP II	Le+	494	(171–1348)	372	(123–749)	0.3
LNFP III	All	363	(269–468)	351	(255–531)	0.8
LNDH I	Se+ Le+	632	(0–1194)	821	(0–1231)	0.5
Σ analyzed HMO		15723	(13137–17176)	15972	(13008–17512)	0.8

* Mann Whitney U-test for independent samples used to compare distributions.

The correlation between growth indices and the 15 HMOs are displayed in Figure 4 (14-days sample) Figure S3 (28-days sample) and Figure S4 (PMW-36 + 0 sample). There were many statistically significant but weak correlations, but some of them were consistent throughout the neonatal period. The sialylated oligosaccharide LSTa correlated positively to the growth of weight and length at all three time points and also to head growth at day 14 of life, while the sialylated oligosaccharides 6SL, LSTb and LSTc correlated negatively to weight and head growth at 14 and 28 days of life.

Milk samples from day 14		Weight gain to day 14	Length gain to day 14	Head growth to day 14	Weight gain to day 28	Length gain to day 28	Head growth to day 28	Weight gain to 36th PMW	Length gain to 36th PMW	Head growth to 36th PMW
3-SL	Correlation Coefficient	0.09	0.11	0.11	0.14	0.13	0.10	0.17	0.18	0.00
	Sig. (2-tailed)	0.40	0.32	0.34	0.19	0.24	0.34	0.11	0.10	0.99
	n	86	86	85	87	85	87	85	85	85
6-SL	Correlation Coefficient	-0.41	-0.05	-0.22	-0.28	-0.11	-0.15	-0.23	-0.12	-0.08
	Sig. (2-tailed)	<0.001	0.66	0.05	0.01	0.30	0.17	0.03	0.27	0.44
	n	86	86	85	87	85	87	85	85	85
LSTa	Correlation Coefficient	0.31	0.13	0.40	0.23	0.20	0.10	0.15	0.14	-0.11
	Sig. (2-tailed)	<0.01	0.22	<0.001	0.03	0.06	0.35	0.18	0.20	0.33
	n	86	86	85	87	85	87	85	85	85
LSTb	Correlation Coefficient	-0.27	-0.03	-0.25	-0.05	0.03	-0.22	-0.17	-0.10	-0.11
	Sig. (2-tailed)	0.01	0.81	0.02	0.66	0.76	0.04	0.12	0.36	0.34
	n	86	86	85	87	85	87	85	85	85
LSTc	Correlation Coefficient	-0.52	0.00	-0.12	-0.48	-0.11	-0.19	-0.24	-0.16	0.01
	Sig. (2-tailed)	<0.001	0.99	0.27	<0.001	0.34	0.08	0.02	0.16	0.95
	n	86	86	85	87	85	87	85	85	85
DSLNT	Correlation Coefficient	-0.09	0.13	-0.04	-0.05	0.14	-0.16	-0.03	0.05	-0.05
	Sig. (2-tailed)	0.41	0.24	0.70	0.65	0.21	0.13	0.76	0.64	0.65
	n	86	86	85	87	85	87	85	85	85
2FL	Correlation Coefficient	0.10	0.06	0.16	0.00	0.14	0.13	0.12	0.20	0.04
	Sig. (2-tailed)	0.38	0.57	0.15	0.99	0.19	0.22	0.29	0.07	0.72
	n	86	86	85	87	85	87	85	85	85
3FL	Correlation Coefficient	-0.15	-0.06	-0.25	-0.11	-0.15	-0.16	-0.13	-0.17	0.04
	Sig. (2-tailed)	0.17	0.61	0.02	0.31	0.17	0.14	0.24	0.13	0.75
	n	86	86	85	87	85	87	85	85	85
LDFT	Correlation Coefficient	0.04	0.23	-0.04	-0.03	0.17	-0.03	0.03	0.17	0.07
	Sig. (2-tailed)	0.74	0.04	0.72	0.76	0.13	0.77	0.75	0.12	0.51
	n	86	86	85	87	85	87	85	85	85
LNT	Correlation Coefficient	-0.17	0.00	-0.04	0.02	0.06	-0.20	-0.20	-0.14	-0.32
	Sig. (2-tailed)	0.12	1.00	0.75	0.87	0.57	0.07	0.07	0.21	<0.01
	n	86	86	85	87	85	87	85	85	85
LNnT	Correlation Coefficient	0.05	0.06	0.27	0.05	0.17	0.09	0.03	0.13	0.07
	Sig. (2-tailed)	0.68	0.61	0.01	0.62	0.13	0.44	0.80	0.25	0.55
	n	86	86	85	87	85	87	85	85	85
LNFP I	Correlation Coefficient	0.134	0.116	0.198	0.098	0.167	0.073	0.102	0.156	-0.025
	Sig. (2-tailed)	0.217	0.286	0.069	0.364	0.127	0.503	0.354	0.155	0.819
	n	86	86	85	87	85	87	85	85	85
LNFP II	Correlation Coefficient	-0.016	-0.015	-0.088	0.027	-0.099	-0.061	-0.112	-0.178	-0.036
	Sig. (2-tailed)	0.885	0.89	0.423	0.803	0.37	0.573	0.309	0.103	0.743
	n	86	86	85	87	85	87	85	85	85
LNFP III	Correlation Coefficient	-0.30	0.01	-0.26	-0.28	-0.07	-0.33	-0.16	-0.11	-0.13
	Sig. (2-tailed)	0.01	0.94	0.02	0.01	0.53	<0.01	0.14	0.31	0.23
	n	86	86	85	87	85	87	85	85	85
LNDH I	Correlation Coefficient	0.07	0.24	0.059	-0.014	0.227	-0.003	0.025	0.131	0.125
	Sig. (2-tailed)	0.52	0.03	0.59	0.90	0.04	0.98	0.82	0.23	0.26
	n	86	86	85	87	85	87	85	85	85
Total HMO content	Correlation Coefficient	-0.13	0.15	0.03	-0.10	0.19	-0.09	-0.04	0.16	-0.07
	Sig. (2-tailed)	0.23	0.17	0.82	0.38	0.09	0.42	0.74	0.15	0.53
	n	86	86	85	87	85	87	85	85	85

Figure 4. Correlations between concentrations of individual human milk oligosaccharide (HMO) (micromol/litre) in milk samples from day 14 and infant growth (change in z-score from birth to measurement on the 14th or 28th day of life or at 36 postmenstrual week (PMW), analysed using Spearman´s rho correlation coefficient. Significant correlations are highlighted with green for positive and red for negative correlations.

4. Discussion

This study in preterm ELBW infants supports the hypothesis that HMO composition in breast milk affect the risk of developing NEC, which is consistent with animal models [14,15,30] and a previous human trial in preterm VLBW infants [16]. The main finding in the present trial was the low diversity of the 15 dominant HMOs in infants developing NEC, which has not been reported in any of the previous trials [14–16]. The study could not confirm the preventive effect of the sialylated HMO DSLNT on NEC found in previous studies [14–16], but instead NEC was associated with low levels of

LNDH I, which is a fucosylated HMO that can only be produced by mothers that are both secretor and Lewis positive.

The HMO composition reflects the mother´s secretor status and Lewis blood group and depends on genetic variation causing different expression of fucosyltransferases. As a consequence, secretor-negative and Lewis-negative mothers cannot produce some of the HMOs. One of them, 2FL, is the most abundant HMO in milk from secretor-positive mothers and has been associated with preventive effects on both NEC [15,30] and infections [31]. There was a trend of lower NEC in infants to secretor and Lewis-positive, as compared to negative, mothers in the present study, and the difference in HMO diversity between NEC and non-NEC cases remained when the material was stratified to include only secretor and Lewis-positive mothers, but disappeared when only secretor and Lewis negative individuals were included. Interestingly, the two infants developing NEC despite high levels of DSLNT had received breast milk from either a secretor-negative or a Lewis-negative mother.

Diversity is crucial for resilience in biological systems [32]. For instance, high microbial diversity in the gut has been associated with reduced risk of developing NEC in preterm infants [33] and asthma in school-age children [34]. The fact that such a high variety of HMOs are produced in human breast milk also suggests that the diversity and composition of the HMOs is more important than single HMOs. However, this does not preclude a preventive effect of administration of a single HMO such as DSNLT [14,15], 2FL [30], or LNDH I in preterm infants, but such an effect still needs to be confirmed in a randomised-controlled trial. The different findings in the human trial on VLBW infants by Autran et al. [16] with a significant correlation between NEC and low DSLNT, but not with total diversity, might be explained by cohort differences: The infants in the present trial were much smaller and immature than in the previous trial [16]. We speculate that the diversity is more important in ELBW than in VLBW infants. Additionally, HMO composition may vary between different countries. Interestingly, Swedish mothers had the lowest DSLNT levels in a previous worldwide study [17].

Human milk oligosaccharides have the potential to influence many of the mechanisms attributed to NEC development such as the immaturity of the immune system, regulation of the microvascular circulation, gut motility, reduced intestinal epithelial barrier function, and aberrant gut microbiota [35,36]. Thus, HMOs have been shown to reduce neutrophil infiltration and activation in vitro [37] and stimulate anti-inflammatory responses in the intestinal epithelium ex vivo [12,13]. The secretor-dependent 2FL modulated CD14 expression in human enterocytes and attenuated LPS-induced inflammation ex vivo [38], and also attenuated the severity of experimental NEC by enhancing mesenteric perfusion in the neonatal intestine via endothelial nitric oxide activation in a murine model [30]. In a murine ex vivo model on gut motility, fucosylated, but not sialylated HMOs diminished colon motor contractions [39]. Moreover, HMOs have structural homology to many cell surface glycans and thus act as decoys by binding to luminal bacteria that are then unable to bind to the surface of the enterocyte [40]. They can mimic carbohydrate-binding motifs of certain enteric pathogens, such as enteropathogenic *E. coli* by acting as a receptor decoy, and prevent adhesion to the apical surface of enterocytes [11]. Low microbial diversity [33] and high abundance of Proteobacteria and *Enterobacteriaceae*, and low abundance of Bacteroidetes have been related to the development of NEC [41]. Bifidobacteria and Bacteroidetes species become dominant intestinal bacteria in healthy breast-fed term infants due to their ability to digest and utilise HMOs via specific glycosidases, while most pathogenic *Enterobacteriaceae* lack these enzymes and are unable to utilize HMOs as a food source [42]. Interestingly, preterm infants to secretor-negative mothers have been shown to have increased abundance of Proteobacteria [43].

Group B Streptococcus (GBS) is the most common pathogen causing neonatal sepsis. The neutral oligosaccharide LNT inhibited growth of GBS in vitro [19], and infants to Lewis-positive mothers were less colonised with GBS in a study in The Gambia [31]. Our study did not confirm these findings.

Breastfeeding has been associated with weight development in infants [44]. There were many but quite weak correlations between growth indices and single HMO in the present study, although some of our findings were consistent throughout the neonatal period. The sialylated LSTa correlated positively to the growth of weight, length and head circumference, which is consistent with a Malawian study in which sialylated HMOs were less abundant in breast milk from mothers to severely stunted infants [18]. Supplementation with sialylated bovine milk oligosaccharide also increased growth in a gnotobiotic animal model [18]. However, not all sialylated HMOs seem to increase growth. In a Gambian study, the sialylated oligosaccharides 3SL and LSTc were positively and negatively correlated, respectively, to weight development [45], while 6SL and LSTc were negatively associated to weight gain in the present study.

Our study has many strengths. It is the largest trial of its kind, although the non-significant associations between NEC and several of the HMOs, such as DSLNT and 2FL, still might be due to insufficient statistical power. Also, the study included only ELBW infants, which is the patient group with the highest risk of developing NEC. The prospective design ensured well-controlled data and precise diagnoses, and samples were obtained longitudinally at three time points during the entire neonatal period. The breast milk sampling was standardised and included all mothers with sufficient breast milk. Fifteen of the most abundant HMOs [46] were measured with an established method, HPAEC-PAD [23,24]. A limitation of the study was the fact that no infants receiving donor milk or formula were included. Moreover, since we collected breast milk samples only at three fixed time points, the duration between sampling and use of the breast milk and the NEC and sepsis onset varied between cases, although most cases started before day 28 of life. However, the variability in HMO composition was higher between mothers than within the same mother over time, and the difference in HMO diversity and LNDH I levels were significantly associated with NEC at all three sampling points. These findings implicate that the duration between the sampling and NEC onset was of minor importance. Like the previous human trial [16], the analyses purely focused on HMO concentrations and not on the absolute HMO amounts received, which depended on the amount milk the infant received. Male gender was significantly more common among the NEC-cases, but there were no differences in HMO diversity in breast milk from mothers of singleton boys and girls. No other potential confounder that we measured differently between NEC and non-NEC cases. However, this does not preclude that some other factors could have influenced the result. A randomized-controlled intervention is needed to prove causality.

5. Conclusions

Our results suggest that the HMO composition in breast milk may be an important factor explaining why exclusively breast milk fed ELBW infants develop NEC. Low HMO diversity and low levels of the HMO LNDH I was associated with NEC development in ELBW infants. A preventive effect of supplementation with single or multiple HMO compounds still needs to be confirmed in future randomised-controlled trials.

Supplementary Materials: The following are available online at http://www.mdpi.com/2072-6643/10/10/1556/s1, Figure S1: NEC among infants to secretor- and Lewis-positive mothers, Figure S2: The HMO diversity in NEC and non-NEC cases stratified by the different secretor groups, Figure S3: The correlation between growth indices and the 15 HMOs at day28, Figure S4: The correlation between growth indices and the 15 HMOs atPMW 36 + 0, Table S1: HMOs at day 28 from mothers to infants who did and did not developed NEC, Table S2: HMOs at day 28 from mothers to infants who did and did not culture-proven sepsis, Table S3: HMOs at PMW 36 + 0 from mothers to infants who did and did not developed NEC. Table S4: HMOs at PMW from mothers to infants who did and did not developed culture-proven sepsis.

Author Contributions: Conceptualization, E.W., G.M., B.J., E.L. and T.A.; Data curation, E.W., M.M., E.L. and T.A.; Formal analysis, E.W., M.M., A.W., E.L. and T.A.; Funding acquisition, G.M., B.J., E.L. and T.A.; Investigation, E.W., M.M., G.M., A.W., B.J., E.L. and T.A.; Methodology, E.W., M.M., G.M., B.J., E.L. and T.A.; Project administration, G.M., B.J. and T.A.; Resources, B.J., E.L. and T.A.; Software, E.W. and M.M.; Supervision, E.L. and T.A.; Validation, E.W., M.M., G.M., B.J., E.L. and T.A.; Visualization, M.M.; Writing—original draft, E.W., M.M., E.L. and T.A.; Writing—review & editing, E.W., M.M., G.M., A.W., B.J., E.L. and T.A.

Funding: This research was funded by Swedish Research Council (grant number 921.2014-7060), The Swedish Society for Medical Research, the Swedish Society of Medicine, the Research Council for the South-East Sweden, ALF Grants, Region Östergötland, the Ekhaga Foundation, and BioGaia AB, Stockholm, Sweden.

Acknowledgments: We thank Fredrik Ingemansson, Josefin Lundström, Anders Palm, Björn Westrup and Laura Österdahl, the study nurses Christina Fuxin and Karin Jansmark for their brilliant and enthusiastic work guiding lactating mothers through the study and all the sampling procedures. We also thank Camilla Janefjord for excellent technical assistance.

Conflicts of Interest: The authors declare no conflict of interest. The funders had no role in the design of the study; in the collection, analyses, or interpretation of data; in the writing of the manuscript, and in the decision to publish the results.

References

1. EXPRESS Group; Fellman, V.; Hellström-Westas, L.; Norman, M.; Westgren, M.; Källén, K.; Lagercrantz, H.; Marsál, K.; Serenius, F.; Wennergren, M. One-year survival of extremely preterm infants after active perinatal care in sweden. *JAMA* **2009**, *301*, 2225–2233. [CrossRef] [PubMed]
2. Boyd, C.A.; Quigley, M.A.; Brocklehurst, P. Donor breast milk versus infant formula for preterm infants: Systematic review and meta-analysis. *Arch. Dis. Child.-Fetal Neonatal Ed.* **2007**, *92*, F169–F175. [CrossRef] [PubMed]
3. Bell, M.J.; Ternberg, J.L.; Feigin, R.D.; Keating, J.P.; Marshall, R.; Barton, L.; Brotherton, T. Neonatal necrotizing enterocolitis. Therapeutic decisions based upon clinical staging. *Ann. Surg.* **1978**, *187*, 1–7. [CrossRef] [PubMed]
4. Lin, P.W.; Stoll, B.J. Necrotising enterocolitis. *Lancet* **2006**, *368*, 1271–1283. [CrossRef]
5. Thomas, J.P.; Raine, T.; Reddy, S.; Belteki, G. Probiotics for the prevention of necrotising enterocolitis in very low-birth-weight infants: A meta-analysis and systematic review. *Acta. Paediatr.* **2017**, *106*, 1729–1741. [CrossRef] [PubMed]
6. Cristofalo, E.A.; Schanler, R.J.; Blanco, C.L.; Sullivan, S.; Trawoeger, R.; Kiechl-Kohlendorfer, U.; Dudell, G.; Rechtman, D.J.; Lee, M.L.; Lucas, A.; et al. Randomized trial of exclusive human milk versus preterm formula diets in extremely premature infants. *J. Pediatr.* **2013**, *163*, 1592–1595. [CrossRef] [PubMed]
7. Roze, E.; Ta, B.D.; van der Ree, M.H.; Tanis, J.C.; van Braeckel, K.N.; Hulscher, J.B.; Bos, A.F. Functional impairments at school age of children with necrotizing enterocolitis or spontaneous intestinal perforation. *Pediatr. Res.* **2011**, *70*, 619–625. [CrossRef] [PubMed]
8. Lönnerdal, B. Bioactive proteins in human milk: Health, nutrition, and implications for infant formulas. *J. Pediatr.* **2016**. [CrossRef] [PubMed]
9. Manti, S.; Lougaris, V.; Cuppari, C.; Tardino, L.; Dipasquale, V.; Arrigo, T.; Salpietro, C.; Leonardi, S. Breastfeeding and il-10 levels in children affected by cow's milk protein allergy: A restrospective study. *Immunobiology* **2017**, *222*, 358–362. [CrossRef] [PubMed]
10. Musilova, S.; Rada, V.; Vlkova, E.; Bunesova, V. Beneficial effects of human milk oligosaccharides on gut microbiota. *Benef. Microbes* **2014**, *5*, 273–283. [CrossRef] [PubMed]
11. Manthey, C.F.; Autran, C.A.; Eckmann, L.; Bode, L. Human milk oligosaccharides protect against enteropathogenic escherichia coli attachment in vitro and epec colonization in suckling mice. *J. Pediatr. Gastroenterol. Nutr.* **2014**, *58*, 165–168. [CrossRef] [PubMed]
12. He, Y.; Liu, S.; Leone, S.; Newburg, D.S. Human colostrum oligosaccharides modulate major immunologic pathways of immature human intestine. *Mucosal. Immunol.* **2014**, *7*, 1326–1339. [CrossRef] [PubMed]
13. Newburg, D.S.; Ruiz-Palacios, G.M.; Morrow, A.L. Human milk glycans protect infants against enteric pathogens. *Annu. Rev. Nutr.* **2005**, *25*, 37–58. [CrossRef] [PubMed]
14. Jantscher-Krenn, E.; Zherebtsov, M.; Nissan, C.; Goth, K.; Guner, Y.S.; Naidu, N.; Choudhury, B.; Grishin, A.V.; Ford, H.R.; Bode, L. The human milk oligosaccharide disialyllacto-n-tetraose prevents necrotising enterocolitis in neonatal rats. *Gut* **2012**, *61*, 1417–1425. [CrossRef] [PubMed]
15. Autran, C.A.; Schoterman, M.H.; Jantscher-Krenn, E.; Kamerling, J.P.; Bode, L. Sialylated galacto-oligosaccharides and 2′-fucosyllactose reduce necrotising enterocolitis in neonatal rats. *Br. J. Nutr.* **2016**, *116*, 294–299. [CrossRef] [PubMed]
16. Autran, C.A.; Kellman, B.P.; Kim, J.H.; Asztalos, E.; Blood, A.B.; Spence, E.C.H.; Patel, A.L.; Hou, J.; Lewis, N.E.; Bode, L. Human milk oligosaccharide composition predicts risk of necrotising enterocolitis in preterm infants. *Gut* **2018**, *67*, 1064–1070. [CrossRef] [PubMed]

17. McGuire, M.K.; Meehan, C.L.; McGuire, M.A.; Williams, J.E.; Foster, J.; Sellen, D.W.; Kamau-Mbuthia, E.W.; Kamundia, E.W.; Mbugua, S.; Moore, S.E.; et al. What's normal? Oligosaccharide concentrations and profiles in milk produced by healthy women vary geographically. *Am. J. Clin. Nutr.* **2017**, *105*, 1086–1100. [CrossRef] [PubMed]
18. Charbonneau, M.R.; O'Donnell, D.; Blanton, L.V.; Totten, S.M.; Davis, J.C.; Barratt, M.J.; Cheng, J.; Guruge, J.; Talcott, M.; Bain, J.R.; et al. Sialylated milk oligosaccharides promote microbiota-dependent growth in models of infant undernutrition. *Cell* **2016**, *164*, 859–871. [CrossRef] [PubMed]
19. Li, M.; Monaco, M.H.; Wang, M.; Comstock, S.S.; Kuhlenschmidt, T.B.; Fahey, G.C., Jr.; Miller, M.J.; Kuhlenschmidt, M.S.; Donovan, S.M. Human milk oligosaccharides shorten rotavirus-induced diarrhea and modulate piglet mucosal immunity and colonic microbiota. *ISME J.* **2014**, *8*, 1609–1620. [CrossRef] [PubMed]
20. Lin, A.E.; Autran, C.A.; Szyszka, A.; Escajadillo, T.; Huang, M.; Godula, K.; Prudden, A.R.; Boons, G.J.; Lewis, A.L.; Doran, K.S.; et al. Human milk oligosaccharides inhibit growth of group b streptococcus. *J. Biol. Chem.* **2017**, *292*, 11243–11249. [CrossRef] [PubMed]
21. Wejryd, E.; Marchini, G.; Frimmel, V.; Jonsson, B.; Abrahamsson, T. Probiotics promoted head growth in extremely low birthweight infants in a double-blind placebo-controlled trial. *Acta. Paediatr.* **2018**, *35*, 802–811. [CrossRef] [PubMed]
22. Niklasson, A.; Albertsson-Wikland, K. Continuous growth reference from 24th week of gestation to 24 months by gender. *BMC Pediatr.* **2008**, *8*, 8. [CrossRef] [PubMed]
23. Gabrielli, O.; Zampini, L.; Galeazzi, T.; Padella, L.; Santoro, L.; Peila, C.; Giuliani, F.; Bertino, E.; Fabris, C.; Coppa, G.V. Preterm milk oligosaccharides during the first month of lactation. *Pediatrics* **2011**, *128*, e1520–e1531. [CrossRef] [PubMed]
24. Nakhla, T.; Fu, D.; Zopf, D.; Brodsky, N.L.; Hurt, H. Neutral oligosaccharide content of preterm human milk. *Br. J. Nutr.* **1999**, *82*, 361–367. [CrossRef] [PubMed]
25. Thurl, S.; Muller-Werner, B.; Sawatzki, G. Quantification of individual oligosaccharide compounds from human milk using high-ph anion-exchange chromatography. *Anal. Biochem.* **1996**, *235*, 202–206. [CrossRef] [PubMed]
26. Landberg, E.; Lundblad, A.; Påhlsson, P. Temperature effects in high-performance anion-exchange chromatography of oligosaccharides. *J. Chromatogr. A* **1998**, *814*, 97–104. [CrossRef]
27. Clarke, K.R.; Green, H.R. Statistical design and analysis for a 'biological effects' study. *Mar. Ecol. Prog. Ser.* **1988**, *46*, 213–226. [CrossRef]
28. Minchin, P.R.; Peter, R. An evaluation of relative robustness of techniques for ecological ordinations. *Vegetation* **1987**, *69*, 89–107. [CrossRef]
29. R-Core-Team. *R: A Language and Environment for Statistical Computing*; R Foundation for Statistical Computing: Vienna, Austria, 2016.
30. Good, M.; Sodhi, C.P.; Yamaguchi, Y.; Jia, H.; Lu, P.; Fulton, W.B.; Martin, L.Y.; Prindle, T.; Nino, D.F.; Zhou, Q.; et al. The human milk oligosaccharide 2′-fucosyllactose attenuates the severity of experimental necrotising enterocolitis by enhancing mesenteric perfusion in the neonatal intestine. *Br. J. Nutr.* **2016**, *116*, 1175–1187. [CrossRef] [PubMed]
31. Andreas, N.J.; Al-Khalidi, A.; Jaiteh, M.; Clarke, E.; Hyde, M.J.; Modi, N.; Holmes, E.; Kampmann, B.; Mehring Le Doare, K. Role of human milk oligosaccharides in group b streptococcus colonisation. *Clin. Transl. Immunol.* **2016**, *5*, e99. [CrossRef] [PubMed]
32. Griffiths, B.S.; Philippot, L. Insights into the resistance and resilience of the soil microbial community. *FEMS Microbiol. Rev.* **2013**, *37*, 112–129. [CrossRef] [PubMed]
33. McMurtry, V.E.; Gupta, R.W.; Tran, L.; Blanchard, E.E.t.; Penn, D.; Taylor, C.M.; Ferris, M.J. Bacterial diversity and clostridia abundance decrease with increasing severity of necrotizing enterocolitis. *Microbiome* **2015**, *3*, 11. [CrossRef] [PubMed]
34. Abrahamsson, T.R.; Jakobsson, H.E.; Andersson, A.F.; Björkstén, B.; Engstrand, L.; Jenmalm, M.C. Low gut microbiota diversity in early infancy precedes asthma at school age. *Clin. Exp. Allergy* **2014**, *44*, 842–850. [CrossRef] [PubMed]
35. Eaton, S.; Rees, C.M.; Hall, N.J. Current research on the epidemiology, pathogenesis, and management of necrotizing enterocolitis. *Neonatology* **2017**, *111*, 423–430. [CrossRef] [PubMed]

36. Marseglia, L.; D'Angelo, G.; Manti, S.; Aversa, S.; Reiter, R.J.; Antonuccio, P.; Centorrino, A.; Romeo, C.; Impellizzeri, P.; Gitto, E. Oxidative stress-mediated damage in newborns with necrotizing enterocolitis: A possible role of melatonin. *Am. J. Perinatol.* **2015**, *32*, 905–909. [PubMed]
37. Bode, L.; Kunz, C.; Muhly-Reinholz, M.; Mayer, K.; Seeger, W.; Rudloff, S. Inhibition of monocyte, lymphocyte, and neutrophil adhesion to endothelial cells by human milk oligosaccharides. *J. Thromb. Haemost.* **2004**, *92*, 1402–1410. [CrossRef] [PubMed]
38. He, Y.; Liu, S.; Kling, D.E.; Leone, S.; Lawlor, N.T.; Huang, Y.; Feinberg, S.B.; Hill, D.R.; Newburg, D.S. The human milk oligosaccharide 2′-fucosyllactose modulates cd14 expression in human enterocytes, thereby attenuating lps-induced inflammation. *Gut* **2016**, *65*, 33–46. [CrossRef] [PubMed]
39. Bienenstock, J.; Buck, R.H.; Linke, H.; Forsythe, P.; Stanisz, A.M.; Kunze, W.A. Fucosylated but not sialylated milk oligosaccharides diminish colon motor contractions. *PLoS ONE* **2013**, *8*, e76236. [CrossRef] [PubMed]
40. Coppa, G.V.; Zampini, L.; Galeazzi, T.; Facinelli, B.; Ferrante, L.; Capretti, R.; Orazio, G. Human milk oligosaccharides inhibit the adhesion to caco-2 cells of diarrheal pathogens: Escherichia coli, vibrio cholerae, and salmonella fyris. *Pediatr. Res.* **2006**, *59*, 377–382. [CrossRef] [PubMed]
41. Pammi, M.; Cope, J.; Tarr, P.I.; Warner, B.B.; Morrow, A.L.; Mai, V.; Gregory, K.E.; Kroll, J.S.; McMurtry, V.; Ferris, M.J.; et al. Intestinal dysbiosis in preterm infants preceding necrotizing enterocolitis: A systematic review and meta-analysis. *Microbiome* **2017**, *5*, 31. [CrossRef] [PubMed]
42. Yu, Z.T.; Chen, C.; Newburg, D.S. Utilization of major fucosylated and sialylated human milk oligosaccharides by isolated human gut microbes. *Glycobiology* **2013**, *23*, 1281–1292. [CrossRef] [PubMed]
43. Underwood, M.A.; Gaerlan, S.; De Leoz, M.L.; Dimapasoc, L.; Kalanetra, K.M.; Lemay, D.G.; German, J.B.; Mills, D.A.; Lebrilla, C.B. Human milk oligosaccharides in premature infants: Absorption, excretion, and influence on the intestinal microbiota. *Pediatr. Res.* **2015**, *78*, 670–677. [CrossRef] [PubMed]
44. Marseglia, L.; Manti, S.; D'Angelo, G.; Cuppari, C.; Salpietro, V.; Filippelli, M.; Trovato, A.; Gitto, E.; Salpietro, C.; Arrigo, T. Obesity and breastfeeding: The strength of association. *Women Birth* **2015**, *28*, 81–86. [CrossRef] [PubMed]
45. Davis, J.C.; Lewis, Z.T.; Krishnan, S.; Bernstein, R.M.; Moore, S.E.; Prentice, A.M.; Mills, D.A.; Lebrilla, C.B.; Zivkovic, A.M. Growth and morbidity of gambian infants are influenced by maternal milk oligosaccharides and infant gut microbiota. *Sci. Rep.* **2017**, *7*, 40466. [CrossRef] [PubMed]
46. Kunz, C.; Meyer, C.; Collado, M.C.; Geiger, L.; Garcia-Mantrana, I.; Bertua-Rios, B.; Martinez-Costa, C.; Borsch, C.; Rudloff, S. Influence of gestational age, secretor, and lewis blood group status on the oligosaccharide content of human milk. *J. Pediatr. Gastroenterol. Nutr.* **2017**, *64*, 789–798. [CrossRef] [PubMed]

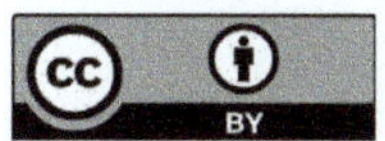

© 2018 by the authors. Licensee MDPI, Basel, Switzerland. This article is an open access article distributed under the terms and conditions of the Creative Commons Attribution (CC BY) license (http://creativecommons.org/licenses/by/4.0/).

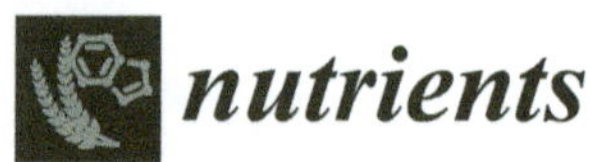

MDPI

Article

Randomized, Double-Blind, Placebo-Controlled Parallel Clinical Trial Assessing the Effect of Fructooligosaccharides in Infants with Constipation

Daniela da Silva Souza [1], Soraia Tahan [1], Thabata Koester Weber [2], Humberto Bezerra de Araujo-Filho [1] and Mauro Batista de Morais [1,*]

[1] Division of Pediatric Gastroenterology, Escola Paulista de Medicina, Universidade Federal de São Paulo, São Paulo 04023-062, Brazil; danielassouza@gmail.com (D.d.S.S.); s.tahan@uol.com.br (S.T.); biogene@gmail.com (H.B.d.A.-F.)

[2] Instituto de Biociências, Universidade Estadual Paulista, Botucatu, São Paulo 18618-689, Brazil; thabataweber@yahoo.com.br

* Correspondence: maurobmorais@gmail.com

Received: 8 September 2018; Accepted: 26 October 2018; Published: 1 November 2018

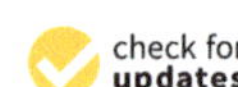

Abstract: Constipation often begins in the first year of life. The aim of this study was to assess the effect of fructooligosaccharides (FOS) in the treatment of infants with constipation. This randomized, double-blind, placebo-controlled clinical trial included infants with constipation who were randomly assigned to one of two parallel groups: FOS or placebo. Either the FOS supplement or the placebo was added to the infant formula. Thirty-six infants completed the 4-week intervention. Therapeutic success occurred in 83.3% of the FOS group infants and in 55.6% of the control group infants ($p = 0.073$; one-tailed test). Compared with the control group, the FOS group exhibited a higher frequency of softer stools ($p = 0.035$) and fewer episodes of straining and/or difficulty passing stools ($p = 0.041$). At the end of the intervention, the mouth-to-anus transit time was shorter (22.4 and 24.5 h, $p = 0.035$), and the Bifidobacterium sp. count was higher ($p = 0.006$) in the FOS group. In conclusion, the use of FOS in infants with constipation was associated with significant improvement in symptoms, but the results showed no statistical significance regarding the success of the therapy compared with the control group. FOS was associated with reduced bowel transit time and higher counts of the genus Bifidobacterium in the stool.

Keywords: constipation; prebiotic; intestinal transit time; infant; *Bifidobacterium*

1. Introduction

Constipation occurs frequently in childhood and accounts for approximately 25% of visits to pediatric gastroenterology outpatient clinics [1–3]. In most cases, symptoms appear during the first year of life [3–5]. This stage of life involves significant changes to the infant's diet, including the introduction of complementary feeding and inappropriate early interruption of breastfeeding [6].

Breastfeeding protects against the development of constipation and is associated with higher stool frequency and softer stools during the first six months of life [5,7,8]. The lower constipation frequency among breastfed infants might be due to the ingestion of prebiotic oligosaccharides, which are the third largest component of breast milk and are absent from nonhuman milk [9]. Oligosaccharides have a bifidogenic effect (contributing to the growth of beneficial bacteria from the genera *Bifidobacterium* and *Lactobacillus*) and modify intestinal metabolic activity by reducing the pH and increasing the short-chain fatty acid concentration. This modulation of the gut microbiota may contribute to increasing the stool bulk and intestinal motility, thus facilitating the passage of stool [10,11].

Considering that human breast milk contains large amounts of oligosaccharides, a mixture of prebiotic oligosaccharides (galactooligosaccharides and fructooligosaccharides) has been added to some infant formulas. The effect of this mixture on the gut microbiota and bowel pattern was assessed. The results indicated an increased stool frequency [12–17] and softer stools [12–17] in the infants who were fed the prebiotic mixture. In addition, the number of fecal *Bifidobacteria* was higher in the group fed the prebiotic mixture than in the control group [13,17]. A recent clinical study conducted in Brazil assessed the effect of galactooligosaccharides on constipation among 6 to 14-year-old children and adolescents. The results showed higher stool frequency, less straining and softer stools during the prebiotic intake period [18].

Although several studies have demonstrated the influence of prebiotics on stool frequency and consistency, no randomized, double-blind, placebo-controlled clinical trial has assessed their use in treating infants with constipation. Therefore, this clinical trial assessed the effect of prebiotic FOS on the bowel pattern of infants (6–24 months old) with constipation as well its effects on mouth-to-anus transit time and stool counts of the genera *Bifidobacterium* and *Lactobacillus*.

2. Materials and Methods

2.1. Study Design

This study was a randomized, double-blind, placebo-controlled, parallel trial that complied with the guidelines formulated by the Consolidated Standards of Reporting Trials (CONSORT) [19]. The trial was registered at the Brazilian Registry of Clinical Trials (registry number RBR-2x8wqc; registry URL: http://www.ensaiosclinicos.gov.br/rg/RBR-2x8wqc/).

Infants aged 6–24 months were assessed for inclusion in the study at basic health units or daycare centers in the cities of Osasco and São Vicente (State of São Paulo, Brazil). Constipation was defined as the elimination of hard stools associated with one of the following characteristics: pain or straining while passing stools, scybalous stools, cylindrical and cracked or cylindrical and thick stools and stool frequency less than three times per week, as per the modified international recommendations [20] used in previous studies [5,21]. After inclusion in the study and before randomization, a daily register of intestinal habits was tracked in a diary for one week and used to confirm the constipation diagnosis.

Infants who fulfilled any of the following criteria were not admitted to the study: (1) exclusively or partially breastfeeding; (2) use of antibiotics, dietary fiber or prebiotic supplements in the past 30 days; (3) iron deficiency anemia (hemoglobin < 11.0 g/dL); 4. current use of medications that can cause constipation (except ferrous sulfate); 5. malnutrition or obesity; 6. infants whose parents were not able to record the infant's bowel pattern during follow-up.

Other exclusion criteria were the clinical need for prescribed laxatives, a diagnosis of fecaloma or FOS or placebo intake below 80%.

2.2. Intervention

Randomization was performed by a health professional who did not participate in the study. A computer-generated random number table was used, and the participants were assigned to blocks by body weight (6.0–8.9 kg, 9.0–11.9 kg and over 12.0 kg). In each weight interval, a block of four participants was assigned to the study and control groups at 2:2 ratios. The prebiotic and placebo were delivered in identical packaging, and the coding was standardized according to the random number table. The participants received the corresponding intervention based on their order of entry into the study. Neither the participants nor the investigators were aware of the intervention (prebiotic or placebo).

The study lasted five weeks with one week for clinical evaluation before randomization. During the intervention, participants received a prebiotic composed of 100% FOS (the FOS polymerization degree ranged from two to six monosaccharide molecules) or a placebo composed of 100% (flavorless) maltodextrin for four weeks. The FOS and placebo doses were 6, 9 or 12 g daily based on the infants' weight groups of 6.0–8.9 kg, 9.0–11.9 kg or over 12.0 kg, respectively. Both were supplied by the same manufacturer (FQF, Farmoquimica, São Paulo, Brazil). Based on the randomization, each patient received the FOS or placebo in two doses. The FOS or placebo supplements were administered in baby bottles and dispersed in infant formula (Milupa^{R}, Danone, Brazil) or cow's milk (Ninhofortificado^{R}, Nestlé, Brazil) for infants aged less than 12 months and older than 12 months, respectively.

2.3. Study Stages

The study involved three stages: baseline, intervention and the last week of the clinical trial. At baseline (first week), clinical interviews were conducted. The interviews included characterization of the infants' bowel patterns and 24-h diet recall; stool samples were also collected, and hemoglobin levels in capillary blood samples and the carmine dye mouth-to-anus transit time were measured. The infants' parents received home monitoring diaries. During the baseline week, the participants received infant formula or iron-fortified cow's milk without supplemental FOS or the placebo. This procedure permitted evaluation of the effect of dietary changes on the infants' bowel patterns. Only infants who continued to experience constipation at the end of the first week were included in the intervention.

The intervention period was conducted over the following four weeks and included one weekly clinical evaluation. Participants received FOS or the placebo as indicated by the randomization. During the intervention, the infants' guardians recorded the bowel patterns and adverse effects in their home monitoring diaries.

During the end-of-study period (the last week of the intervention period), a second stool sample was collected, the carmine dye mouth-to-anus transit time was measured, and 24-h diet recall was recorded.

2.4. Study Procedures

The infants' bowel patterns were assessed based on data provided by their guardians at clinical interviews based on their home monitoring diaries.

Hemoglobin concentration in the capillary blood samples was measured using a photometer (HemoCue, Angelholm, Sweden). Infants with anemia (hemoglobin concentration less than 11 g/dL per the World Health Organization [21]) were excluded. Anemia was evaluated and treated by pediatricians at basic health units. The guardians of infants without anemia who were receiving ferrous sulfate at prophylactic doses were directed to discontinue the medication during the study period.

The mouth-to-anus transit time, expressed in hours, was measured using carmine dye (Certistain, Merck, Brazil). The dye was administered at a dose of 0.25 g dissolved in 50 mL of water [22]. Guardians were directed to record the dates and times at which the infants ingested the dye and first expelled red-stained stools.

The infants' typical diets were assessed using the 24-h recall method [23]. Energy, macronutrient (carbohydrate, fat and protein) and micronutrient (calcium and iron) intake estimates were calculated using Nutrition Decision Making Support System software (version 2.5) (Universidade Federal de São Paulo, São Paulo, Brazil). Dietary fiber intake was calculated using the Brazilian Food Composition Table (Tabela Brasileira de Composição de Alimentos) [24], which lists the dietary fiber content of foods according to the Association of Official Analytical Chemists' (AOAC) enzymatic-gravimetric method [25].

Body weight and height were measured at all clinical evaluations. Infants were weighed without clothes using digital scales (Filizola, São Paulo, Brazil) with 15-kg capacities and 5-g sensitivities. Body length was measured using a portable, horizontal 100-cm stadiometer with 0.1-cm precision. The weights and lengths of the infants are expressed as weight-per-age, length-per-age and weight-per-length z-scores. Z-scores were calculated using the World Health Organization's Anthro software, version 3.2.2 (Geneva, Switzerland) [26].

The guardians who received instructions on delivering the FOS or placebo were also asked to record the infants' bowel patterns (stool frequency and consistency, pain, crying, straining or difficulty passing stools) and adverse effects (excessive crying, regurgitation or vomiting) each day in their home monitoring diaries. To facilitate description of stool shape and consistency, a scale with four figures illustrating infant stools was appended to the home monitoring diary.

For determining the number of *Bifidobacterium* and *Lactobacillus*, stool samples were collected by the guardians according to established guidelines. Approximately 1 g of each stool sample was transferred to a microtube containing ASL buffer from the DNA extraction QIAamp Mini Stool Kit, and the sample was stored at −20 °C until the DNA was to be extracted. The bacterial genomic DNA was extracted according to the protocol recommended by the extraction kit manufacturer (Qiagen, Hilden, Germany), and the purified DNA was diluted in a buffer solution to a final volume of 200 μL. The DNA concentration was measured using a NanoDrop 1000 spectrophotometer (Thermo Scientific, Waltham, MA, USA). All DNA samples were diluted to a final concentration of 20 ng/μL and stored at −20 °C.

DNA from all fecal samples was subjected to real-time polymerase chain reaction (qPCR). The primers used were selected to identify and quantify *Lactobacillus* spp. [27] and *Bifidobacterium* spp. [28]. All reactions were performed in duplicate in a final volume of 10 μL that included 5 μL of Rotor-gene SYBR Green PCR Master Mix (Qiagen, Hilden, Germany). Thermocycling was performed in a Rotor-gene Q device (Qiagen, Hilden, Germany) with the following parameters: 5 min at 95 °C and 40 cycles of 95 °C for 10 s and 60 °C for 15 s. The dissociation protocol used to obtain the melting curve was 95 °C for 1 min followed by variation of the temperature from 70 °C to 95 °C with a temperature increase of 1 °C/s. The negative control contained all the ingredients except the DNA sample. The standard curve for all of the analyses was created by amplifying a Topo TA plasmid (Invitrogen, ThermoFisher, Waltham, MA, USA) carrying a fragment of the reference gene previously amplified by conventional PCR, and its specificity was confirmed by sequencing and BLAST system alignment. With the molecular mass of the plasmid and insert known, it is possible to calculate the copy number as follows: mass in daltons (g/mol) = (size of double-stranded (ds) product in base pairs (bp)) (330 Da × 2 nucleotides (nt)/bp) [29–31]. If the copy number and the concentration of the plasmid DNA are known, the number of molecules added to subsequent real-time PCR runs can be calculated, thus providing a standard for determining the copy numbers of specific genes [29–31]. The real-time PCR results are expressed as log CFU per gram of stool (log CFU/g) using the average number of copies of 16S rRNA genes in each bacterium to normalize the counts [29–31].

2.5. Outcomes

The primary outcome was therapeutic success defined as a normal bowel pattern at the end of the study, i.e., predominantly soft, amorphous or cylindrical stools without cracks as well as the absence of pain or difficulty passing stools (a pattern incompatible with the criteria adopted herein for characterizing constipation). Therapeutic failure was defined as the persistence of a bowel pattern indicating constipation at the end of the study or a clinical need for laxatives during the intervention period.

Secondary outcomes were stool frequency, stool consistency, pain and/or crying when passing stools, and difficulty and/or straining while passing stools during the last week of the clinical trial. The mouth-to-anus transit time and *Bifidobacterium* spp. and *Lactobacillus* spp. counts were measured before and at the end of the intervention.

2.6. Ethical Issues

The study protocol was approved by the Research Ethics Committee of the Universidade Federal de São Paulo (Federal University of São Paulo). Written informed consent was obtained from the parents of the infants prior to inclusion in the study.

2.7. Statistical Analysis

Sample size was calculated based on the primary outcome (therapeutic success). A success rate of 70% was assumed for the group that received FOS, and a success rate of 20% was assumed for the control group. For $\alpha = 0.05$ and $\beta = 0.20$ (power = 0.80), each group should include 19 individuals.

To compare the mean and median values between groups, parametric (Student's *t*-test) or non-parametric (Mann–Whitney U) tests were used based on the data distribution. A chi-squared test was used to compare proportions. For the variables therapeutic success, stool frequency, stool consistency, and occurrence of pain and/or crying when passing stools or difficulty and/or straining when passing stools, the study goal was to establish whether the FOS performed better than the placebo. Therefore, p-values from one-tailed tests were used to compare those variables. Calculations were performed using SigmaStat 3.1 (Systat, San Jose, CA, USA) and EpiInfo (CDC, Atlanta, GA, USA). Differences between groups were considered significant when $p < 0.05$.

3. Results

3.1. Patients

Seventy-five infants were eligible for inclusion in the study; however, the constipation diagnosis was unconfirmed in 26 (34.7%) cases during the first week's assessment, five guardians dropped out during the baseline period, and six did not consent to participate. Thus, 38 infants were randomly assigned to the two groups. The study group ($n = 19$) received FOS, and the control group ($n = 19$) received the placebo. No statistically significant differences were found between the groups at the time of inclusion in the study (after the end of the baseline period) (Table 1). During the intervention period, one participant in the FOS group dropped out for medical reasons (pneumonia), and one participant in the control group dropped out due to a family trip. Therefore, 36 infants completed the clinical trial: 18 in the FOS group and 18 in the control group (Figure 1).

Table 1. Demographic and clinical characteristics at baseline.

	FOS Group ($n = 19$)	Control Group ($n = 19$)	p
Age (months)	12.77 ± 4.37	13.00 ± 5.19	0.890 †
Sex			
Female	10 (52.6%)	10 (52.6%)	1.000 *
Male	9 (47.4%)	9 (47.4%)	
Number of bowel movements per week	6.27 ± 1.32	5.66 ± 1.87	0.133 †
Predominant stool shape and consistency			
Cylindrical with cracks	13 (68.4%)	8 (42.1%)	0.191 *
Scybalous	6 (31.6%)	11 (57.9%)	
Straining and/or difficulty in more than 50% of bowel movements	16 (84.2%)	16 (84.2%)	1.000 *
Pain and/or crying in more than 50% of bowel movements	11 (57.9%)	12 (63.2%)	1.000 *

FOS: fructooligosaccharide; Consistency and shape: predominant occurrence (more than four times per week); * Two-tailed chi-squared test with Yates' correction; † Two-tailed Student's *t*-test, mean ± standard deviation.

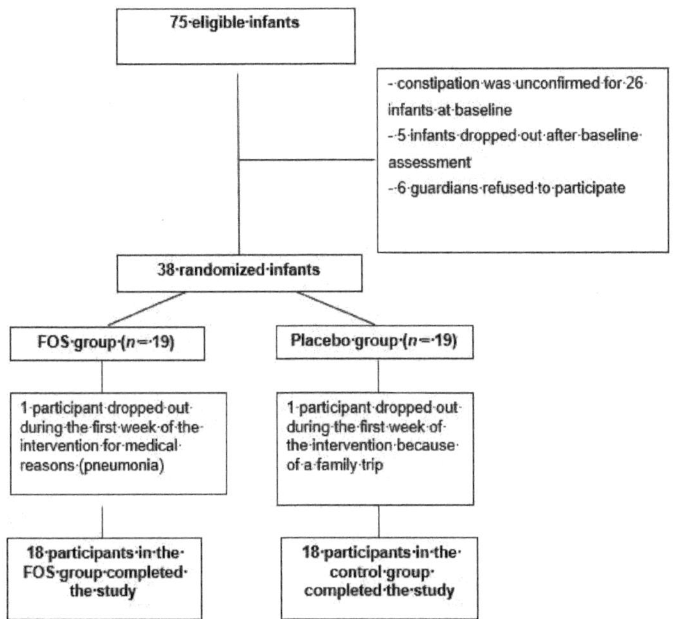

Figure 1. Flowchart showing the study participants. FOS: fructooligosaccharide.

3.2. Primary Outcome

Therapeutic success occurred more frequently in the FOS group (15/18, 83.3%) than in the control group (10/18, 55.6%); however, this difference was not statistically significant ($p = 0.073$, one-tailed chi-squared test).

3.3. Secondary Outcome

For the secondary outcomes, all variables were similar at admission (Table 2). The weekly stool frequencies in the last week of the study were similar in both groups, and no statistically significant increment in the number of bowel movements occurred between the baseline and the last week of the study. Both groups presented fewer ($p < 0.05$) bowel movements with pain/crying or straining/difficulty when passing stool and increments ($p < 0.05$) in the percentages of bowel movements with soft stool. At the last week of the study, the FOS group presented fewer bowel movements with straining/difficulty ($p = 0.041$) and a higher percentage of passing soft stools than the control group ($p = 0.035$).

The median mouth-to-anus transit times for the FOS and control groups were similar ($p = 0.740$, two-tailed Mann-Whitney test) upon admission in the study, at 23.3 h (percentiles 25 and 75: 22.2; 25.6) and 23.5 h (percentiles 25 and 75: 21.9; 27.0), respectively. At the end of the study, the mouth-to-anus transit time was lower ($p = 0.035$; one-tailed Mann–Whitney test) in the FOS group (median: 22.4 h; percentiles 25 and 75: 18.3; 25.7) than in the control group (median: 24.5 h; percentiles 25 and 75: 23.0; 33.3).

Table 2. Clinical secondary outcomes at baseline and at the end of the study (stool frequency, percentage of straining, difficulty, pain, crying during defecation and percentage of soft stools).

	FOS Group (n = 18)	Control Group (n = 18)	p *
Number of bowel movements per week			
Baseline week	6.27 ± 1.32	5.66 ± 1.87	0.133
Last week of the study	6.33 ± 1.28	6.11 ± 1.53	0.320
Pain/crying when passing stools (percent of bowel movements)			
Baseline week	55.13 ± 44.07	60.09 ± 44.44	0.369
Last week of the study	14.68 ± 29.15	28.39 ± 43.82	0.138
Straining/difficulty when passing stools (percent of bowel movements)			
Baseline week	84.47 ± 29.39	79.47 ± 37.63	0.330
Last week of the study	29.65 ± 41.73	55.07 ± 43.44	0.041
Soft stool consistency (percent of bowel movements)			
Baseline week	12.12 ± 15.91	16.92 ± 15.07	0.180
Last week of the study	73.38 ± 29.38	55.38 ± 36.32	0.035

* The data are presented as mean ± standard deviation (One-tailed Student's t-test).

At the end of the study, the number of bacteria of the genus *Bifidobacterium* was higher in the FOS group than in the control group (Table 3).

Table 3. Secondary outcome: *Bifidobacterium and Lactobacillus* genus counts (log CFU/g).

	FOS Group (n = 18)	Control Group (n = 18)	p
Bifidobacterium			
Baseline	6.39 (5.25–8.36)	6.61 (4.48–7.99)	0.301
End of the study	7.37 (5.86–8.43)	5.60 (4.46–6.42)	0.006
Lactobacillus			
Baseline	6.27 (4.33–7.54)	6.03 (2.95–7.23)	0.248
End of the study	6.45 (4.83–7.61)	5.39 (3.37–6.73)	0.095

The data are presented as median values with the 25th and 75th percentile values in parentheses (Mann-Whitney test).

The z-scores (weight-for-height, weight-for-age, height-for-age and body mass index-for-age) and the food intake as per the 24-h food recall method were similar in the FOS and control groups at baseline and at the end of the study (data not shown). Dietary fiber intake (excluding the FOS supplement used in the intervention) was 6.6 ± 2.1 g/day and 7.4 ± 2.4 g/day at admission (p = 0.269) in the FOS and control groups, respectively. At the end of the study, these values were 6.5 ± 2.3 g/day and 7.1 ± 2.2 g/day (p = 0.457), respectively.

3.4. Adverse Effects

All participants who completed the 4-week intervention (n = 36) consumed more than 80% of the delivered amount of FOS or placebo. Adverse effects were reported only in the FOS group (two infants with abdominal distension and flatulence), but the treatment was continued. One of the infants in the FOS group had two vomiting episodes during the first week of intervention.

4. Discussion

This clinical trial showed that FOS intake contributed to relieving infant constipation (increased frequency of softer stools) and reducing the number of defecation events with straining and/or difficulty passing stools. FOS also reduced the bowel transit time and increased the number of *Bifidobacterium* in constipated infants who were treated with FOS relative to the control group. The stool frequencies in the two groups were similar at baseline and at the last week of the study. Although the difference did not reach statistical significance, therapeutic success was more frequently achieved in the group treated with FOS than in the control group.

Per the 2014 ESPGHAN/NASPGHAN guideline for constipation, routine use of prebiotics is not recommended for treating childhood constipation. Recently, a clinical trial performed in

Brazil [17] showed a positive effect of galactooligosaccharide probiotics on constipation in children and adolescents aged 4–16 years. That study showed softer stools, increased stool frequency and less pain or difficulty when passing stools during the prebiotic intake period. The present study showed similar results except for stool frequency. However, the defecation frequency of constipated infants included in our study was not reduced; therefore, no increase in the bowel movement frequency was expected.

Prebiotics were administered to healthy bottle-fed infants in previous clinical trials [12–16] to assess their influence on bowel patterns. Infants who received prebiotic mixtures of galacto- and fructooligosaccharides exhibited softer stools. Our results agreed with these studies, as the frequency of softer stools increased after four weeks of intervention only with FOS. Additionally, the mixture used in the infant formula contained 90% galactooligosaccharides and only 10% FOS.

The increased frequency of softer stools and the consequent reduction in defecation events with straining and/or difficulty when passing stools in the FOS-treated group might be related to the effect of this prebiotic on the gut microbiota. Prebiotics are carbohydrates that are not digested in the gastrointestinal tract and are used as an energy source by the gut bacteria [10]. Other studies found that consumption of a mixture of galacto- and fructooligosaccharides increased the number of *Bifidobacterium* [12,13]. Our results showed that at the end of the study *Bifidobacterium* numbers were higher in the FOS group. Thus, only FOS had a prebiotic effect as observed for the galacto- and fructooligosaccharide mixture. This effect might be associated with the short-chain fatty acids produced by the fermentation of prebiotics. The modulation of gut microbiota may contribute to increasing the stool bulk and may stimulate intestinal motility, thus facilitating stool expulsion [10,32].

The daily FOS dose varied between 6 g and 12 g according to the infants' weights. Infant formula containing 8 g/L of the galacto- and fructooligosaccharide mixture provides 6 g of prebiotic in 750 mL. Therefore, the dose of FOS used in the present study was similar to or higher than the amount that would be provided by regular daily intake of 750 mL of infant formula containing 8 g/L of the galacto- and fructooligosaccharide mixture. The supplemented FOS was well tolerated since only one infant presented two vomiting episodes during the first week of intervention. Mild flatulence and abdominal distension were observed in two FOS group patients; however, the treatment was continued. Therefore, the FOS supplementation was well tolerated, with mild adverse effects in few infants.

The limitations of the present study include the following. The sample may have been insufficient to demonstrate statistical significance for therapeutic success in the FOS and control groups. The therapeutic success observed in the FOS group (83.3%) was similar to the expected value (80%) used to estimate the sample size. The number of infants included in the trial complied with the calculated sample size; however, the proportion of constipated infants in the control group who had therapeutic success (55.6%) was much higher than the value (20%) used in the sample size estimate. The guidance for healthy eating for infants provided at the time of inclusion in the study and the substitution of cow's milk for infant formula in patients younger than 12 months likely had an effect on improving the constipation. This might also explain the high number of infants (26/75; 34.7%; Figure 1) who were not confirmed to have constipation after the first week of clinical observation (prior to randomization). The macronutrient intake, including dietary fiber, assessed by the 24-h food recall method was similar in the FOS and control groups before and at the end of the intervention. The dietary fiber intake (soluble and insoluble) varied between 6.5 and 7.4 g/day. The suggested daily intake of dietary fiber for this age group is 5–10 g [33]. Notably, neither the American Health Foundation [34] nor the Dietary Recommended Intake [35] recommend specific amounts of dietary fiber intake during the first year of life. Therefore, the quantity of macronutrients, including dietary fiber, consumed by the participants in this study may not explain the decreased constipation. Additionally, the type of milk consumed by all infants was changed at the beginning of the first week, corresponding to the baseline of the clinical trial. Most infants had been fed cow's milk containing added starch and sugar, which is a frequent feeding habit for infants in Brazil [36,37]. The change in infant formula or the use of fortified cow's milk in the correct dilution may explain the decreased constipation in the first week and in the control group during the intervention period. These results should not be extrapolated to severely constipated infants since this clinical trial did not include infants requiring other laxatives or fecal disimpaction.

5. Conclusions

In conclusion, the use of FOS in infants with constipation was associated with significant improvement in symptoms, but the results showed no statistical significance regarding the success of the therapy compared with the control group. However, the improved stool consistency, the reduced number of episodes of straining and/or difficulty passing stools and the reduced bowel transit time detected among the infants fed FOS are relevant findings that will contribute to preventing more severe constipation symptoms among constipated infants. Additional clinical trials assessing the effect of prebiotics on infant constipation are needed to confirm the results of this study and to provide data for a future meta-analysis.

Author Contributions: D.d.S.S. designed the study, performed the clinical study and data collection, performed data analysis and interpretation, wrote the first draft of the manuscript and revised the manuscript. S.T. designed the study, performed data analysis and revised the manuscript, T.K.W. designed the study, performed the clinical study, performed data analysis and interpretation, wrote the first draft of the manuscript and revised the manuscript. H.B.d.A.-F. contributed to sample analysis and review of the manuscript. M.B.d.M. designed the study, performed data analysis and interpretation, wrote the first draft of the manuscript and revised the manuscript. All authors meet the ICMJE criteria for authorship and have read and approved the final version of the manuscript.

Funding: This study and D.d.S.S. were supported by CNPq–Conselho Nacional de Desenvolvimento Científico e Tecnológico and CAPES–Coordenação de Aperfeiçoamento de Pessoal de Nível Superior.

Acknowledgments: FQM: Farmoquimica, Brazil supplied the active product (FOS) and placebo. No funder had any role in the study design, data collection, data analysis or interpretation, or writing of the manuscript.

Conflicts of Interest: The authors declare no conflict of interest.

References

1. Mugie, S.M.; Benninga, M.A.; Di Lorenzo, C. Epidemiology of constipation in children and adults: A systematic review. *Best Pract. Res. Clin. Gastroenterol.* **2011**, *25*, 3–18. [CrossRef] [PubMed]
2. Benninga, M.A.; Faure, C.; Hyman, P.E.; St James Roberts, I.; Schechter, N.L.; Nurko, S. Childhood functional gastrointestinal disorders: Neonate/Toddler. *Gastroenterology* **2016**, *150*. [CrossRef] [PubMed]
3. Tabbers, M.M.; DiLorenzo, C.; Berger, C.; Langendam, M.W.; Nurko, S.; Staiano, A.; Vandenplas, Y.; Benninga, M.A. Evaluation and treatment of functional constipation in infants and children: Evidence-based recommendations from ESPGHAN and NASPGHAN. *J. Pediatr. Gastroenterol. Nutr.* **2014**, *58*, 258–274. [CrossRef] [PubMed]
4. Loening-Baucke, V. Constipation in early childhood: Patient characteristics, treatment, and long-term follow up. *Gut* **1993**, *34*, 1400–1404. [CrossRef] [PubMed]
5. Aguirre, A.N.; Vitolo, M.R.; Puccini, R.F.; de Morais, M.B. Constipation in infants: Influence of type of feeding and dietary fiber intake. *J. Pediatr.* **2002**, *78*, 2002–2008. [CrossRef]
6. Agostoni, C.; Decsi, T.; Fewtrell, M.; Goulet, O.; Kolacek, S.; Koletzko, B.; Michaelson, K.F.; Moreno, L.; Puntis, J.; Rigo, J.; et al. Complementary feeding: A commentary by the ESPGHAN Committee on Nutrition. *J. Pediatr. Gastroenterol. Nutr.* **2008**, *46*, 99–110. [CrossRef] [PubMed]
7. Weaver, L.T.; Ewing, G.; Taylor, L.C. The bowel habit of milk-fed infants. *J. Pediatr. Gastroenterol. Nutr.* **1998**, *7*, 568–571. [CrossRef]
8. Tunc, V.T.; Camurdan, A.D.; Ilhan, M.N.; Sahin, F.; Beyazova, U. Factors associated with defecation patterns in 0–24 month-old children. *Eur. J. Pediatr.* **2008**, *167*, 1357–1362. [CrossRef] [PubMed]
9. Chen, X. Human milk oligosaccharides (HMOS): Structure, function, and enzyme-catalyzed synthesis. *Adv. Carbohydr. Chem. Biochem.* **2015**, *72*, 1013–1090. [CrossRef]
10. Scholtens, P.A.M.J.; Goossens, D.A.M.; Staiano, A. Stool characteristics of infants receiving short-chain galacto-oligosaccharides and long-chain fructooligosaccharides: A review. *World J. Gastroenterol.* **2014**, *20*, 13446–13452. [CrossRef] [PubMed]

11. Vandenplas, Y.; Abkar, A.; Bellaiche, M.; Benninga, M.; Chouraqui, J.P.; Çokura, F.; Harb, T.; Hegar, B.; Lifschitz, C.; Ludwig, T.; et al. Prevalence and health outcomes of functional gastrointestinal symptoms in infants from birth to 12 months of age. *J. Pediatr. Gastroenterol. Nutr.* **2015**, *61*, 531–537. [CrossRef] [PubMed]
12. Boehm, G.; Lidestri, M.; Casetta, P.; Jelinek, J.; Negretti, F.; Stahl, B.; Marini, A. Supplementation of a bovine milk formula with an oligosaccharide mixture increases counts of faecalbifidobacteria in preterm infants. *Arch. Dis. Child. Fetal Neonatal Ed.* **2002**, *86*, 178–181. [CrossRef]
13. Moro, G.; Minoli, I.; Mosca, M.; Fanaro, S.; Jelinek, J.; Stahl, B.; Boehm, G. Dosagerelated bifidogenic effects of galacto- and fructooligosaccharides in formula-fed term infants. *J. Pediatr. Gastroenterol. Nutr.* **2002**, *34*, 291–295. [CrossRef] [PubMed]
14. Moro, G.; Arslanoglu, S.; Stahl, B.; Jelinek, J.; Wahn, U.; Boehm, G. A mixture of prebiotic oligosaccharides reduces the incidence of atopic dermatitis during the first six months of age. *Arch. Dis. Child.* **2006**, *91*, 814–819. [CrossRef] [PubMed]
15. Costalos, C.; Kapiki, A.; Apostolou, M.; Papathoma, E. The effect of a prebiotic supplemented formula on growth and stool microbiology of term infants. *Early Hum. Dev.* **2008**, *84*, 45–49. [CrossRef] [PubMed]
16. Bisceglia, M.; Indrio, F.; Riezzo, G.; Poerio, V.; Corapi, U.; Raimondi, F. The effect of prebiotics in the management of neonatal hyperbilirubinaemia. *Acta Paediatr.* **2009**, *98*, 1579–1581. [CrossRef] [PubMed]
17. Veereman-Wauters, G.; Staelens, S.; Van de Broek, H.; Plaskie, K.; Wesling, F.; Roger, L.C.; McCartney, A.L.; Assam, P. Physiological and bifidogenic effects of prebiotic supplements in infant formulae. *J. Pediatr. Gastroenterol. Nutr.* **2011**, *52*, 763–771. [CrossRef] [PubMed]
18. Beleli, C.A.V.; Antonio, M.A.R.G.; Santos, R.; Pastore, G.M.; Lomazi, E.A. Effect of 4′ galactooligosaccharide on constipation symptoms. *J. Pediatr.* **2015**, *91*, 567–573. [CrossRef] [PubMed]
19. Schulz, K.F.; Altman, D.G.; Moher, D.; CONSORT Group. CONSORT 2010 statement: Updated guidelines for reporting parallel group randomised trials. *BMJ* **2010**, *340*, c332. [CrossRef] [PubMed]
20. Hyams, J.; Colleti, R.; Faure, C.; Gabriel-Martinez, E.; Maffei, H.V.; Morais, M.B.; Vandenplas, Y. Functional gastrointestinal disorders: Working group report of the first world congress of pediatric gastroenterology, hepatology and nutrition. *J. Pediatr. Gastroenterol. Nutr.* **2002**, *3*, 110–117. [CrossRef]
21. Maffei, H.V.L.; Vicentini, A.P. Prospective evaluation of dietary treatment in childhood constipation: High dietary fiber and wheat bran intake are associated with constipation amelioration. *J. Pediatr. Gastroenterol. Nutr.* **2011**, *52*, 55–59. [CrossRef] [PubMed]
22. Dimson, S.B. Carmine as an index of transit time in children with simple constipation. *Arch. Dis. Child.* **1970**, *45*, 232–235. [CrossRef] [PubMed]
23. Thompson, F.E.; Byers, T. Dietary assessment resource manual. *J. Nutr.* **1994**, *124*, 2245–2301. [CrossRef]
24. Núcleo de Estudos e Pesquisasem Alimentação (NEPA); UniversidadeEstadual de Campinas (UNICAMP). *Tabela Brasileira de Composição de Alimentos (TACO)*, 2nd ed.; UNICAMP: Campinas, Brazil, 2006; Available online: http://www.cfn.org.br/wp-content/uploads/2017/03/taco_4_edicao_ampliada_e_revisada.pdf (accessed on 30 October 2018).
25. Association of Official Analytical Chemists (AOAC). *Official Methods of Analysis of AOAC International*, 17th ed.; AOAC International: Gaithersburg, MD, USA, 2000.
26. World Health Organization (WHO). *Anthro Manual*, Version 3.2.2: Software for Assessing Growth and Development of the World's Children; 2011. Available online: http://www.who.int/childgrowth/software/en/ (accessed on 30 October 2018).
27. Rinttilä, T.; Kassinen, A.; Malinen, E.; Krogius, L.; Palva, A. Development of an extensive set of 16S rDNA-targeted primers for quantification of pathogenic and indigenous bacteria in faecal samples by real-time PCR. *J. Appl. Microbiol.* **2004**, *97*, 1166–1177. [CrossRef] [PubMed]
28. Langendijk, P.S.; Schut, F.; Jansen, G.J.; Raangs, G.C.; Kamphuis, G.R.; Wilkinson, M.H.; Welling, G.M. Quantitative fluorescence in situ hybridization of Bifidobacterium spp. with genus-specific 16S rRNA-targeted probes and its application in fecal samples. *Appl. Environ. Microbiol.* **1995**, *61*, 3069–3075. [PubMed]
29. De Araujo-Filho, H.B.; Carmo-Rodrigues, M.S.; Mello, C.S.; Melli, L.C.; Tahan, S.; Pignatari, A.C.; Morais, M.B. Children living near a sanitary landfill have increased breath methane and Methanobrevibactersmithii in their intestinal microbiota. *Archaea* **2014**, *2014*, 576249. [CrossRef] [PubMed]

30. Mello, C.S.; Rodrigues, M.S.D.C.; Araujo-Filho, H.B.A.; Melli, L.C.F.L.; Tahan, S.; Pignatari, A.C.C.; de Morais, M.B. Fecal microbiota analysis of children with small intestinal bacterial overgrowth among residents of an urban slum in Brazil. *J. Pediatr.* **2018**, *94*, 483–490. [CrossRef] [PubMed]
31. Mello, C.S.; Carmo-Rodrigues, M.S.; Araujo-Filho, H.B.; Melli, L.C.; Tahan, S.; Pignatari, A.C.; de Morais, M.B. Gut microbiota differences in children from distinct socioeconomic levels living in the same urban area in Brazil. *J. Pediatr. Gastroenterol. Nutr.* **2016**, *63*, 460–465. [CrossRef] [PubMed]
32. Vandenplas, Y.; Zakharova, I.; Dmitrieva, Y. Oligosaccharides in infant formula: More evidence to validate the role of prebiotics. *Br. J. Nutr.* **2015**, *113*, 1339–1344. [CrossRef] [PubMed]
33. Agostoni, C.; Riva, E.; Giovannini, M. Dietary fiber in weaning foods of young children. *Pediatrics* **1995**, *96*, 1002–1005. [PubMed]
34. Williams, C.L.; Bollella, M.; Wynder, E.L. A new recommendation for dietary fiber in childhood. *Pediatrics* **1995**, *96*, 985–988. [PubMed]
35. National Research Council (NRC). *Dietary Reference Intakes for Energy, Carbohydrate, Fiber, Fat, Fatty Acids, Cholesterol, Protein, and Amino Acids*; National Academy Press: Washington, DC, USA, 2002.
36. Morais, T.B.; Sigulem, D.M.; Maranhão, H.S.; de Morais, M.B. Bacterial contamination and nutrient content of home-prepared milk feeding bottles of infants attending a public outpatient clinic. *J. Trop. Pediatr.* **2005**, *51*, 87–92. [CrossRef] [PubMed]
37. Penna de Carvalho, M.F.; Morais, T.B.; de Morais, M.B. Home-made feeding bottles have inadequacies in their nutritional composition regardless of socioeconomic class. *J. Trop. Pediatr.* **2013**, *59*, 286–291. [CrossRef] [PubMed]

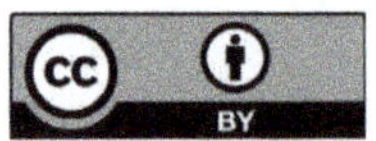

© 2018 by the authors. Licensee MDPI, Basel, Switzerland. This article is an open access article distributed under the terms and conditions of the Creative Commons Attribution (CC BY) license (http://creativecommons.org/licenses/by/4.0/).

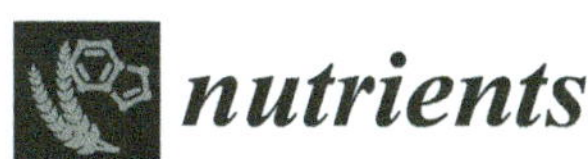

MDPI

Article

Efficacy of *Lactobacillus* Administration in School-Age Children with Asthma: A Randomized, Placebo-Controlled Trial

Chian-Feng Huang [1,2], Wei-Chu Chie [1] and I-Jen Wang [3,4,5,*]

1 Institute of Epidemiology and Preventive Medicine, College of Public Health, National Taiwan University, Taipei 10055, Taiwan; davidbee416@gmail.com (C.-F.H.); weichu@ntu.edu.tw (W.-C.C.)
2 Taoyuan Psychiatric Center, Ministry of Health and Welfare, Taoyuan 33058, Taiwan
3 Department of Pediatrics, Taipei Hospital, Ministry of Health and Welfare, No. 127, Su-Yuan Road, Hsin-Chuang Dist., Taipei 242, Taiwan
4 College of Public Health, China Medical University, Taichung 40402, Taiwan
5 School of Medicine, National Yang-Ming University, Taipei 112, Taiwan
* Correspondence: wij636@gmail.com; Tel.: +886-2-2276-5566 (ext.2532); Fax: +886-2-2998-8028

Received: 29 September 2018; Accepted: 29 October 2018; Published: 5 November 2018

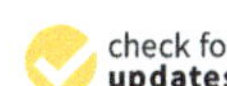

Abstract: Probiotics may have immunomodulatory effects. However, these effects in asthma remain unclear and warrant clinical trials. Here, we evaluated the effects of *Lactobacillus paracasei* (LP), *Lactobacillus fermentum* (LF), and their combination (LP + LF) on the clinical severity, immune biomarkers, and quality of life in children with asthma. This double-blind, prospective, randomized, placebo-controlled trial included 160 children with asthma aged 6–18 years (trial number: NCT01635738), randomized to receive LP, LF, LP + LF, or a placebo for 3 months. Their Global Initiative for Asthma–based asthma severity, Childhood Asthma Control Test (C-ACT) scores, Pediatric Asthma Severity Scores, Pediatric Asthma Quality of Life Questionnaire scores, peak expiratory flow rates (PEFRs), medication use, the levels of immune biomarkers (immunoglobulin E (IgE), interferon γ, interleukin 4, and tumor necrosis factor α) at different visits, and the associated changes were evaluated. Compared with the placebo group by generalized estimating equation model, children receiving LP, LF, and LP + LF had lower asthma severity ($p = 0.024$, 0.038, and 0.007, respectively) but higher C-ACT scores ($p = 0.005$, < 0.001, and < 0.001, respectively). The LP + LF group demonstrated increased PEFR ($p < 0.01$) and decreased IgE levels ($p < 0.05$). LP, LF, or their combination (LP + LF) can aid clinical improvement in children with asthma.

Keywords: *Lactobacillus*; probiotics; asthma; Childhood Asthma Control Test; peak expiratory flow rate; immunoglobulin E

1. Introduction

Asthma, a chronic complex disease of the airways, is characterized by reversible airflow obstruction, bronchial hyperresponsiveness, and underlying inflammation [1]. The prevalence of asthma has increased in the past decades. A potential mechanism underlying this high prevalence is the microbial hypothesis [2], which argues that less microbial exposure upregulates the cytokine production of T-helper cell type 2 (Th2), leading to an increase in allergic diseases. According to this hypothesis, probiotic administration is an alternative treatment for atopic disease, which when administered in adequate amounts, can confer a health benefit to the host [3]. The researchers found that probiotics have some health effects in atopic disease patients through immunity balancing of T-helper cell type 1 (Th1) and Th2, particularly in those with atopic dermatitis (AD). However, relevant studies focusing on asthma patients are limited.

A meta-analysis found that, although perinatal and early-life probiotic administration reduces atopic sensitization risk and total immunoglobulin E (IgE) levels in children, it may not reduce their asthma risk [4]. However, some studies have reported the benefit of using probiotics, in addition to standard care, for treating children with asthma. A randomized, placebo-controlled trial for 7-week *Enterococcus faecalis* treatment demonstrated decreased peak flow variability in children with asthma [5]. Lee et al. also reported significant improvements in the pulmonary function of children with asthma after a regimen of vegetable, fish oil, and fruit supplementation along with probiotic administration [6]. However, these aforementioned studies were designed as mixed interventions with relatively small sample sizes.

In the present study, we thus included participants representing a population of school-age children with asthma randomized to receive pure strains of *Lactobacillus paracasei* GMNL-133 (BCRC 910520, CCTCC M2011331) (LP), *Lactobacillus fermentum* GM-090 (BCRC 910259, CCTCC M204055) (LF), or their mixture (LP + LF). We focused on the therapeutic effects of the probiotics on the disease severity, quality of life, immune biomarkers, and fecal microbial composition in school-age children with asthma.

2. Materials and Methods

2.1. Participants

This double-blind, randomized, placebo-controlled trial was conducted between December 2011 and September 2013 at the pediatric outpatient clinics of Taipei Hospital, Ministry of Health and Welfare. The inclusion criteria were 6–18 years of age with a history of intermittent to moderate persistent asthma (Global Initiative for Asthma (GINA) steps 1–3) for at least 1 year. We excluded children who had received immunosuppressants, antibiotics, systemic corticosteroids, or antimycotics within 4 weeks before study enrolment or antihistamines within 3 days before study enrolment. The children who had an immunodeficiency disease, other major medical problems, or used probiotic preparations within 4 weeks before study enrolment were also excluded. We acquired written informed consent from all the parents in compliance with the principles of the Helsinki Declaration. The Taipei hospital's Institutional Review Board ratified the study protocol (TH-IRB-10-14). The study was registered under trial number NCT01635738.

2.2. Protocol

An investigator enrolled the children and sequentially assigned them a patient number associated with a code. Capsules were prepared and coded by GenMont Biotech Inc. (in their Current Good Manufacturing Practice–certified facilities, Tainan, Taiwan) and dispensed by a study nurse. The children were randomized using computer-generated 4-block design lists created by a statistician, with stratification according to age, sex, severity, and current medication use. We assessed the eligibility of 160 recruited children and randomly allocated them to four groups, with 40 participants in each group (Figure 1). The groups were then randomized to receive LP, LF, LP + LF, or placebo for 3 months. All the investigators, study nurses, and participants were blinded to treatment assignment over the study duration. A capsule count was performed monthly to ensure that the capsules were taken as applicable. Randomization code was deciphered only at the end of the trial.

2.3. Outcome Measures

The primary outcome was the changes in asthma severity and Childhood Asthma Control Test (C-ACT) scores over 3 months of the intervention compared with baseline. At baseline and follow-up visits at 0, 1, 2, 3, and 4 months of intervention, we determined GINA-based asthma severity and recorded C-ACT scores, Pediatric Asthma Quality of Life Questionnaire (PAQLQ) scores, Pediatric Asthma Severity Scores (PASSs), peak expiratory flow rates (PEFRs), and medication use. Skin prick test and blood serum analysis were performed at 0 and 3 months of intervention. In addition, fecal microbial analysis was performed for comprehensive evaluation before and after the 3-month treatment course. The changes in PAQLQ score, PASS, PEFR, skin prick test reactivity, serum immune biomarker levels, and fecal probiotic microbial composition were the secondary outcomes (Figure 2).

2.4. Laboratory Methods

Skin prick tests using commercial extracts were performed to detect asthma-causing allergens, including mite, cockroach, animal dander, egg, milk, and crab allergens [7]. The levels of IgE and other serum immune biomarkers, such as interferon (IFN) γ, interleukin (IL) 4, and tumor necrosis factor (TNF) α, were measured through enzyme-linked immunosorbent assay [8]. Specific intestinal bacterial strains in the feces were quantified using conventional culture techniques [9].

2.5. Sample Size Estimation

Using nQuery Advisor + nTerim 3.0 (Statistical Solutions Ltd., Cork, Ireland), we calculated the number of participants required to detect the presence of any significant differences in C-ACT scores. According to previous data [10], to detect significant differences in the effects of probiotics on C-ACT scores with 90% power and a 5% significance level, each study group must include at least 22 participants. To allow for a 20% loss from ineligibility or withdrawal, we decided to enroll 30 children in each group. After power assessment, we estimated that 120 total participants would suffice and thus scheduled recruitment of 160 children.

2.6. Statistical Analysis

The baseline demographic data of the four groups were compared using analysis of variance. Intragroup comparisons for severity, C-ACT scores, PASSs, PAQLQ scores, and immune biomarker levels at baseline and 3 months of treatment were performed using the paired t test. Differences in outcome variables between the treatment and placebo groups over the five visits were evaluated using a generalized estimating equation (GEE) model after adjustment for potential confounders. All children who completed the study were included in the analysis, regardless of their compliance. All reasons for dropouts or premature withdrawal from the study as well as missing values were recorded. Significance was set at a two-tailed α at 0.05, and all analyses were performed on SPSS (version 21).

3. Result

3.1. Baseline Characteristics of Participants

Of 160 recruited children, 152 were finally enrolled and randomly assigned to receive LP, LF, LP + LF, or placebo. Figure 1 shows the relevant patient consort diagram, and Table 1 presents the baseline demographic characteristics of 147 children who completed the entire evaluation. The randomization process ensured adequate comparability between the treatment and placebo groups. No statistically significant differences were observed for any demographic, clinical, or functional variables. Moreover, the clinical manifestation of asthma was similar between the two groups. No significant differences were observed in the severity, total serum IgE level, the rate of sensitization to various allergens, the PEFR, or other parameters between the groups at baseline (Table 2).

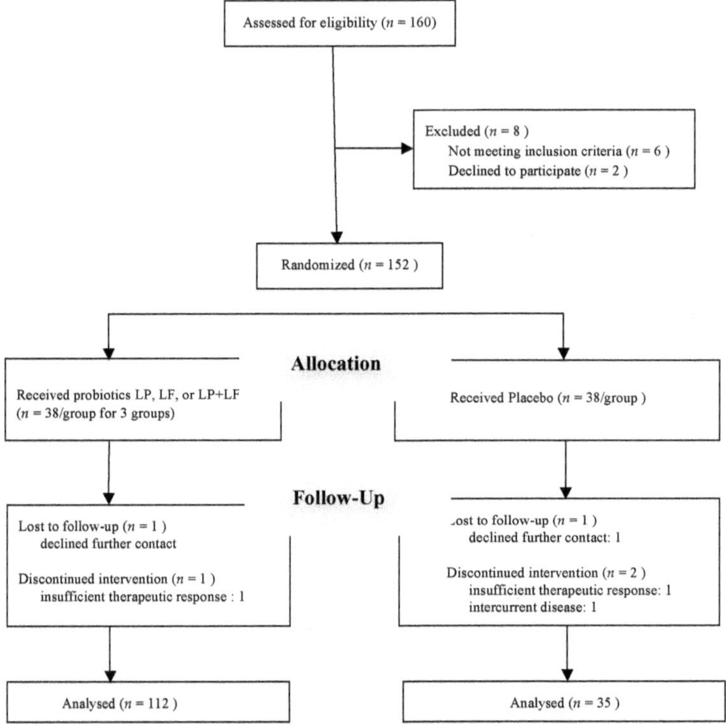

Figure 1. Consort diagram.

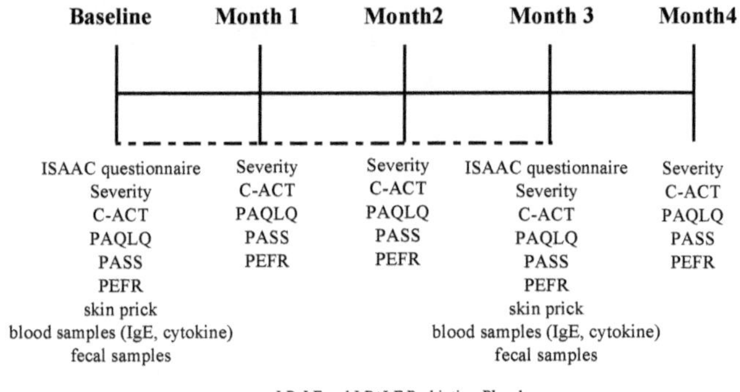

Figure 2. Study protocol.

Table 1. Baseline demographic characteristics of study participants (N = 147).

Characteristics	LP (n = 38)	LF (n = 38)	LP + LF (n = 36)	Placebo Group (n = 35)
Male, N (%)	22 (57.9)	24 (63.2)	19 (52.8)	18 (51.4)
Age (years), Mean (SD)	7.68 (2.21)	7.37 (2.34)	7.00 (1.79)	7.86 (2.50)
Height (cm), Mean (SD)	121.24 (18.49)	117.81 (17.21)	117.51 (15.89)	122.23 (18.94)
Weight (Kg), Mean (SD)	26.45 (10.08)	25.14 (10.16)	24.75 (10.29)	26.30 (11.76)
IgE (kU/I), Mean (SD)	611.26 (511.83)	600.23 (739.18)	748.22 (896.40)	493.06 (773.52)
Combine with allergic rhinitis (AR), N (%)	31 (81.6)	31 (81.6)	32 (88.9)	28 (80.0)
Combine with atopic dermatitis (AD), N (%)	15 (39.5)	10 (26.3)	11 (30.6)	9 (25.7)

Table 1. *Cont.*

Characteristics	LP (*n* = 38)	LF (*n* = 38)	LP + LF (*n* = 36)	Placebo Group (*n* = 35)
Allergic sensitization, *N* (%)				
Mite	33 (86.8)	32 (84.2)	30 (83.3)	29 (82.9)
Cockroach	3 (7.9)	2 (5.3)	1 (2.8)	0 (0)
Animal dander	2 (5.3)	2 (5.3)	1 (2.8)	1 (2.9)
Milk	2 (5.3)	3 (7.9)	1 (2.8)	0 (0)
Egg	2 (5.3)	2 (5.3)	1 (2.8)	1 (2.9)
Crab	2 (5.3)	3 (7.9)	1 (2.8)	0 (0)
Maternal history of atopic disease, *N* (%)	21 (55.3)	22 (57.9)	12 (33.3)	15 (42.9)
Paternal history of atopic disease, *N* (%)	21 (55.3)	21 (55.3)	20 (55.6)	17 (48.6)

LP, *Lactobacillus paracasei*; LF, *Lactobacillus fermentum*.

Table 2. Subscale measures at baseline (N = 147).

Subscale	LP (*n* = 38) Mean (SD)	LF (*n* = 38) Mean (SD)	LP + LF (*n* = 36) Mean (SD)	Placebo (*n* = 35) Mean (SD)	*p*-Value 4 Groups
Severity	2.16 (0.64)	2.13 (0.62)	2.28 (0.62)	2.20 (0.58)	0.757
C-ACT	19.89 (4.28)	17.87 (5.54)	19.81 (4.72)	20.77 (4.75)	0.074
PAQLQ	5.44 (1.17)	5.40 (1.41)	5.90 (0.85)	5.58 (1.16)	0.268
PASS	16.84 (5.27)	16.29 (5.79)	15.71 (4.85)	15.60 (5.16)	0.738
IFN-γ (ng/uL)	170.73 (188.44)	150.75 (158.12)	156.97 (167.18)	145.28 (162.26)	0.954
IL-4 (ng/uL)	36.05 (29.63)	48.48 (85.06)	61.10 (117.67)	55.38 (86.94)	0.773
TNF-α (ng/uL)	292.95 (425.14)	324.71 (512.82)	231.88 (187.97)	207.51 (340.37)	0.690
IgE (kU/I)	611.26 (511.83)	600.23 (739.18)	748.22 (896.40)	493.06 (773.52)	0.547
Fecal cell count Log10 (CFU/g)					
Lactobacillus	8.07 (0.87)	7.90 (0.95)	7.49 (1.15)	7.71 (0.92)	0.101
Bifidobacterium	8.81 (0.91)	8.74 (0.85)	8.75 (1.12)	8.90 (0.72)	0.872
Clostridium	7.19 (0.78)	6.63 (1.09)	6.84 (1.18)	6.79 (1.11)	0.133

LP, *Lactobacillus paracasei*; LF, *Lactobacillus fermentum*; C-ACT, Childhood Asthma Control Test; PAQLQ, Pediatric Asthma Quality of Life Questionnaire; PASS, Pediatric Asthma Severity Scores.

3.2. *Effects of Probiotics on Severity of Asthma and Quality of Life*

Significant intragroup differences were detected in C-ACT scores, the primary outcome, in all groups, except the placebo group (Figure 3). Compared with the placebo group, both asthma severity and C-ACT scores significantly improved in the LP, LF, and LP + LF groups according to our age- and sex-adjusted GEE model (Table 3). No significant difference was noted on both asthma severity and C-ACT scores between the LP + LF and the LP and LF groups, respectively. The PAQLQ scores and PASSs demonstrated no significant group-by-time effects. In the LP + LF group, PEFRs improved significantly ($p < 0.01$).

Table 3. The p values and effect sizes (β) compared with the placebo group (n = 35) using a generalized estimating equation model.

Measure	LP Group (*n* = 38)		LF Group (*n* = 38)		LP + LF Group (*n* = 36)	
	β (95% CI)	*P* Value	β (95% CI)	*P* Value	β (95% CI)	*P* Value
Severity	−0.34 (−0.63, −0.04)	0.024 *	−0.30 (−0.59, −0.02)	0.038 *	−0.43 (−0.74, −0.12)	0.007 *
C-ACT	3.13 (−0.95, 5.31)	0.005 *	4.54 (2.44, 6.65)	< 0.001 *	3.83 (1.78, 5.89)	< 0.001 *
PAQLQ	−0.32 (−0.86, 0.23)	0.256	−0.30 (−0.89, 0.28)	0.310	−0.43 (−0.96, 0.09)	0.104
PASS	−1.39 (−4.09, 1.30)	0.311	−1.14 (−3.79, 1.51)	0.400	−0.48 (−3.17, 2.20)	0.725
PEFR	8.77 (−11.74, 29.27)	0.402	28.83 (−3.55, 61.21)	0.081	33.81 (8.62, 59.00)	0.009 *

Adjusted for age and sex, * $p < 0.05$. LP, *Lactobacillus paracasei*; LF, *Lactobacillus fermentum*; C-ACT, Childhood Asthma Control Test; PAQLQ, Pediatric Asthma Quality of Life Questionnaire; PASS, Pediatric Asthma Severity Scores; PEFR, peak expiratory flow rate.

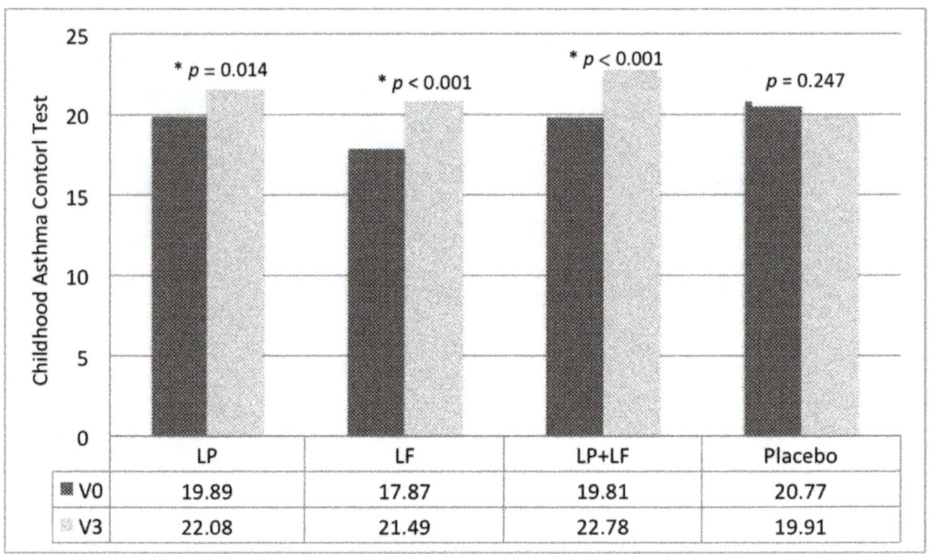

Figure 3. Intragroup differences in Childhood Asthma Control Test scores. * $p < 0.05$.

3.3. Effects of Probiotics on Sensitization and Immune Biomarker Levels

At the end of treatment, the total serum IgE levels significantly decreased only in the LP + LF group ($p < 0.05$; Table 4). Nevertheless, among all groups, significant intragroup differences, but no intergroup differences, were noted in the skin prick test reactivity to mite allergens. However, no such significant differences were noted for other allergens between before and after the intervention (Table S1). Moreover, serum IFN-γ, IL-4, and TNF-α levels did not demonstrate any significant changes (Table 4).

Table 4. Immune biomarker levels at baseline and subsequent changes ($N = 147$).

Subscale	Examination	LP ($n = 38$) Mean (SD)	LF ($n = 38$) Mean (SD)	LP + LF ($n = 36$) Mean (SD)	Placebo Group($n = 35$) Mean (SD)	p-Value 4 Groups
IgE	Baseline	611.26 (511.83)	600.23 (739.18)	748.22 (896.40)	493.06 (773.52)	0.547
(kU/I)	month 3	482.42 (371.68)	496.40 (622.51)	377.29 (268.51) *	577.81 (705.94)	0.448
IFN-γ	Baseline	170.73 (188.44)	150.75 (158.12)	156.97 (167.18)	145.28 (162.26)	0.954
(ng/uL)	month 3	158.01 (164.61)	182.75 (373.50)	221.41 (426.21)	166.21 (197.61)	0.886
IL-4	Baseline	36.05 (29.63)	48.4 (85.06)	61.10 (117.67)	55.38 (86.94)	0.773
(ng/uL)	month 3	51.16 (85.33)	49.58 (67.82)	55.09 (109.40)	104.13 (215.39)	0.366
TNF-α	Baseline	292.95 (425.14)	324.71 (512.82)	231.88 (187.97)	207.51 (340.37)	0.690
(ng/uL)	month 3	315.23 (625.85)	777.92 (1731.71)	584.30 (959.98)	550.48 (1059.83)	0.514

LP, *Lactobacillus paracasei*; LF, *Lactobacillus fermentum*. * $p < 0.05$ (Intragroup comparisons).

3.4. Fecal Microbial Composition, Rescue Medication Use and Compliance

All intervention groups showed lower counts of *Clostridium* than did the placebo group. However, these intergroup differences were nonsignificant (Table S2). The frequencies of oral steroid (Table S3), bronchodilator (Table S4), and antihistamine use (Table S5) demonstrated no significant intergroup differences. The compliance of each group is more than 93% without intergroup differences (Table S6).

4. Discussion

The present study effectively resolves the debate regarding whether pure probiotics are beneficial to children with asthma. Using a GEE model, we found that LP, LF, and LP + LF interventions along with standard asthma therapy effectively reduced asthma severity and increased C-ACT scores. Furthermore, LP + LF increased both serum IgE levels and PEFRs, implying the existence of a dose-dependent effect.

Consistent with the present study results, a randomized clinical trial by Chen et al. [10] revealed the beneficial effects of probiotics on the severity of asthma and clinical symptoms, but they included participants with asthma accompanied by persistent allergic rhinitis. By contrast, studies have demonstrated the significant effects of various probiotics on some parameters of asthma, but not on its clinical severity, in children with asthma [11,12]. In addition to probiotics containing a single bacterial strain, the clinical advantage of applying a mixture of bacterial strains [13] or using mixed therapy that includes a probiotic regimen [6] has been demonstrated in asthma patients. The reasons for inconsistencies in the aforementioned results may be the variabilities in genetic backgrounds, disease severity, culture, and diet of the participants; moreover, the differences in the study designs, mixed regimens, and strain doses and combinations may also affect the results because the effects of probiotics are strain-specific [14].

We selected LP for this trial because it previously demonstrated beneficial effects in airway hypersensitivity patients [15]. Moreover, it can inhibit related Th2 cytokine production and rebalance the Th1/Th2 immune response by increasing IFN-γ levels, as noted in murine bronchoalveolar lavage samples [16]. We also used LF, which can increase IFN-γ levels in patients with AD [17] and ameliorate oxidative damage, food allergies, and food-derived infections [18,19]. The present study is the first one in a clinical setting that compared the effects of both single- and mixed-strain probiotics.

Regarding the effects on serum immune biomarker levels, a clinical trial applied single-strain *Lactobacillus gasseri* A5 probiotics to school children with asthma and allergic rhinitis and reported a nonsignificant reduction in total IgE levels [10]. In the current study, the administration of LF + LP was associated with a significant decrease in IgE levels, while the administration of LP or LF alone showed a tendency to decrease IgE levels, albeit without reaching statistical significance. Similarly, the significant decrease was noted in PEFRs in the LP + LF group. These results may be explained by the synergistic interactions or dose-dependent effects, which were also noted in other probiotic-related trials [20,21]; however, the mechanisms underlying these effects remain unclear.

Studies reporting intragroup differences in the effects of probiotics on IgE levels in children with asthma are limited [22]. However, the significance of probiotic-elicited reduction in IgE levels in children with AD has been reported by several studies [23]. Notably, studies have also revealed that, in addition to regulating IgE levels, probiotics can regulate cytokine levels in patients with AD. For instance, in some AD studies [24,25], probiotics significantly reduced serum IL-4 levels, which were compatible with less Th2 responses. However, such cytokine-related findings in the context of asthma are required. The few studies mentioning the related measurement lack consistency in results [10,22].

Notably, based on the preceding comparison of different allergic diseases, gastrointestinal probiotic administration is more efficient at alleviating AD than at alleviating respiratory tract allergic diseases, namely, asthma and allergic rhinitis. Furthermore, the sensitization pattern for asthma allergens, as observed in the current study using the skin prick test, was also different from that for AD allergens. Consistent with previous studies, mites are the predominant aeroallergen of asthma [26–28]. We noted significant postintervention changes in mite sensitization among all groups; however, no intergroup differences were observed. Due to the difference between AD and respiratory tract allergic diseases, it might be useful to consider an alternative method for probiotic administration in children with asthma, such as the intranasal route, which demonstrated effective results in a murine model [29]; however, related human studies are warranted.

Considering the pathogenesis, asthma might be viewed as atopic processes later in life, implying a more systemic level. A review article summarized current experimental data and gave the interpretation of the allergy march; epidermal barrier dysfunction in early life was found to initiate systemic sensitization, which later facilitates the further development of asthma and allergic rhinitis [30]. Another longitudinal study suggested that children with early atopic AD have higher risk of asthma than do those with nonatopic AD [31]. Therefore, the administration of a high probiotic dose, probiotic strain mixture, or mixed therapy including probiotics appears suitable for children with asthma compared to other atopic disease; this inference is partly supported by previous trials [6,13].

Regarding fecal intestinal microbiota, the numbers of *Lactobacillus*, *Bifidobacterium*, and *Clostridium* before and after intervention demonstrated no intergroup differences among all four groups. The LP + LF group demonstrated a tendency to elevate the fecal colony counts of *Lactobacillus* and *Bifidobacterium* compared to the placebo group, but without reaching statistical significance. It may be explained by the dose-dependent effect: only the combination group received adequate probiotics against consumption. In addition to *Lactobacillus*, we analyzed the numbers of *Bifidobacterium* and *Clostridium* because asthma is associated with a higher amount of *Clostridium* [32] and a lower level of *Bifidobacterium* [33] in previous studies, respectively. We found the numbers of *Clostridium* in LP group tended to decrease after intervention, but without reaching statistical significance. This was probably because *Lactobacillus* reestablished gut microbiota, as suggested by Durack et al. [34]. The authors asserted that *Lactobacillus* supplements may recompose gut microbiota, thus preventing atopy and asthma. Furthermore, decreases in *Clostridium* counts may facilitate colonization by other microorganisms, thus increasing the gut microbial diversity, potentially another protective factor against asthma [35].

This study has some limitations. First, the children with asthma continued receiving standard therapy along with the probiotics, impeding the potential delineation of the effects of probiotics alone. However, the interference is ethical and unavoidable. Moreover, no group differences were noted in oral steroid or bronchodilator use between before and after the intervention. Additionally, these treatments may mask the therapeutic effects of probiotics, which make the results toward the null and strengthen our positive finding. Second, the compliance of the children was another concern. To ensure compliance, we used the capsule counting method rather than the patient record method; this method was easier and less expensive than detection of the study probiotic strains in the feces. Finally, some confounders, including selection bias, host factors (e.g., genetic backgrounds and original microbiota), and environmental factors (e.g., diet and lifestyle) existed. To mitigate this limitation, randomization was performed.

Nevertheless, our study has several strengths: relatively large sample size, comprehensive outcome measures (including C-ACT scores, PAQLQ scores, PASSs, and skin prick testing), and longitudinal repeated measures. We collected different types of data, specifically various serum biomarker levels and fecal microbial compositions. Moreover, a novelty of our study was that we combined two probiotic strains (LP + LF) and noted superior effects in lowering IgE and elevating PEFR than single stain alone. This topic can provide pediatricians, immunologists, and other health care professionals evidence of *Lactobacillus* administration for childhood asthma. Furthermore, it can also inspire public health experts.

5. Conclusions

Our study supports that *Lactobacillus* is beneficial to children with asthma. We found that both LP and LF can reduce asthma severity and improve asthma control in school-age children. The combination of LP plus LF appears to be more effective in childhood asthma than either LP or LF alone. LP, LF, and their combination were well tolerated with fair compliance and without adverse effects reported.

Supplementary Materials: The following are available online at http://www.mdpi.com/2072-6643/10/11/1678/s1, Table S1: Skin prick test reactivity, Table S2: Fecal bacterial colony counts, Table S3: Oral steroid use frequency at baseline and during follow-up visits, Table S4: Oral bronchodilator use frequency at baseline and during follow-up visits, Table S5: Oral anti-histamine use frequency at baseline examination and on follow-up visits, Table S6: Probiotics capsules mean taken days monthly record.

Author Contributions: C.-F.H. analyzed and interpreted the data, and wrote the manuscript. W.-C.C. interpreted the data and revised the manuscript. I.-J.W. collected, analyzed, and interpreted the data. I.-J.W. designed the research and revised the manuscript. All authors read and approved the final manuscript.

Funding: This study was supported by funding from the GenMont Biotec Inc. and by the grants from the National Science Council (NSC 97-2314-B-192-001-MY2) in Taiwan.

Acknowledgments: We thank Miss Ya-Hui Chen and Mr Yi-Hsing Chen for help in the laboratory analysis and related working staff for clinical examination and data collection.

Conflicts of Interest: The Taipei Hospital, the Ministry of Health and Welfare Authority, has a contract with GenMont Biotec Inc. whereby GenMont Biotec Inc. provided the study costs for probiotics. The authors declare no conflict of interest.

References

1. Shifren, A.; Witt, C.; Christie, C.; Castro, M. Mechanisms of remodeling in asthmatic airways. *J. Allergy (Cairo)* **2012**, *2012*. [CrossRef] [PubMed]
2. Kim, H.J.; Kim, H.Y.; Lee, S.Y.; Seo, J.H.; Lee, E.; Hong, S.J. Clinical efficacy and mechanism of probiotics in allergic diseases. *Korean J. Pediatr.* **2013**, *56*, 369–376. [CrossRef] [PubMed]
3. Schlundt, J. *Report of a Joint FAO/WHO Expert Consultation on Evaluation of Health and Nutritional Properties of Probiotics in Food Including Powder Milk with Live Lactic Acid Bacteria*; Food and Agriculture Organization of the United Nations: Córdoba, Argentina, 2001.
4. Ta, V.; Laubach, S. Probiotic administration in early life, atopy, and asthma: A Meta-analysis of clinical trials. *Pediatrics* **2013**, *132*, e666–e676. [CrossRef] [PubMed]
5. Stockert, K.; Schneider, B.; Porenta, G.; Rath, R.; Nissel, H.; Eichler, I. Laser acupuncture and probiotics in school age children with asthma: A randomized, placebo-controlled pilot study of therapy guided by principles of Traditional Chinese Medicine. *Pedriatr. Allergy Immunol.* **2007**, *18*, 160–166. [CrossRef] [PubMed]
6. Lee, S.C.; Yang, Y.H.; Chuang, S.Y.; Huang, S.Y.; Pan, W.H. Reduced medication use and improved pulmonary function with supplements containing vegetable and fruit concentrate, fish oil and probiotics in asthmatic school children: A randomised controlled trial. *Br. J. Nutr.* **2013**, *110*, 145–155. [CrossRef] [PubMed]
7. Duotip-Test®II Package Insert. Available online: https://www.penallergytest.com/wp-content/uploads/Duo-Tip-2-Package-Insert.pdf (accessed on 16 September 2018).
8. Shyur, S.-D.; Jan, R.-L.; Webster, J.R.; Chang, P.; Lu, Y.J.; Wang, J.Y. Determination of multiple allergen-specific IgE by microfluidic immunoassay cartridge in clinical settings. *Pediatr. Allergy Immunol.* **2010**, *21*, 623–633. [CrossRef] [PubMed]
9. Tsai, C.C.; Chiu, T.H.; Ho, C.Y.; Lin, P.P.; Wu, T.Y. Effects of anti-hypertension and intestinal micro-flora of spontaneously hypertensive rats fed gammaaminobutyric acid-enriched Chingshey purple sweet potato fermented milk by lactic acid bacteria. *Afr. J. Microbiol. Res.* **2013**, *7*, 932–940.
10. Chen, Y.S.; Jan, R.L.; Lin, Y.L.; Chen, H.H.; Wang, J.Y. Randomized placebo-controlled trial of lactobacillus on asthmatic children with allergic rhinitis. *Pediatr. Pulmonol.* **2010**, *45*, 1111–1120. [CrossRef] [PubMed]
11. Miraglia Del Giudice, M.; Maiello, N.; Decimo, F.; Fusco, N.; D'Agostino, B.; Sullo, N.; Capasso, M.; Salpietro, V.; Gitto, E.; Ciprandi, G.; et al. Airways allergic inflammation and *L. reuterii* treatment in asthmatic children. *J. Biol. Regul. Homeost. Agents* **2012**, *26*, S35–S40. [PubMed]
12. Giovannini, M.; Agostoni, C.; Riva, E.; Salvini, F.; Ruscitto, A.; Zuccotti, G.V.; Radaelli, G. A randomized prospective double blind controlled trial on effects of long-term consumption of fermented milk containing lactobacillus casei in pre-school children with allergic asthma and/or rhinitis. *Pediatr. Res.* **2007**, *62*, 215–220. [CrossRef] [PubMed]
13. Miraglia Del Giudice, M.; Indolfi, C.; Capasso, M.; Maiello, N.; Decimo, F.; Ciprandi, G. Bifidobacterium mixture (B longum BB536, B infantis M-63, B breve M-16V) treatment in children with seasonal allergic rhinitis and intermittent asthma. *Ital. J. Pediatr.* **2017**, *43*. [CrossRef] [PubMed]
14. Wickens, K.; Black, P.N.; Stanley, T.V.; Mitchell, E.; Fitzharris, P.; Tannock, G.W.; Purdie, G.; Crane, J. A differential effect of 2 probiotics in the prevention of eczema and atopy: A double-blind, randomized, placebo-controlled trial. *J. Allergy Clin. Immunol.* **2008**, *122*, 788–794. [CrossRef] [PubMed]
15. Fujiwara, D.; Wakabayashi, H.; Watanabe, H. A double blind trial of Lactobacillus paracasei strain KW3110 administration for immunomodulation in patients with pollen allergy. *Allergol. Int.* **2005**, *54*, 143–149. [CrossRef]

16. Wang, X.; Hui, Y.; Zhao, L.; Hao, Y.; Guo, H.; Ren, F. Oral administration of lactobacillus paracasei 19 attenuates PM2.5-induced enhancement of airway hyperresponsiveness and allergic airway response in murine model of asthma. *PLoS ONE* **2017**, *12*. [CrossRef] [PubMed]
17. Prescott, S.L.; Dunstan, J.A.; Hale, J.; Breckler, L.; Lehmann, H.; Weston, S. Clinical effects of probiotics are associated with increased interferon-gamma responses in very young children with atopic dermatitis. *Clin. Exp. Allergy* **2005**, *35*, 1557–1564. [CrossRef] [PubMed]
18. El-Ghaish, S.; Rabesona, H.; Choiset, Y.; Sitohy, M.; Haertle, T.; Chobert, J.M. Proteolysis by Lactobacillus fermentum IFO3956 isolated from Egyptian milk products decreases immuno-reactivity of αS1-casein. *J. Dairy Res.* **2011**, *78*, 203–210. [CrossRef] [PubMed]
19. Mikelsaar, M.; Zilmer, M. Lactobacillus fermentum ME-3 an antimicrobial and antioxidative probiotic. *Microb. Ecol. Health Dis.* **2009**, *21*, 1–27. [CrossRef] [PubMed]
20. Chang, Y.S.; Trivedi, M.K.; Jha, A.; Lin, Y.F.; Dimaano, L.; Garcia-Romero, M.T. Synbiotics for prevention and treatment of atopic dermatitis: a meta-analysis of randomized clinical trials. *JAMA Pediatr.* **2016**, *170*, 236–242. [CrossRef] [PubMed]
21. Szulińska, M.; Łoniewski, I.; van Hemert, S.; Sobieska, M.; Bogdański, P. Dose-dependent effects of multispecies probiotic supplementation on the lipopolysaccharide (LPS) level and cardiometabolic profile in obese postmenopausal women: A 12-week randomized clinical trial. *Nutrients* **2018**, *10*, 773. [CrossRef] [PubMed]
22. Lin, J.; Zhang, Y.; He, C.; Dai, J. Probiotics supplementation in children with asthma: A systematic review and meta-analysis. *J. Paediatr. Child Health* **2018**, *54*, 953–961. [CrossRef] [PubMed]
23. Kim, S.O.; Ah, Y.M.; Yu, Y.M.; Choi, K.H.; Shin, W.G.; Lee, J.Y. Effects of probiotics for the treatment of atopic dermatitis: A meta-analysis of randomized controlled trials. *Ann. Allergy Asthma Immunol.* **2014**, *113*, 217–226. [CrossRef] [PubMed]
24. Wang, I.J.; Wang, J.Y. Children with atopic dermatitis show clinical improvement after Lactobacillus exposure. *Clin. Exp. Allergy* **2015**, *45*, 779–787. [CrossRef] [PubMed]
25. Prakoeswa, C.R.; Herwanto, N.; Prameswari, R.; Astari, L.; Sawitri, S.; Hidayati, A.N.; Indramaya, D.M.; Kusumowidagdo, E.R.; Surono, I.S. Lactobacillus plantarum IS-10506 supplementation reduced SCORAD in children with atopic dermatitis. *Benef. Microbes* **2017**, *8*, 833–840. [CrossRef] [PubMed]
26. Oncham, S.; Udomsubpayakul, U.; Laisuan, W. Skin prick test reactivity to aeroallergens in adult allergy clinic in Thailand: A 12-year retrospective study. *Asia Pac. Allergy* **2018**, *8*. [CrossRef] [PubMed]
27. Arshad, S.H.; Tariq, S.M.; Matthews, S.; Hakim, E. Sensitization to common allergens and its association with allergic disorders at age 4 years: A whole population birth cohort study. *Pediatrics* **2001**, *108*. [CrossRef]
28. Vidal, C.; Lojo, S.; Juangorena, M.; Gonzalez-Quintela, A. Association between asthma and sensitization to allergens of Dermatophagoides pteronyssinus. *J. Investig. Allergol. Clin. Immunol.* **2016**, *26*, 304–309. [CrossRef] [PubMed]
29. Spacova, I.; Petrova, M.; Fremau, A.; Pollaris, L.; Vanoirbeek, J.; Ceuppens, J.L.; Seys, S.; Lebeer, S. Intranasal administration of probiotic Lactobacillus rhamnosus GG prevents birch pollen-induced allergic asthma in a murine model. *Allergy* **2018**. [CrossRef] [PubMed]
30. Spergel, J.M. From atopic dermatitis to asthma: The atopic march. *Ann. Allergy Asthma Immunol.* **2010**, *105*, 99–106. [CrossRef] [PubMed]
31. Novembre, E.; Cianferoni, A.; Lombardi, E.; Bernardini, R.; Pucci, N.; Vierucci, A. Natural history of "intrinsic" atopic dermatitis. *Allergy* **2001**, *56*, 452–453. [CrossRef] [PubMed]
32. Stiemsma, L.T.; Arrieta, M.C.; Dimitriu, P.A.; Cheng, J.; Thorson, L.; Lefebvre, D.L.; Azad, M.B.; Subbarao, P.; Mandhane, P.; Becker, A.; et al. Shifts in *Lachnospira* and *Clostridium* sp. in the 3-month stool microbiome are associated with preschool age asthma. *Clin. Sci.* **2016**, *130*, 2199–2207. [CrossRef] [PubMed]
33. Hevia, A.; Milani, C.; López, P.; Donado, C.D.; Cuervo, A.; González, S.; Suarez, A.; Turroni, F.; Gueimonde, M.; Ventura, M.; et al. Allergic patients with long-term asthma display low levels of Bifidobacterium adolescentis. *PLoS ONE* **2016**, *11*. [CrossRef] [PubMed]

34. Durack, J.; Kimes, N.E.; Lin, D.L.; Rauch, M.; McKean, M.; McCauley, K.; Panzer, A.R.; Mar, J.S.; Cabana, M.D.; Lynch, S.V. Delayed gut microbiota development in high-risk for asthma infants is temporarily modifiable by *Lactobacillus* supplementation. *Nat. Commun.* **2018**, *9*. [CrossRef] [PubMed]
35. Abrahamsson, T.R.; Jakobsson, H.E.; Andersson, A.F.; Bjorksten, B.; Engstrand, L.; Jenmalm, M.C. Low gut microbiota diversity in early infancy precedes asthma at school age. *Clin. Exp. Allergy* **2014**, *44*, 842–850. [CrossRef] [PubMed]

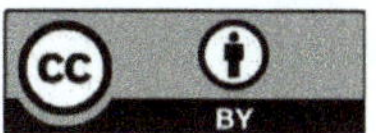

© 2018 by the authors. Licensee MDPI, Basel, Switzerland. This article is an open access article distributed under the terms and conditions of the Creative Commons Attribution (CC BY) license (http://creativecommons.org/licenses/by/4.0/).

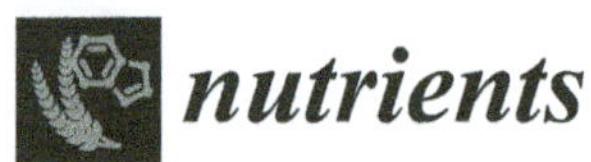

MDPI

Review

Rationale of Probiotic Supplementation during Pregnancy and Neonatal Period

Maria Elisabetta Baldassarre [1,*], Valentina Palladino [1], Anna Amoruso [1], Serena Pindinelli [1], Paola Mastromarino [2], Margherita Fanelli [3], Antonio Di Mauro [1] and Nicola Laforgia [1]

1 Neonatology and Neonatal Intensive Care Unit, Department of Biomedical Science and Human Oncology, "Aldo Moro" University of Bari, P.zza Giulio Cesare 11, 70124 Bari, Italy; valentinapalladino@hotmail.it (V.P.); amorusoanna@hotmail.it (A.A.); stefsere@alice.it (S.P.); antonio.dimauro@uniba.it (A.D.M.); nicola.laforgia@uniba.it (N.L.)

2 Section of Microbiology, Department of Public Health and Infectious Diseases, Sapienza University, Piazzale Aldo Moro 5, 00185 Rome, Italy; paola.mastromarino@uniroma1.it

3 Department of Interdisciplinary Medicine, "Aldo Moro" University of Bari, 70100 Bari, Italy; margherita.fanelli@uniba.it

* Correspondence: mariaelisabetta.baldassarre@uniba.it; Tel.: +39-080-5592220 or +39-3296114818

Received: 24 September 2018; Accepted: 3 November 2018; Published: 6 November 2018

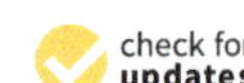

Abstract: Probiotics are living microorganisms that confer a health benefit when administered in adequate amounts. It has been speculated that probiotics supplementation during pregnancy and in the neonatal period might reduce some maternal and neonatal adverse outcomes. In this narrative review, we describe the rationale behind probiotic supplementation and its possible role in preventing preterm delivery, perinatal infections, functional gastrointestinal diseases, and atopic disorders during early life.

Keywords: "Probiotics"[Mesh]; "Pregnancy"[Mesh]; "Infant, Newborn"[Mesh]

---

1. Introduction

Gut microbiota is a heterogeneous microbial community that includes 10^{14} microorganisms comprising predominantly bacteria, but also viruses, archaeans, and protozoa, and is considered as a super-organ that dynamically interacts with the host in a mutual relationship [1,2]. Gut microbiota plays a significant role in human immunology, nutrition, and pathological processes. Despite inter-individual variability, in adults, 80% of gut microbiota is composed of three dominant phyla: *Bacteroidetes*, *Firmicutes*, and *Actinobacteria* [3]. The final composition of the intestinal microbiota is influenced by multiple factors such as genetic heritage, type of delivery, mode of feeding, administration of probiotics or antibiotics, stress, and infections [4]. The neonatal microbiota is highly different compared to the adult one, since the first is characterized by rapid changes [5]. At birth, the newborn is exposed to a set of bacteria including *staphylococci*, *enterobacteria*, and *enterococci* that immediately colonize the gastrointestinal tract. In the first days of life, the gut is inhabited mainly by *Bifidobacterium*, *Lactobacillus*, *Clostridium*, and *Bacteroides*. From one to five months of life, the population of the gastrointestinal tract consists of *Bifidobacteriales*, *Lactobacillales*, and *Clostridiales*. At one year of age, the microbiota is similar to the adult one [6,7]

Traditionally, babies have been considered sterile in utero while microbes colonize their gut during delivery and after the birth [8]. Several studies suggest that the placenta and amniotic fluid are involved in this process. In fact, the fetus incorporates an initial microbiome before birth [9,10]. Placental microbiome composition has been recently characterized, and includes non-pathogenic strains of *Bacteroidetes Firmicutes*, *Fusobacteria*, *Proteobacteria*, and *Tenericutes* [11]. During pregnancy, the ingestion of bacteria present in the amniotic fluid influences the foetal gut microbiome. Further, maternal microorganisms are present in the meconium and in the cord blood [12,13] in the total absence of chorioamnionitis.

The microbiota colonizes the host before birth and matures definitively during the twelve months following delivery [14]. During this moment, the fetus comes into contact with maternal vaginal bacteria that immediately reach the newborn gastrointestinal tract. The gut of infants born vaginally are colonized prevalently with *Bifidobacterium* and *Streptococcus*. In contrast, caesarean delivery is associated with a decrease of *Bifidobacteria*, while *Clostridium* and *Bacteroides* prevail [15–17]. There is some evidence that *Bifidobacteria* influence the development of very common allergic disorders such as atopic eczema and asthma [18,19]. Additionally, cesarean sections, especially as elective procedures, seem to represent a risk factor for autoimmunity and metabolic disorders [20,21]. Moreover, *bifidobacteria* are the most represented bacteria in the gastrointestinal tract of healthy infants. Beside the type of delivery, other factors affect microbial colonization in newborns. The abuse of antibiotics during pregnancy or after birth seems to reduce the number of *bifidobacteria* [22]. Schumann at al. have recently demonstrated a severe decrease of intestinal aerobic and anaerobic bacteria in rats treated with daily intragastric gavage of amoxicillin [23]. The gestational age at the birth is one of main factors that delineates the profile of gut microbiota. In fact, preterm newborns, in comparison to term births, have higher rates of anaerobic bacterial colonization, in particular *Enterobacteriaceae* [24] and *Enterococcaceae* [25,26]. During a premature delivery, it is not guaranteed that close contact with the vaginal mucosa and a smaller amount of bacteria are ingested. Additionally, in neonatal intensive care units, the wide use of antibiotics contributes to reduced growth indexes of gut bacteria, creating a restricted microbial population [27]. Abnormal vaginal microbiota or active bacterial infection during pregnancy alter the acquisition of neonatal flora promoting preterm delivery [28]. The presence of pathogenic bacteria in the amniotic fluid activates the innate immune response, and the production of prostaglandins increases uterine contractility, promoting premature birth [29].

Moreover, breastfeeding is another important determining factor in establishing the gut microbiome, and is a source of short- and long-term health benefits for the child. In the short term, it has been observed that it decreases the risk of infections, diarrhoea, type-1 diabetes, and necrotizing enterocolitis; while the long term benefits of breastfeeding include protection from the development of diseases like type-2 diabetes, inflammatory bowel disease, and obesity [30]. Breast milk contains fats, proteins, cytokines, enzymes, antibodies, and nutrients that influence the growth of the child and the development of his/her immune system [31]. Other components are antimicrobial agents like lactoferrin, lysozyme, peroxidase, defensins, IgAs, and oligosaccharides. The rich composition of human milk provides passive immunoprotection against infections and inflammation [32].

Among these components, lactoferrin is an important protein in breast milk, mostly in colostrum, and is involved in the regulation of the immune system and inflammatory response. A recent study suggests that during breastfeeding, lactoferrin is transferred to the intestine of the newborn. The fecal concentration of this protein progressively increases in the first month after birth, promoting the growth and differentiation of the immature intestine. Therefore, lactoferrin seems to promote the proliferation of enterocytes and closure of enteric gap junctions regulating the postnatal intestinal development [33]. Finally, lactoferrin is considered as a growth promoter for *bifidobacteria*, the predominant beneficial microorganism of human gut [34].

Furthermore, there is accumulating evidence that human milk is not sterile, but contains maternally-delivered bacteria, i.e., mainly lactobacilli and bifidobacteria. The number of bacteria ingested by an infant per 800 mL of milk consumed daily is estimated at 1×10^5–1×10^7 [35].

Microorganisms present in the breast milk are transferred from the mother's intestine to the mammary gland through the lymphatic system by dendritic cells by openings in the tight junctions of the intestinal epithelium [36]. The bacteria contained in the breast milk affect the composition of the gut microbiota in infants, and they could protect against infectious diseases and promote the maturation of the immune system. [37,38]. Additionally, other factors in breast milk including oligosaccharides, s-IgA, and lactoferrin influence the proliferation of healthy microbiota [7,39]. Intestinal bacteria stimulate endogenous production of s-IgA [40], activation of T regulatory cells [41,42] and anti-inflammation response [43,44]. Therefore, appropriate gut colonization through breastfeeding is involved in the correct development of immune system and in prevention of diseases.

Gastrointestinal flora composition differs mostly in breast- and formula-fed infants. Several studies conducted on stool samples of newborns have shown that bifidobacteria are present in the flora of both groups, but their number is higher in breastfed infants in comparison to formula-fed infants; instead, the number of *E. coli* and *Bacteroides* is higher in formula-fed infants [6]. These differences remain, even after breastfeeding is discontinued [7].

Current evidence supports a link between the activity and composition of the gut microbiota and human health and disease. The correct development of gut microbiota composition affects many organs, including neural, immune, and gastrointestinal systems. The gut microbiota composition is altered in many diseases, like disorders of the gut-brain axis [45], immune and gastrointestinal disorders [46,47], and allergic diseases [48]. The potential modulation of the gut microbiota through the administration of probiotics is very prominent in the prevention of human diseases starting from pregnancy.

2. Methods

An exhaustive search for eligible studies was performed in PubMed, Embase, Medline, Cochrane library and Web of Science database.

The following subject MeSH headings were used: "Probiotics"[Mesh], "Pregnancy"[Mesh], "Lactation"[Mesh], "Breast Feeding"[Mesh], "Premature Birth"[Mesh], "Infection"[Mesh], "Gastrointestinal Diseases"[Mesh]. Furthermore, free text for "allergy", "atopy", "gut-brain axis", and proper Boolean operators "AND" "OR" were also included to be as comprehensive as possible. Additional studies were sought using references in articles retrieved from searches.

Search limits were set for RCT, involving only human subjects, and published between October 2008 and October 2018. The review was limited to studies written in English.

3. Role of Probiotics Administration in the Prevention of Infection and Preterm Delivery during Pregnancy

Vaginal microbiota alterations and infections during pregnancy lead to a greater possibility of preterm delivery; this is related to the development of neonatal infections, sepsis, and necrotising entercocolitis. The use of probiotics seems to modulate the composition of vaginal microflora. Vitali et al. have conducted a pilot, non-randomized, controlled, and perspective study that demonstrated the influence on the vaginal microbiota of pregnant women of dietary supplementation with a probiotic mixture containing *L. paracasei* DSM 24733, *L. plantarum* DSM 24730, *L. acidophilus* DSM 24735, and *L. delbrueckii* subsp. *bulgaricus* DSM 24734), three strains of bifidobacteria (*B. longum* DSM 24736, *B. breve* DSM 24732, and *B. infantis* DSM 24737), and one strain of *Streptococcus thermophilus* DSM 24731, produced at Danisco-Dupont, WI, USA and currently sold in Continental Europe and USA under the brand Vivomixx® and Visbiome®, respectively. The characterization of vaginal bacteria in women supplemented with this multistrain probiotic showed an increase of *bifidobacteria* and a reduction of *Atopobium vaginae,* resulting in the prevention of bacterial vaginosis. Furthermore, IL-4 and IL-10 levels are influenced by alteration in the vaginal microbial environment. The decline of cytokines involved in the antiphlogistic process were noticed in a control women group that did not consume the probiotic mixture [49]. In contrast, Gille et al. in a recent trial demonstrated that the supplementation with *Lactobacillus rhamnosus GR-1* and *L reuteri RC-14* for two months during pregnancy does not improve the normal composition of vaginal microbiota compared to the placebo group [50].

Group B Streptococcal (GBS) vaginal colonization is considered a principal cause of neonatal sepsis, pneumonia, and meningitis [51]. The Centres for Disease Control and Prevention (CDC) suggest parenteral antibiotic administration during delivery as preventive therapy for women diagnosed with GBS at 35 and 37 weeks of gestation [52]. The possible impact of probiotic administration on prevention of infections during pregnancy has been investigated.

Recently, Olsen at al. performed a randomized pilot study to determine a potential causal relationship between probiotic administration during pregnancy and vaginal Group B Streptococcal (GBS) colonization. There was no significant difference in the incidence of GBS vaginal infections between the women supplemented with probiotics and the control group. However, a greater proportion of commensal bacteria was found in pregnant women who had used probiotics [53]. Besides Ho M. et al. conducted a randomized controlled trial to examine the effect of the oral administration of *Lactobacillus reuteri RC-14* and *Lactobacillus rhamnosus GR-1* in pregnant women with a vaginal and rectal GBS colonization. Compared to the placebo group, women treated with probiotics had significantly-reduced rectal and vaginal GBS colonization rates [54].

Bacterial vaginosis increases the risk of spontaneous preterm delivery and neonatal complications [55]. Few studies have tested the efficacy of probiotics in the prevention of preterm births. A prospective cohort study recently showed that the administration of a milk supplemented with probiotics during pregnancy reduced preeclampsia and preterm delivery risk [56]. Furthermore, a randomised controlled trial tested the early administration effect of *Lactobacillus rhamnosus GR-1* and *Lactobacillus reuteri RC-14* in women during gestation affected by low/intermadiate grade of vaginosis, to have a reduce premature delivery risk [57].

In a randomized clinical trial, the use of a yoghurt that contained *Lactobacillus bulgaris, Streptococcus thermophilus, Probiotic lactobacillus,* and *Bifidobacterium lactis* has been investigated in pregnant women in the treatment of bacterial vaginosis versus the use of clindamycin. Compared to the use of clindamycin, the administration of probiotics has a significant effect only on the reduction of vaginal pH, which seems to be associated with a lower risk of preterm delivery [58]. Therefore, there is no determinant evidence from clinical trials that confirms role of probiotics in the prevention of preterm delivery (Table 1). A recent metanalysis including 21 studies confirms that there is no evidence that the administration of probiotics in pregnant women reduces the risk of preterm delivery [59].

The potential role of probiotics in the prevention of infections during pregnancy and in preterm infants remains unclear, and requires further research.

Table 1. Role of probiotics administration in the prevention of infection and preterm delivery during pregnancy.

Author, Year	Study Design	Study Population	Intervention Strain Dose (D) Start of Treatment (S) End of Treatment (E)	Placebo	Outcomes Evaluations	Follow-Up	Side Effects
Gille et al., 2016 [50]	Randomized, placebo-controlled, triple-blind, parallel group trial	320 pregnant women	*L. rhamnousus*, GR-1® and *L. reuteri*, RC-14® D: 1 × 10^9 colony-forming unit (CFU) of each strain S: first trimester of pregnancy E: after 8 weeks of treatment	Indistinguishable placebo capsule	- Proportion of normal vaginal microbiota Main outcome: probiotics not improve the normal composition of vaginal microbiota compared to the placebo group	No available	Not observed
Olsen et al., 2010 [53]	Pilot randomised controlled trial	34 Group B streptococcus—positive pregnant women	*Lactobacillus rhamnosus* GR-1 (GR- 1) and *Lactobacillus fermentum/reuteri* RC-14 (RC-14) D: 1 × 10^8 CFU viable strain S: 36 weeks of gestation E: for three weeks or until the birth	No probiotics in control group	- Incidence of vaginal Group B streptococcus colonization Main outcome: no significant difference in the incidence of GBS vaginal infections between the women supplemented with probiotics and the control group	6 months after delivery	Not observed
Ho et al., 2016 [54]	Prospective, double-blind randomized clinical trial	110 GBS-positive pregnant women	*L. rhamnosus* GR-1 and *L. reuteri* RC-14 D: 1 × 10^9 CFU of both strain S: at 35 e 37 weeks of gestation E: at delivery	Indistinguishable placebo capsule	- Incidence of vaginal GBS colonization - Cause of admittance to the neonatal Unit Main outcome: Probiotics administration significantly reduced rectal and vaginal GBS colonization rate	No available	Not observed
Krauss-Silva Krauss-Silva et al., 2011 [57]	Prospective Double blind Randomized Controlled	664 pregnant women	*Lactobacillus rhamnosus* GR-1 and *Lactobacillus reuteri* RC-14 D: 2 × 10^6 CFU of each strain S: 20 weeks of gestation E: at delivery	Indistinguishable placebo capsule	- Incidence of spontaneous preterm delivery - Neonatal morbidities Main outcome: no conclusive results on the efficacy of probiotics in the prevention of preterm birth	No available	adverse events minor and non-specific of probiotics use
Hantoushzadeh et al., 2012 [58]	Double-blind, placebo-controlled, parallel-group randomized clinical trial	310 pregnant women with symptomatic BV	Probiotic yogurt: *lactobacillus bulgaris, streptococcus thermophilus, probiotic lactobacillus, and bifidobacterium lactis* D: 100 g twice a day for one week S: third trimester of pregnancy E: for one week	Orally-administered clindamycin (300 mg twice a day for 1 week)	- BV cure rate after one week of treatment - Preterm birth, Premature rupture of membranes, pH decrease and recurrence Main outcome: reduction of vaginal pH in women supplemented with probiotics	Until delivery	Not observed

4. Role of Probiotics Administration in the Prevention of Allergic Diseases

At birth, the lymphoid system of the newborn is not yet mature and Th1 response is inhibited. Therefore, it is necessary that the immune system clear the gap between Th1 and Th2 response. Microbiota has a crucial role during this critical phase [60]. There is a relationship between gut microbiome patterns and the potential role of modulation of innate immune signaling in the prevention of allergic diseases. West et al. have shown that after the birth, the maturation of the intestinal microbiota influences the innate immune response and the development of atopic eczema. This study suggests that alteration of gut microbial population increases the risk of the development of atopic-eczema due to a lack of modulation on inflammatory cytokines mediated by the microbiome [61]. Moreover, antibiotics, caesarean section, and infant formula are factors that modify microbiome composition and are related to the development of allergic diseases [62].

Probiotic supplementation to mothers during breastfeeding positively influences the microbial composition of breast milk and positively modulates the neonatal immune system mainly through the regulation of both Th1- and Th2-type response and by the stimulation of tolerance [63]. It has been observed that administration to mothers of a probiotic mixture containing *L. paracasei* DSM 24733, *L. plantarum* DSM 24730, *L. acidophilus* DSM 24735, and *L. delbrueckii* subsp. *bulgaricus* DSM 24734), three strains of *bifidobacteria* (*B. longum* DSM 24736, *B. breve* DSM 24732, and *B. infantis* DSM 24737), and one strain of *Streptococcus thermophilus* DSM 24731 (Danisco-Dupont, WI, USA and currently sold in Continental Europe and USA under the brand Vivomixx® and Visbiome®, respectively) resulted in an increase of lactobacilli and bifidobacteria in both colostrum and mature milk [7]. This probiotic mixture seems to play a key role in the regulation of the immune response which is influenced by the type of delivery; by comparing women with vaginal delivery under probiotics or placebo, an increase in bifidobacteria and lactobacilli was observed in the colostra and mature milk in the first group; no difference, however, was observed between the two groups of women who underwent caesarean section [63]. Maternal probiotic supplementation before and after delivery seems to prevent atopic eczema in children (Table 2), but further studies are requested to confirm this relation with other allergic disorders.

In a randomized, double-blind trial, women were given probiotic milk or placebo from the 36th week of gestational age to 3rd month after delivery during breastfeeding. At 2 years of age, all infants were tested for atopic dermatitis, asthma, and other allergic diseases. The study demonstrates that administration of probiotics to mothers during pregnancy decreases the incidence of atopic dermatitis, but has no effect on asthma [64]. Enomoto et al., in an open trial, confirmed that the administration of a combination of Bifidobacteria from 1 month before delivery to mothers and 6 months after birth to babies significantly reduced the incidence of cutaneous allergic diseases (eczema/atopic dermatitis). Moreover, women in the study group exhibit lower fecal Proteobacteria concentrations; this is related to higher children fecal concentration of Bacterioidetes at 4 months of age [65].

In contast, a recent randomized placebo-controlled trial demonstrated that the administration of *Lactobacillus rhamnosus* HN001 to pregnant woman before and after delivery during breastfeeding seems not to prevent the development of infant eczema, wheeze, and atopic sensitization during the first year of life [66]. In addition, another clinical trial shows that the supplementation of *Lactobacillus* GG in women from the 6th month of pregnancy and after birth (to mothers during breastfeeding or to infants for 6 months) does not reduce the incidence of developing allergic diseases in children followed up to 36 months of age [67].

Rautava et al. found that maternal supplementation of a mixture of probiotics 2 months before delivery and 2 months after lactation reduces the risk of developing eczema in infants in the first 2 years of life [68]. Furthermore, Kim et al. prove that the maternal supplementation of *Bifidobacterium bifidum*, *B. lactis*, and *Lactobacillus acidophilus* 4–8 weeks before delivery and until 6 months after the birth reduces the prevalence of eczema in the first year of life in children [69].

In a pAnda study, a mixture of probiotics (*Bifidobacterium bifidum*, *Bifidobacterium lactis*, and *Lactococcus lactis*) administrated to mothers before delivery and to infants for the first year of life reduced the incidence of eczema during the first 3 months of life compared to placebo group [70].

Simpson et al. have confirmed the long-term protective effect on the baby of probiotic maternal administration: children assessed at 6 years of age have a lower incidence of the development of atopic dermatitis, while this has not been confirmed for other allergic diseases [71]. Therefore, several studies have confirmed the role of probiotics in the early prevention of eczema in children, and these benefits were shown to persist over time. A recent randomized, controlled study (Probiotics in the Prevention of Allergy among Children in Trondheim, ProPACT) in part explains how perinatal maternal probiotics supplementation can play a protective role in the development of atopic dermatitis. In this study T-regs, Th-1, Th-2, and Th-17 lymphocyte or the Th-1/Th-2 ratio seem not to be influenced by a mixture of LGG, La-5, and Bb-12, but this reduces the proportion of Th-22 number [72].

The World Allergy Organization (WAO) convened a guideline panel to develop evidence-based recommendations about the use of probiotics in the prevention of allergies. The WAO guideline panel suggests:

- that by using probiotics in pregnant women at high risk for allergy in their children, there is a net benefit resulting primarily from prevention of eczema (conditional recommendation, very low-quality evidence).
- that by using probiotics in women who breastfeed infants at high risk of developing allergy, there is a net benefit resulting primarily from prevention of eczema (conditional recommendation, very low-quality evidence).
- using probiotics in infants at high risk of developing allergies, because there is a net benefit resulting primarily from prevention of eczema (conditional recommendation, very low-quality evidence).

Currently-available evidence does not indicate that probiotic supplementation reduces the risk of developing allergies in children, but there is a net benefit primarily in the prevention of eczema [73].

Table 2. Probiotics administration during pregnancy and after delivery in prevention of allergic disorders.

Author, Year	Study Design	Study Population	Intervention Strain Dose (D) Start of Treatment (S) End of Treatment (E)	Placebo	Outcomes Evaluations	Follow-Up	Side Effects
Dotterud et al., 2015 [64]	Randomized, double-blind trial	415 pregnant women	Probiotic milk: Biola ® (Tine BA, Oslo, Norway), contained *Lactobacillus rhamnosus* GG (LGG), *Bifidobacterium animalis subsp. lactis* Bb-12 (Bb-12) and *L. acidophilus* La-5 (La-5). D: 5×10^{10} CFU of LGG and Bb-12, and 5×10^9 colony-forming unit (CFU) of La-5 daily S: 4 weeks before the expected delivery date (to mothers) E: 3 weeks after delivery(to mothers during breastfeeding)	Indistinguishable placebo milk	- Development of atopic diseases in children (asthma, atopic dermatitis and allergic rhinoconjunctivitis) Main outcome: probiotics administration reduces the incidence of AD in children	24 months after delivery	Not observed
Enomoto et al., 2014 [65]	Open-trial study	166 pregnant women	*B. longum* BB536 [ATCC BAA-999] and *B. breve* M-16V [LMG 23729] D: two sachets, each containing approximately 5×10^9 CFU of both probiotics S: 4 weeks before the expected delivery date (to mothers) E: 6 months after delivery(to infants)	The control group no received probiotics	- Development of allergic symptoms in children - Composition of faecal samples (mothers and infants) Main outcome: probiotics administration reduces the incidence of AD/eczema in children	36 months after delivery	Not observed
Wickens et al., 2018 [66]	Randomized placebo-controlled trial	423 pregnant women	*Lactobacillus rhamnosus* HN001 (HN001) D: 6×10^9 CFU S: from 14–16 weeks gestation (to mothers) E: 6 months post-partum (to mothers during breast-feeding)	Indistinguishable placebo capsules	- Development of atopic diseases in children - Immunomodulatory factors in breast milk (TGF-β1, TGF-β2) Main outcome: probiotic supplementation not prevent infant eczema	12 months after delivery	Not observed
Ou et al., 2012 [67]	Prospective, double-blind, placebo-controlled clinical trial	191 pregnant women	*Lactobacillus GG;* ATCC 53103; D: 1×10^{10} CFU daily S: From the second trimester of pregnancy (to mothers) E: 6 months post-partum (to mothers during breastfeeding and to infants)	microcrystalline cellulose	- Development of allergic diseases in children. - Improvement of maternal allergic symptom score and plasma immune parameters Main outcome: probiotic supplementation not prevent infant allergic disease	36 months after delivery	Not observed
Rautava et al., 2012 [68]	Parallel, double-blind placebo-controlled trial	241 pregnant women	(1) *Lactobacillus rhamnosus LPR* and *Bifidobacterium longum BL999 (LPR+BL999)* (2) *L paracasei ST11* and *B longum BL999 (ST11+BL999)* D: 1×10^9 CFU for each probiotic S: 2 months before delivery (to mothers) E: 2 months post-partum (to mother during breast-feeding)	Indistinguishable placebo	- Development of allergic diseases in children. Main outcome: probiotic supplementation prevents infant eczema	24 months after delivery	Not observed

Table 2. *Cont.*

Author, Year	Study Design	Study Population	Intervention Strain Dose (D) Start of Treatment (S) End of Treatment (E)	Placebo	Outcomes Evaluations	Follow-Up	Side Effects
Kim et al., 2010 [69]	Randomized, double-blind, placebo-controlled trial	112 pregnant women	*Bifidobacterium bifidum* BGN4, *B. lactis* AD011, and *Lactobacillus acidophilus* AD031 D: 1.6×10^9 CFU for each probiotic S: 4–8 weeks before delivery (to mothers) E: until 6 months after delivery (to mothers during breastfeeding and to infants)	Indistinguishable powder	Assess the occurrence of eczema Main outcome: probiotics administration reduces the incidence of eczema in children	12 months after delivery	adverse events minor and non-specific of probiotics use
Niers et al., 2009 [70]	Double-blind, randomized, placebo-controlled trial	136 pregnant women	*Bifidobacterium bifidum*, *Bifidobacterium lactis*, and *Lactococcus lactis* D: 1×10^9 CFU of each strain S: last 6 weeks of pregnancy (to mothers) E: 12 months after delivery (to infants)	Indistinguishable powder	- Development of allergic diseases in infants - Molecular analysis of fecal microbiota in infants - Cytokine analysis in infants Main outcome: probiotics administration reduces the incidence of eczema in children at 3rd month of life	24 months after delivery	Not observed
Simpson et al., 2015 [71]	Randomised controlled trial	415 pregnant women	Probiotic milk: *Lactobacillus rhamnosus* GG, *L. acidophilus* La-5 and *Bifidobacterium animalis* subsp. lactis Bb-12 D: 5×10^{10} CFU of *Lactobacillus rhamnosus* and *Bifidobacterium animalis* and 5×10^9 CFU of L. acidophilus La-5 S: from 36 weeks gestation (to mothers) E: until 3 months postpartum (during breast-feeding)	Placebo milk	Development of allergic diseases in infants Main outcome: probiotics administration reduces the incidence of atopic dermatitis	6 years after delivery	Not observed

5. Brain-Gut Microbiota Axis

The microbiota plays an important role in the interaction between the brain and the enteric nervous system, known as the "brain-gut microbiota axis". Thanks to this axis, information from the Central nervous system can influence the motor, secretory, and sensitive functions of the gastrointestinal tract; conversely, visceral signals from the gut can modulate brain activity, mood, and behavior [7]. The gut-brain dialogue involves neuro-immuno-endocrine mediators [74].

It is believed that alterations in the microbiota gut-brain axis are associated with the onset of irritable bowel syndrome (IBS) or functional gastrointestinal (GI) disorders [75], and might be implicated in autism spectrum disorders (ASDs) [76–78], anxiety-depressive behaviors [76,79–81], and chronic pain [82]. However, the sites, the pathways and molecular mechanisms responsible for these alterations must be better defined.

Different models have been used to define the gut brain axis (GBA), including gut microbial perturbation by antibiotics and probiotics, fecal microbial transplantation, and mice who lived without any exposure to microorganisms (germ-free, GF) [83]. GF animals were born by Caesarean section and lived in aseptic conditions.

There is supporting evidence that metabolites derived from maternal gut microbiome modulate the neurotransmitter, synaptic, and neurotrophic signaling systems, thus influencing fetal brain development [84]. Petterson et al. underline that "healthy" intestinal microbiota is crucial for the programming of mammalian neurodevelopment and later adult behavior. This study suggests that early microbial colonization influences the expression of synaptic-related proteins (e.g., synaptophysin, which is an indicator of synaptogenesis), signaling pathways, and neurotransmitter turnover, that could modulate the synaptic transmission influencing motor control and emotional behavior in adults [85].

It has also been reported that maternal separation (MS) in rodents induced dysbiosis and brain and behavioral changes [86]. MS triggers depression and anxiety-like behavior [87,88], hyper-responsiveness of the HPA axis [89], increased intestinal permeability [90–92], and visceral hypersensitivity [93].

Maternal stress and MS might be implicated with modifications of gut brain axis [94,95] and probiotics seem to improve those gut and brain changes caused by perinatal stressors [96–98]. In different studies, it was observed that postnatal microbial colonization regulates an adequate HPA response to stress [99] and the hippocampal serotoninergic system [100]. It was also described a decrease in depression and anxiety-like behavior after the administration of oral probiotics in mice [96,101,102] and humans [103,104] with normal gut microbiota.

Furthermore, the short-chain fatty acids (SCFA s) generated by the colonic microbiota represent a significant source of energy for the gastrointestinal cells. In this regard, colonocytes from germ-free C57BL/6 rodents showed lower energy statuses than normally-raised mice [105].

Additionally, the loss of intestinal-generated SCFAs induces metabolic changes that may affect neurodevelopment and alter mechanisms associated with feeding behavior and metabolism [83].

Indeed, recent studies compare ingestive behavior between mice with gut microbial composition and GF, suggesting that gut microbioma modulate feeding behavior. GF mice showed lower blood levels of leptin and ghrelin, and a higher inclination for lipids, justified by the increased expression of oral receptors for fats and a decreased one for gut fatty-acid receptors [106].

Furthermore, it was observed that *bifidobacterium B. longum 1714* improves cognition in mice [107]. Additionally, the administration of a probiotic mixture containing *L. paracasei* DSM 24733, *L. plantarum* DSM 24730, *L. acidophilus* DSM 24735, and *L. delbrueckii* subsp. *bulgaricus* DSM 24734), three strains of bifidobacteria (*B. longum* DSM 24736, *B. breve* DSM 24732, and *B. infantis* DSM 24737), and one strain of *Streptococcus thermophilus* DSM 24731 (Danisco-Dupont, WI, USA, currently sold in Continental Europe and USA under the brand Vivomixx® and Visbiome®, respectively) to aged animals induced a reduction of the age-related attenuation of LTP through modifications of the gut microbiota [108]. These results are interesting but translational studies in humans are necessary.

6. Probiotics and Functional Gastrointestinal Disorders

Probiotics have an important role in the maturation and health of the intestinal tract. The composition of gut microbiota is involved in the development of gastrointestinal functions, particularly in the gut-brain axis, and participates in emitting and receiving signals to and from the brain [109]. This connection occurs with different mechanisms: through the release of cytokines and chemokine (immune pathway), through neural pathways, and through the production of intestinal neuroendocrine factors (endocrine pathway) [6]. Therefore, through changes of the microbiota, bidirectional relationships between the gut and brain are modified, thus influencing the pathogenesis of functional gastrointestinal disorders. The most common diseases in early life are infantile colic, a benign and functional gastrointestinal disorder that affects around 20% of young infants. Colic is associated with parental frustration and anxiety, and resolves spontaneously after the first three to four months of life. Although infantile colic is a self-resolving condition, it implies long-term effects on a child's behavior, sleep, and allergies [110].

According to the Rome IV criteria for functional gastrointestinal disorders, infantile colic is diagnosed in infants younger than 4 months of age if the following symptoms occur: paroxysms of irritability, fussing or crying that starts and stops without obvious cause; episodes lasting 3 or more hours per day and occurring at least 3 days per week for at least 1 week; and no failure to thrive [111].

Infantile colic presents a multifactorial aetiology, but the cause remains unclear. However, some causative mechanisms have been suggested like behavioral, food allergies and hypersensitivities, immaturity of gut function, and dysmotility [112].

An extensive number of possible factors have been hypothesized, like increased painful intestinal contractions, lactose intolerance, food hypersensitivity, gas, parental misinterpretation of the normal crying pattern, and altered gut microbiota (dysbiosis). In the management of infantile colic, many therapies are used, such as dietary, pharmacological, and behavioral interventions. However, data on their effectiveness are limited. Dysbiosis may play an important role in the pathogenesis of infantile colic, and gut microbiota modification with probiotics can have advantages on the management of infantile colic [113].

Partty et al. have conducted a randomized, double-blind, prospective study based on the administration of *L. rhamnosus* GG (ATCC 53103) or placebo to mothers daily for 4 weeks before expected delivery, and subsequently to the child or the mother, if breast-feeding, for 6 months, to evaluate the influence on the appearance of functional gastrointestinal disorders.

They hypothesized that colic crying, typical of the perinatal period, was associated with functional gastrointestinal disorders later in childhood.

Their 13-year follow-up study showed that administration of *L. rhamnosus* GG (ATCC 53103) does not affect the appearance of functional gastrointestinal disorders later in childhood, but suggests that different probiotics or probiotic combinations may be needed [114]. (Table 3).

It has been shown that probiotic administration to women during pregnancy and lactation can change the composition of breast milk, and consequently, its immunomodulatory molecular composition, bestowing benefits on the child in the form of reduced instances of gastrointestinal disorders.

A study conducted in 2013 showed an increase in breast milk of anti-inflammatory molecules such as TGF-B and IL-10 in supplemented mothers compared to the control group. Indeed, maternal probiotic supplementation leads to an increase of the TGF-B, which stimulates gut maturity, influencing IgA production and oral tolerance induction, and that seems to improve gastrointestinal functional symptoms in infants [115].

In a recent study, Baldassarre et al. have demonstrated that the use of a probiotic mixture (*L. paracasei* DSM 24733, *L. plantarum* DSM 24730, *L. acidophilus* DSM 24735, and *L. delbrueckii* subsp. *bulgaricus* DSM 24734), three strains of bifidobacteria (*B. longum* DSM 24736, *B. breve* DSM 24732, and *B. infantis* DSM 24737), and one strain of *Streptococcus thermophilus* DSM 24731, Vivomixx®,

Danisco-Dupont, WI, USA) appears safe and reduces inconsolable crying in exclusively breastfed infants with infantile colic [116].

Many studies have also been conducted on the prophylactic use of probiotics in the first months of life to treat breastfed infants with colic. In particular, benefits of the use of *Lactobacillus reuteri* on functional gastrointestinal disorders have been studied.

Gutiérrez-Castrellón et al. [117] have demonstrated the superiority of the use of *L. reuteri DSM 17938* with a dose of 10^8 CFU/day for 21 to 28 days to significantly reduce the duration of crying episodes during the day.

Recently, Indrio et al. [118] have suggested that oral supplementation of *L. reuteri,* for the first three months of life, not only reduces the probability of colic episodes and other functional gastrointestinal disorders, like gastroesophageal reflux and constipation, but also the number of visits and hospitalizations.

In conclusion, *L. reuteri DSM17938* is effective, and may be recommended for breastfed infants with colic, while its role in formula-fed infants requires further study [119].

7. Safety of Probiotics in Pregnancy and Neonatal Period

The early supplementation of probiotics in the perinatal and postnatal periods seems to have a positive impact on future health of infants. In this article we have shown the beneficial effects of probiotics in preventing infections before and after delivery and atopy in children. However, to define the possible role of the early administration of probiotics on the development of the nervous system of newborns, future studies and randomized trials are required. The use of probiotics is usually considered safe, even in first months of life. Despite the large use of probiotics during pregnancy and perinatal period, there are few studies that tested their safety during this period. Development of infections or other adverse effects in adult patients after the use of probiotics are rarely reported and often involve immunocompromised patients [120,121]. Allen et al., in a randomized, double-blinded, placebo-controlled trial, have tested the possible adverse effects of the administration of a probiotics mixture to pregnant women and to their infants after the birth. In this study, none of the adverse effects was attributed to the supplementation of probiotics [122]. Moreover, Baldassarre et al., in a prospective, double-blinded, randomized, controlled trial, confirmed that the early administration of probiotics during pregnancy has no side effects in mothers or in infants [115]. In addition, Luoto et al. in a clinical trial, involving 256 pregnant women and their offspring, showed no side effects in mothers and children after the administration of *Lactobacillus rhamnosus* GG and *Bifidobacterium lactis Bb12* probiotics mixture [123]. In contrast, Kuitunen et al. have suggested that the early supplementation of probiotics negatively influences hematologic values in infants. In this trial, children supplemented with probiotics before and after the birth have significantly lower haemoglobin levels compared to the placebo group at 6th month of life. This effect is transient, and may be due to a potential inflammation of the intestinal mucosa probably caused by probiotics [124] (Table 4). Future studies are needed to confirm the total safety of the use of probiotics during pregnancy and in the early stages of life.

Table 3. Probiotics and functional gastrointestinal disorders.

Author, Year	Study Design	Study Population	Intervention Strain Dose (D) Start of Treatment (S) End of Treatment (E)	Placebo	Outcomes Evaluations	Follow-Up	Side Effects
Partty et al., 2013 [114]	Randomized Double-blind Prospective Follow up	159 women	*L. rhamnosus GG* (ATCC 53103) D: not available S: 4 weeks before expected delivery E: 6 months after delivery to child or to the mother if breast-feeding	Indistinguishable powder	Functional gastrointestinal disorders Main outcome: administration of *L. rhamnosus GG* (ATCC 53103) does not affect the appearance of functional gastrointestinal disorders later in childhood	13 years	Not observed
Baldassarre et al., 2016 [115]	Prospective Double-blind Randomized Controlled	66 women aged 18–44	Probiotic mixture: *L. paracasei* DSM 24733, *L. plantarum* DSM 24730, *L. acidophilus* DSM 24735, *L. delbrueckii* subsp. *bulgaricus* DSM 24734, *B. longum* DSM 24736, *B. breve* DSM 24732, *B. infantis* DSM 24737, *Streptococcus thermophilus* DSM 24731 D: 900 billion S: 4 weeks before expected delivery E: 4 weeks after delivery	Indistinguishable powder	- cytokine profile and secretory IgA in breast milk - lactoferrin and sIgA levels in stool samples of newborns - newborn gastrointestinal symptoms - neonatal growth pattern Main outcome: maternal supplementation with probiotic modulates breast milk cytokines pattern in newborns and improves gastrointestinal functional symptoms	4 weeks after delivery	Not observed

Table 4. Safety of probiotics in pregnancy and neonatal period.

Author, Year	Study Design	Study Population	Intervention Strain Dose (D) Start of Treatment (S) End of Treatment (E)	Placebo	Outcomes Evaluations	Follow-Up	Side Effects
Luoto et al., 2010 [123]	Double-blind, placebo-controlled study	256 pregnant women	*Lactobacillus rhamnosus* GG and *Bifidobacterium lactis* Bb12 D: 10^{10} colony-forming unit (CFU)/d each S: first trimester of pregnancy (to mothers) E: to the end of exclusive breastfeeding	Indistinguishable placebo capsule	- Safety and efficacy of probiotic in mothers and infants Main outcome: probiotics supplementation reduced the frequency of gestational diabetes mellitus with a normal duration of pregnancies and no adverse events in mothers or children	24 months after delivery	Not observed
Allen et al., 2010 [122]	Randomized, double-blinded, placebo-controlled trial	454 pregnant women	Two strains of lactobacilli (*Lactobacillus salivarius CUL61 and Lactobacillus paracasei CUL08*) and bifidobacteria (*Bifidobacterium animalis subsp. lactis CUL34 and Bifidobacterium bifidum CUL20)* D: a total of 1×10^{10} CFU/d S: last month of pregnancy (to mother) E: until 6 months of life (to infants)	Indistinguishable placebo capsule	- Symptoms and adverse effects in mother and infants Main outcome: No side effects were attributed to probiotics supplementation	24 months after delivery	Not observed
Kuitunen et al., 2009 [124]	Prospective randomized controlled trial	1223 pregnant women	*Lactobacillus rhamnosus GG (ATCC 53103)* 5×10^9 CFU, *L rhamnosus LC705* *(DSM 7061)* 5×10^9 CFU, *Bifidobacterium breve Bb99* *(DSM 13692)* 2×10^8 CFU, and *Propionibacterium freudenreichii ssp* *shermanii JS (DSM 7076)* 2×10^9 CFU S: 4 weeks before delivery (to mothers) E: until 6 months of life (to infants)	Indistinguishable placebo	- Safety and efficacy of probiotic in mothers and infants - Blood and faecal samples taken from children Main outcome: Infants in the probiotic group have lower haemoglobin levels compared to the placebo group at 6th month of life	24 months after delivery	lower haemoglobin levels at 6th month of life

8. Conclusions

In the last 20 years, it has been shown that the constitution of the human microbiome is conditioned by multiple elements such as genetic heritage, prematurity, cesarean section, kind of infant nutrition, administration of probiotics or antibiotics, perinatal stressors, and infections. Further studies demonstrated that a normal intestinal microbiota takes part in the induction of the immune tolerance [125,126]. Alterations of the microbiota are associated with the development of many pathological states like infantile colic, inflammatory bowel disease, necrotizing enterocolitis, asthma, atopic diseases, celiac disease, diabetes, mood disorders, and autism spectrum disorders. Additional studies are needed to attest that probiotics could have a protective function against the onset and the progression of these diseases. Nowadays there is no standard recommendation for performing targeted supplementation in individual patients.

Studies suggest that the microbiota may influence immunologic and inflammatory systemic responses, and thus, modulate the onset of sensitization and allergy.

In 2015, the WAO guidelines on the prevention of allergies recommends using probiotics in: (a) pregnant women at high risk for having an allergic child; (b) women who breastfeed infants at high risk of developing allergies; and (c) infants at high risk of developing allergies [73].

These are the only recommendations by the Scientific Community for using probiotics as a preventive intervention for diseases during pregnancy and perinatal period, despite the many studies demonstrating clinical benefits from the administration of probiotics in pregnancy and the perinatal period. So, it is important to obtain more data about the exact composition of microbiomes and the alterations which occur in specific diseases. It is also important to underline that the security and effectiveness of findings attributable to one single probiotic product cannot be applied to other probiotic formulations, especially if the product is administered to patients such as pregnant women and newborns; this is a serious task, and therapeutic discomfort that multi-strain probiotic formulations lack generic names, because they are food supplements. Many clinicians and patients are unaware that deficiencies in the regulation of probiotics mean that the formulations sold under these medically-recognized brand names may no longer be the same as the original products on which the clinical efficacy and safety evidence is based. FAO/WHO guidelines for probiotics state that proper nomenclature and strain designation are required on a probiotic product. Without proper identification of the strains and/or of the clarification of the origin of the product such as manufacturing site, the clinical evidence is erroneously transferred from one product to another. This is the reason why limiting the information to probiotic genera/species is not the best choice [127], and more stringent quality control of probiotics is required [128].

Author Contributions: M.E.B. and V.P. drafted the initial manuscript and revised the final manuscript. A.A. and S.P. made substantial contributions to data acquisition. A.D.M., P.M., M.F. and N.L. reviewed and revised the manuscript. All authors approved the final manuscript as submitted.

Funding: This research received no external funding.

Conflicts of Interest: The authors declare no conflict of interest.

References

1. Hillman, E.T.; Yao, H.L.T.; Nakatsu, C.H. Microbial Ecology along the Gastrointestinal Tract. *Microbes Environ.* **2017**, *32*, 300–313. [CrossRef] [PubMed]
2. O'Hara, A.M.; Shanahan, F. The gut flora as a forgotten organ. *EMBO Rep.* **2006**, *7*, 688–693. [CrossRef] [PubMed]
3. Lay, C.; Sutren, M.; Rochet, V.; Saunier, K.; Doré, J.; Rigottier-Gois, L. Design and validation of 16S rDNA probes to enumerate members of the Clostridium leptum subgroup in human faecal microbiota. *Environ. Microbiol.* **2005**, *7*, 933–946. [CrossRef] [PubMed]

4. Gill, S.R.; Pop, M.; Deboy, R.T.; Eckburg, P.B.; Turnbaugh, P.J.; Samuel, B.S.; Gordon, J.I.; Relman, D.A.; Fraser-Liggett, C.M.; Nelson, K.E. Metagenomic analysis of the human distal gut microbiome. *Science* **2006**, *312*, 1355–1359. [CrossRef] [PubMed]
5. Pickard, J.M.; Zeng, M.Y.; Caruso, R.; Núñez, G. Gut microbiota: Role in pathogen colonization, immune responses, and inflammatory disease. *Immunol. Rev.* **2017**, *279*, 70–89. [CrossRef] [PubMed]
6. Indrio, F.; Riezzo, G.; Raimondi, F.; Di Mauro, A.; Francavilla, R. Microbiota Involvement in the Gut-Brain Axis. *JPGN* **2013**, *57*, S11–S15. [CrossRef]
7. Baldassarre, M.E.; Bellantuono, L.; Mastromarino, P.; Miccheli, A.; Fanelli, M.; Laforgia, N. Gut and Breast Milk Microbiota and Their Role in the Development of the Immune Function. *Curr. Pediatr. Rep.* **2014**, *2*, 218–226. [CrossRef]
8. Escherich, T. The intestinal bacteria of the neonate and breast-fed infant 1885. *Rev. Infect. Dis.* **1989**, *11*, 352–356. [CrossRef] [PubMed]
9. Jiménez, E.; Marín, M.L.; Martín, R.; Odriozola, J.M.; Olivares, M.; Xaus, J.; Fernández, L.; Rodríguez, J.M. Is meconium from healthy newborns actually sterile? *Res. Microbiol.* **2008**, *159*, 187–193. [CrossRef] [PubMed]
10. Collado, M.C.; Rautava, S.; Aakko, J.; Isolauri, E.; Salminen, S. Human gut colonisation may be initiated in utero by distinct microbial communities in the placenta and amniotic fluid. *Sci. Rep.* **2016**, *6*, 23129. [CrossRef] [PubMed]
11. Aagaard, K.; Ma, J.; Antony, K.M.; Ganu, R. The placenta harbors a unique microbiome. *Sci. Transl. Med.* **2014**, *6*, 237ra65. [CrossRef] [PubMed]
12. Perez, P.F.; Doré, J.; Leclerc, M.; Levenez, F.; Benyacoub, J.; Serrant, P.; Segura-Roggero, I.; Schiffrin, E.J.; Donnet-Hughes, A. Bacterial imprinting of the neonatal immune system: Lessons from maternal cells? *Pediatrics* **2007**, *119*, e724–e732. [CrossRef] [PubMed]
13. Ardissone, A.N.; de la Cruz, D.M.; Davis-Richardson, A.G.; Rechcigl, K.T.; Li, N.; Drew, J.C.; Murgas-Torrazza, R.; Sharma, R.; Hudak, M.L.; Triplett, E.W.; et al. Meconium microbiome analysis identifies bacteria correlated with premature birth. *PLoS ONE* **2014**, *9*, e90784. [CrossRef] [PubMed]
14. Walker, W.A. The importance of appropriate initial bacterial colonization of the intestine in newborn, child and adult health. *Pediatr. Res.* **2017**, *82*, 387–395. [CrossRef] [PubMed]
15. Sirilun, S.; Takahashi, H.; Boonyaritichaikij, S.; Chaiyasut, C.; Lertruangpanya, P.; Koga, Y.; Mikami, K. Impact of maternal bifidobacteria and the mode of delivery on Bifidobacterium microbiota in infants. *Benef. Microbes* **2015**, *6*, 767–774. [CrossRef] [PubMed]
16. Lundgren, S.N.; Madan, J.C.; Emond, J.A.; Morrison, H.G.; Christensen, B.C.; Karagas, M.R.; Hoen, A.G. Maternal diet during pregnancy is related with the infant stool microbiome in a delivery mode-dependent manner. *Microbiome* **2018**, *6*, 109. [CrossRef] [PubMed]
17. Azad, M.B.; Konya, T.; Maughan, H.; Guttman, D.S.; Field, C.J.; Chari, R.S.; Sears, M.R.; Becker, A.B.; Scott, J.A.; Kozyrskyj, A.L. Gut microbiota of healthy Canadian infants: Profiles by mode of delivery and infant diet at 4 months. *CMAJ* **2013**, *185*, 385–394. [CrossRef] [PubMed]
18. Wopereis, H.; Oozeer, R.; Knipping, K.; Belzer, C.; Knol, J. The first thousand days—Intestinal microbiology of early life: Establishing a symbiosis. *Pediatr. Allergy Immunol.* **2014**, *25*, 428–438. [CrossRef] [PubMed]
19. Van Zwol, A.; Van Den Berg, A.; Knol, J.; Twisk, J.W.; Fetter, W.P.; Van Elburg, R.M. Intestinal microbiota in allergic and nonallergic 1 year-old very low birth weight infants after neonatal glutamine supplementation. *Acta Paediatr.* **2010**, *99*, 1868–1874. [CrossRef] [PubMed]
20. Mårild, K.; Stephansson, O.; Montgomery, S.; Murray, J.A.; Ludvigsson, J.F. Pregnancy outcome and risk of celiac disease in offspring: A nationwide case-control study. *Gastroenterology* **2012**, *142*, 39–45. [CrossRef] [PubMed]
21. Thavagnanam, S.; Fleming, J.; Bromley, A.; Shields, M.D.; Cardwell, C.R. A meta-analysis of the association between Caesarean section and childhood asthma. *Clin. Exp. Allergy* **2008**, *38*, 629–633. [CrossRef] [PubMed]
22. Imoto, N.; Morita, H.; Amanuma, F.; Maruyama, H.; Watanabe, S.; Hashiguchi, N. Maternal antimicrobial use at delivery has a stronger impact than mode of delivery on bifidobacterial colonization in infants: A pilot study. *J. Perinatol.* **2018**, *15*, 16. [CrossRef] [PubMed]
23. Schumann, A.; Nutten, S.; Donnicola, D.; Comelli, E.M.; Mansourian, R.; Cherbut, C.; Corthesy-Theulaz, I.; Garcia-Rodenas, C. Neonatal antibiotic treatment alters gastrointestinal tract developmental gene expression and intestinal barrier transcriptome. *Physiol. Genom.* **2005**, *23*, 235–245. [CrossRef] [PubMed]

24. Taft, D.H.; Ambalavanan, N.; Schibler, K.R.; Yu, Z.; Newburg, D.S.; Ward, D.V.; Morrow, A.L. Intestinal microbiota of preterm infants differ over time and between hospitals. *Microbiome* **2014**, *2*, 36. [CrossRef] [PubMed]
25. Gritz, E.C.; Bhandari, V. The Human Neonatal Gut Microbiome: A Brief Review. *Front. Pediatr.* **2015**, *3*, 17. [PubMed]
26. Magne, F.; Abély, M.; Boyer, F.; Morville, P.; Pochart, P.; Suau, A. Low species diversity and high interindividual variability in faeces of preterm infants as revealed by sequences of 16S rRNA genes and PCR-temporal temperature gradient gel electrophoresis profiles. *FEMS Microbiol. Ecol.* **2006**, *57*, 128–138. [CrossRef] [PubMed]
27. Neu, J. Gastrointestinal development and meeting the nutritional needs of premature infants. *Am. J. Clin. Nutr.* **2007**, *85*, 629S–634S. [CrossRef] [PubMed]
28. Meis, P.J.; Goldenberg, R.L.; Mercer, B.; Moawad, A.; Das, A.; McNellis, D.; Johnson, F.; Iams, J.D.; Thom, E.; Andrews, W.W. The preterm prediction study: Significance of vaginal infections. National Institute of Child Health and Human Development Maternal-Fetal Medicine Units Network. *Am. J. Obstet. Gynecol.* **1995**, *173*, 1231–1235. [CrossRef]
29. Goldenberg, R.L.; Hauth, J.C.; Andrews, W.W. Intrauterine infection and preterm delivery. *N. Engl. J. Med.* **2000**, *342*, 1500–1507. [CrossRef] [PubMed]
30. Le Huërou-Luron, I.; Blat, S.; Boudry, G. Breast-v. formula-feeding: Impacts on the digestive tract and immediate and long-term health effects. *Nutr. Res. Rev.* **2010**, *23*, 23–36. [CrossRef] [PubMed]
31. Mastromarino, P.; Capobianco, D.; Campagna, G.; Laforgia, N.; Drimaco, P.; Dileone, A.; Baldassarre, M.E. Correlation between lactoferrin and beneficial microbiota in breast milk and infant's feces. *BioMetals* **2014**, *27*, 1077–1086. [CrossRef] [PubMed]
32. Buccigrossi, V.; de Marco, G.; Bruzzese, E.; Ombrato, L.; Bracale, I.; Polito, G.; Guarino, A. Lactoferrin induces concentration-dependent functional modulation of intestinal proliferation and differentiation. *Pediatr. Res.* **2007**, *61*, 410–414. [CrossRef] [PubMed]
33. Oda, H.; Wakabayashi, H.; Yamauchi, K.; Abe, F. Lactoferrin and bifidobacteria. *Biometals* **2014**, *27*, 915–922. [CrossRef] [PubMed]
34. Arrieta, M.C.; Stiemsma, L.T.; Dimitriu, P.A.; Thorson, L.; Russell, S.; Yurist-Doutsch, S.; Kuzeljevic, B.; Gold, M.J.; Britton, H.M.; Lefebvre, D.L.; et al. Early infancy microbial and metabolic alterations affect risk of childhood asthma. *Sci. Transl. Med.* **2015**, *7*, 307ra152. [CrossRef] [PubMed]
35. Donnet-Hughes, A.; Perez, P.F.; Doré, J.; Leclerc, M.; Levenez, F.; Benyacoub, J.; Serrant, P.; Segura-Roggero, I.; Schiffrin, E.J. Potential role of the intestinal microbiota of the mother in neonatal immune education. *Proc. Nutr. Soc.* **2010**, *69*, 407–415. [CrossRef] [PubMed]
36. Fernández, L.; Langa, S.; Martin, V.; Maldonado, A.; Jiménez, E.; Martin, R.; Rodríguez, J.M. The human milk microbiota: Origin and potential roles in health and disease. *Pharmacol. Res.* **2013**, *69*, 1–10. [CrossRef] [PubMed]
37. Bergmann, H.; Rodríguez, J.M.; Salminem, S.; Szajewska, H. Probiotics in human milk and prebiotico supplementation in infant nutrition: A workshop report. *Br. J. Nutr.* **2014**, *112*, 1119–1128. [CrossRef] [PubMed]
38. Newburg, D.S.; Walker, W.A. Protection of the neonate by the immune system of developing gut and of human milk. *Pediatr. Res.* **2007**, *61*, 2–8. [CrossRef] [PubMed]
39. Gregory, K.E.; Walker, W.A. Immunologic factors in human milk and disease prevention in the preterm infant. *Curr. Pediatr. Rep.* **2013**, *1*, 222–228. [CrossRef] [PubMed]
40. Jost, T.; Lacroix, C.; Braegger, C.P.; Chassard, C. New insights in gut microbiota establishment in healthy breast fed neonates. *PLoS ONE* **2012**, *7*, e44595. [CrossRef] [PubMed]
41. Schwartz, S.; Friedberg, I.; Ivanov, I.V.; Davidson, L.A.; Goldsby, J.S.; Dahl, D.B.; Herman, D.; Wang, M.; Donovan, S.M.; Chapkin, R.S. A metagenomic study of diet-dependent interaction between gut microbiota and host in infants reveals differences in immune response. *Genome Biol.* **2012**, *13*, r3. [CrossRef] [PubMed]
42. Furuta, G.; Walker, W.A. Non-immune defense mechanisms of the gastrointestinal tract. In *Infections of the Gastrointestinal Tract*; Blaser, M.J., Smith, P.D., Ravdin, J.I., Greenberg, H.B., Guerrant, R.L., Eds.; Raven Press Ltd.: New York, NY, USA, 1995; pp. 89–98.

43. Chichlowski, M.; De Lartigue, G.; German, J.B.; Raybould, H.E.; Mills, D.A. Bifidobacteria isolated from infants and cultured on human milk oligosaccharides affect intestinal epithelial function. *J. Pediatr. Gastroenterol. Nutr.* **2012**, *55*, 321–327. [CrossRef] [PubMed]
44. Rautava, S.; Walker, W.A. Breatfeeding—An extrauterine link between mother and child. *Breastfeed. Med.* **2009**, *4*, 3–10. [CrossRef] [PubMed]
45. Arneth, B.M. Gut-brain axis biochemical signalling from the gastrointestinal tract to the central nervous system: Gut dysbiosis and altered brain function. *Postgrad. Med. J.* **2018**, *94*, 446–452. [CrossRef] [PubMed]
46. Lazar, V.; Ditu, L.M.; Pircalabioru, G.G.; Gheorghe, I.; Curutiu, C.; Holban, A.M.; Picu, A.; Petcu, L.; Chifiriuc, M.C. Aspects of Gut Microbiota and Immune System Interactions in Infectious Diseases, Immunopathology, and Cancer. *Front. Immunol.* **2018**, *9*, 1830. [CrossRef] [PubMed]
47. Konturek, P.C.; Haziri, D.; Brzozowski, T.; Hess, T.; Heyman, S.; Kwiecien, S.; Konturek, S.J.; Koziel, J. Emerging role of fecal microbiota therapy in the treatment of gastrointestinal and extra-gastrointestinal diseases. *J. Physiol. Pharmacol.* **2015**, *66*, 483–491. [PubMed]
48. Hua, X.; Goedert, J.J.; Pu, A.; Yu, G.; Shi, J. Allergy associations with the adult fecal microbiota: Analysis of the American Gut Project. *EBioMedicine* **2015**, *3*, 172–179. [CrossRef] [PubMed]
49. Vitali, B.; Cruciani, F.; Baldassarre, M.E.; Capursi, T.; Spisni, E.; Valerii, M.C.; Candela, M.; Turroni, S.; Brigidi, P. Dietary supplementation with probiotics during late pregnancy: Outcome on vaginal microbiota and cytokine secretion. *BMC Microbiol.* **2012**, *12*, 236. [CrossRef] [PubMed]
50. Gille, C.; Böer, B.; Marschal, M.; Urschitz, M.S.; Heinecke, V.; Hund, V.; Speidel, S.; Tarnow, I.; Mylonas, I.; Franz, A.; et al. Effect of probiotics on vaginal health in pregnancy. EFFPRO, a randomized controlled trial. *Am. J. Obstet. Gynecol.* **2016**, *215*, 608-e1. [PubMed]
51. Russell, N.J.; Seale, A.C.; O'Sullivan, C.; Le Doare, K.; Heath, P.T.; Lawn, J.E.; Bartlett, L.; Cutland, C.; Gravett, M.; Ip, M.; et al. Risk of Early-Onset Neonatal Group B Streptococcal Disease with Maternal Colonization Worldwide: Systematic Review and Meta-analyses. *Clin. Infect. Dis.* **2017**, *65* (Suppl. 2), S152–S159. [CrossRef] [PubMed]
52. Verani, J.R.; McGee, L.; Schrag, S.J. Prevention of perinatal group B streptococcal disease–revised guidelines from CDC, 2010. *MMWR Recomm. Rep.* **2010**, *59*, 1–32. [PubMed]
53. Olsen, P.; Williamson, M.; Traynor, V.; Georgiou, C. The impact of oral probiotics on vaginal Group B Streptococcal colonisation rates in pregnant women: A pilot randomised control study. *Women Birth* **2018**, *31*, 31–37. [CrossRef] [PubMed]
54. Ho, M.; Chang, Y.Y.; Chang, W.C.; Lin, H.C.; Wang, M.H.; Lin, W.C.; Chiu, T.H. Oral Lactobacillus rhamnosus GR-1 and Lactobacillus reuteri RC-14 to reduce Group B Streptococcus colonization in pregnant women: A randomized controlled trial. *Taiwan J. Obstet. Gynecol.* **2016**, *55*, 515–518. [CrossRef] [PubMed]
55. Nelson, D.B.; Hanlon, A.; Nachamkin, I.; Haggerty, C.; Mastrogiannis, D.S.; Liu, C.; Fredricks, D.N. Early pregnancy changes in bacterial vaginosis-associated bacteria and preterm delivery. *Paediatr. Perinat. Epidemiol.* **2014**, *28*, 88–96. [CrossRef] [PubMed]
56. Myhre, R.; Brantsæter, A.L.; Myking, S.; Gjessing, H.K.; Sengpiel, V.; Meltzer, H.M.; Haugen, M.; Jacobsson, B. Intake of probiotic food and risk of spontaneous preterm delivery. *Am. J. Clin. Nutr.* **2011**, *93*, 151–157. [CrossRef] [PubMed]
57. Krauss-Silva, L.; Moreira, M.E.L.; Alves, M.B.; Braga, A.; Camacho, K.G.; Batista, M.R.R.; Almada-Horta, A.; Rebello, M.R.; Guerra, F. A randomised controlled trial of probiotics for the prevention of spontaneous preterm delivery associated with bacterial vaginosis: Preliminary results. *Trials* **2011**, *12*, 239. [CrossRef] [PubMed]
58. Hantoushzadeh, S.; Golshahi, F.; Javadian, P.; Khazardoost, S.; Aram, S.; Hashemi, S.; Mirarmandehi, B.; Borna, S. Comparative efficacy of probiotic yoghurt and clindamycin in treatment of bacterial vaginosis in pregnant women: A randomized clinical trial. *J. Matern. Fetal Neonatal Med.* **2012**, *25*, 1021–1024. [CrossRef] [PubMed]
59. Jarde, A.; Lewis-Mikhael, A.M.; Moayyedi, P.; Stearns, J.C.; Collins, S.M.; Beyene, J.; McDonald, S.D. Pregnancy outcomes in women taking probiotics or prebiotics: A systematic review and meta-analysis. *BMC Pregnancy Childbirth* **2018**, *18*, 14. [CrossRef] [PubMed]
60. De Brito, C.A.; Goldoni, A.L.; Sato, M.N. Immune adjuvants in early life: Targeting the innate immune system to overcome impaired adaptive response. *Immunotherapy* **2009**, *1*, 883–895. [CrossRef] [PubMed]

61. West, C.; Rydén, P.; Lundin, D.; Engstrand, L.; Tulic, M.K.; Prescott, S.L. Gut microbiome and innate immune response patterns in IgE-associated eczema. *Clin. Exp. Allergy* **2015**, *45*, 1419–1429. [CrossRef] [PubMed]
62. Azad, M.B.; Kozyrskyj, A.L. Perinatal programming of asthma: The role of gut microbiota. *Clin. Dev. Immunol.* **2012**, *2012*, 932072. [CrossRef] [PubMed]
63. Mastromarino, P.; Capobianco, D.; Miccheli, A.; Praticò, G.; Campagna, G.; Laforgia, N.; Capursi, T.; Baldassarre, M.E. Administration of a multistrain probiotic product (VSL#3) to women in the perinatal period differentially affects breast milk beneficial microbiota in relation to mode of delivery. *Pharmacol Res.* **2015**, *95–96*, 63–70.
64. Dotterud, C.K.; Storrø, O.; Johnsen, R.; Oien, T. Probiotics in pregnant women to prevent allergic disease: A randomized, double-blind trial. *Br. J. Dermatol.* **2010**, *163*, 616–623. [CrossRef] [PubMed]
65. Enomoto, T.; Sowa, M.; Nishimori, K.; Shimazu, S.; Yoshida, A.; Yamada, K.; Furukawa, F.; Nakagawa, T.; Yanagisawa, N.; Iwabuchi, N.; et al. Effects of bifidobacterial supplementation to pregnant women and infants in the prevention of allergy development in infants and on fecal microbiota. *Allergol. Int.* **2014**, *63*, 575–585. [CrossRef] [PubMed]
66. Wickens, K.; Barthow, C.; Mitchell, E.A.; Stanley, T.V.; Purdie, G.; Rowden, J.; Kang, J.; Hood, F.; van den Elsen, L.; Forbes-Blom, E.; et al. Maternal supplementation alone with Lactobacillus rhamnosus HN001 during pregnancy and breastfeeding does not reduce infant eczema. *Pediatr. Allergy Immunol.* **2018**, *29*, 296–302. [CrossRef] [PubMed]
67. Ou, C.Y.; Kuo, H.C.; Wang, L.; Hsu, T.Y.; Chuang, H.; Liu, C.A.; Chang, J.C.; Yu, H.R.; Yang, K.D. Prenatal and postnatal probiotics reduces maternal but not childhood allergic diseases: A randomized, double-blind, placebo-controlled trial. *Clin. Exp. Allergy* **2012**, *42*, 1386–1396. [CrossRef] [PubMed]
68. Rautava, S.; Kainonen, E.; Salminen, S.; Isolauri, E. Maternal probiotic supplementation during pregnancy and breast-feeding reduces the risk of eczema in the infant. *J. Allergy Clin. Immunol.* **2012**, *130*, 1355–1360. [CrossRef] [PubMed]
69. Kim, J.Y.; Kwon, J.H.; Ahn, S.H.; Lee, S.I.; Han, Y.S.; Choi, Y.O.; Lee, S.Y.; Ahn, K.M.; Ji, G.E. Effect of probiotic mix (*Bifidobacterium bifidum, Bifidobacterium lactis, Lactobacillus acidophilus*) in the primary prevention of eczema: A double-blind, randomized, placebo-controlled trial. *Pediatr. Allergy Immunol.* **2010**, *21*, e386–e393. [CrossRef] [PubMed]
70. Niers, L.; Martín, R.; Rijkers, G.; Sengers, F.; Timmerman, H.; van Uden, N.; Smidt, H.; Kimpen, J.; Hoekstra, M. The effects of selected probiotic strains on the development of eczema (the PandA study). *Allergy* **2009**, *64*, 1349–1358. [CrossRef] [PubMed]
71. Simpson, M.R.; Dotterud, C.K.; Storrø, O.; Johnsen, R.; Øien, T. Perinatal probiotic supplementation in the prevention of allergy related disease: 6 year follow up of a randomised controlled trial. *BMC Dermatol.* **2015**, *15*, 13. [CrossRef] [PubMed]
72. Rø, A.D.B.; Simpson, M.R.; Rø, T.B.; Storrø, O.; Johnsen, R.; Videm, V.; Øien, T. Reduced Th22 cell proportion and prevention of atopic dermatitis in infants following maternal probiotic supplementation. *Clin. Exp. Allergy* **2017**, *47*, 1014–1021. [CrossRef] [PubMed]
73. Fiocchi, A.; Pawankar, R.; Cuello-Garcia, C.; Ahn, K.; Al-Hammadi, S.; Agarwal, A.; Beyer, K.; Burks, W.; Canonica, G.W.; Ebisawa, M.; et al. World Allergy Organization-McMaster University Guidelines for allergic disease prevention (GLAD-P): Probiotics. *World Allergy Organ J.* **2015**, *8*, 4. [CrossRef] [PubMed]
74. Carabotti, M.; Maselli, M.A.; Severi, C. The gut-brain axis: Interactions between enteric microbiota, central and enteric nervous systems. *Ann. Gastroenterol.* **2015**, *28*, 203–209. [PubMed]
75. Mayer, E.A.; Savidge, T.; Shulman, R.J. Brain Gut Microbiome Interactions and Functional Bowel Disorders. *Gastroenterology* **2014**, *146*, 1500–1512. [CrossRef] [PubMed]
76. Cryan, J.F.; Dinan, T.G. Mind-altering microorganisms: The impact of the gut microbiota on brain and behavior. *Nat. Rev. Neurosci.* **2012**, *13*, 701–712. [CrossRef] [PubMed]
77. Mayer, E.A.; Padua, D.; Tillisch, K. Altered brain-gut axis in autism: Comorbidity or causative mechanisms? *Bioessays* **2014**, *36*, 933–939. [CrossRef] [PubMed]
78. Roman, P.; Rueda-Ruzafa, L.; Cardona, D.; Cortes-Rodriguez, A. Gut brain axis in the executive function of autism spectrum disorder. *Behav. Pharmacol.* **2018**, *29*, 654–663. [CrossRef] [PubMed]
79. Park, A.J.; Collins, J.; Blennerhassett, P.A.; Ghia, J.E.; Verdu, E.F.; Bercik, P.; Collins, S.M. Altered colonic function and microbiota profile in a mouse model of chronic depression. *Neurogastroenterol. Motil.* **2013**, *25*. [CrossRef] [PubMed]

80. Foster, J.A.; McVey Neufeld, K.A. Gut-brain axis: How the microbiome influences anxiety and depression. *Trends Neurosci.* **2013**, *36*, 305–312. [CrossRef] [PubMed]
81. Crumeyrolle-Arias, M.; Jaglin, M.; Bruneau, A.; Vancassel, S.; Cardona, A.; Daugé, V.; Naudon, L.; Rabot, S. Absence of the gut microbiota enhances anxiety-like behavior and neuroendocrine response to acute stress in rats. *Psychoneuroendocrinology* **2014**, *42*, 207–217. [CrossRef] [PubMed]
82. Amaral, F.A.; Sachs, D.; Costa, V.V.; Fagundes, C.T.; Cisalpino, D.; Cunha, T.M.; Ferreira, S.H.; Cunha, F.Q.; Silva, T.A.; Nicoli, J.R.; et al. Commensal microbiota is fundamental for the development of inflammatory pain. *Proc. Natl. Acad. Sci. USA* **2008**, *105*, 2193–2197. [CrossRef] [PubMed]
83. Mayer, E.A.; Tillisch, K.; Gupta, A. Gut/brain axis and microbiota. *J. Clin. Investig.* **2015**, *125*, 926–938. [CrossRef] [PubMed]
84. Arentsen, T.; Qian, Y.; Gkotzis, S.; Femenia, T.; Wang, T.; Udekwu, K.; Forssberg, H.; Heijtz, R.D. The bacterial peptidoglycan-sensing molecule Pglyrp2 modulates brain development and behavior. *Mol. Psychiatry* **2017**, *22*, 257–266. [CrossRef] [PubMed]
85. Heijtz, R.D.; Wang, S.; Anuar, F.; Quian, F.; Bjorkholm, B.; Samuelsson, A.; Hibberd, M.; Forssberg, H.; Petterson, S. Normal gut microbiota modulates brain development and behavior. *Proc. Natl. Acad. Sci. USA* **2011**, *108*, 3047–3052. [CrossRef] [PubMed]
86. De Palma, G.; Blennerhassett, P.; Lu, J.; Deng, Y.; Park, A.J.; Green, W.; Denou, E.; Silva, M.A.; Santacruz, A.; Sanz, Y.; et al. Microbiota and host determinants of behavioural phenotype in maternally separated mice. *Nat. Commun.* **2015**, *6*, 7735. [CrossRef] [PubMed]
87. Varghese, A.K.; Verdú, E.F.; Bercik, P.; Khan, W.I.; Blennerhassett, P.A.; Szechtman, H.; Collins, S.M. Antidepressants attenuate increased susceptibility to colitis in a murine model of depression. *Gastroenterology* **2006**, *130*, 1743–1753. [CrossRef] [PubMed]
88. Lippmann, M.; Bress, A.; Nemeroff, C.B.; Plotsky, P.M.; Monteggia, L.M. Long-term behavioural and molecular alterations associated with maternal separation in rats. *Eur. J. Neurosci.* **2007**, *25*, 3091–3098. [CrossRef] [PubMed]
89. Gareau, M.G.; Silva, M.A.; Perdue, M.H. Pathophysiological mechanisms of stress-induced intestinal damage. *Curr. Mol. Med.* **2008**, *8*, 274–281. [CrossRef] [PubMed]
90. Barreau, F.; Ferrier, L.; Fioramonti, J.; Bueno, L. Neonatal maternal deprivation triggers long term alterations in colonic epithelial barrier and mucosal immunity in rats. *Gut* **2004**, *53*, 501–506. [CrossRef] [PubMed]
91. Gareau, M.G.; Jury, J.; Perdue, M.H. Neonatal maternal separation of rat pups results in abnormal cholinergic regulation of epithelial permeability. *Am. J. Physiol. Gastrointest. Liver Physiol.* **2007**, *293*, G198–G203. [CrossRef] [PubMed]
92. Oines, E.; Murison, R.; Mrdalj, J.; Gronli, J.; Milde, A.M. Neonatal maternal separation in male rats increases intestinal permeability and affects behavior after chronic social stress. *Physiol. Behav.* **2012**, *105*, 1058–1066. [CrossRef] [PubMed]
93. Hyland, N.P.; Julio-Pieper, M.; O'Mahony, S.M.; Bulmer, D.C.; Lee, K.; Quigley, E.M.; Dinan, T.G.; Cryan, J.F. A distinct subset of submucosal mast cells undergoes hyperplasia following neonatal maternal separation: A role in visceral hypersensitivity? *Gut* **2009**, *58*, 1029–1030. [CrossRef] [PubMed]
94. O'Mahony, S.M.; Marchesi, J.R.; Scully, P.; Codling, C.; Ceolho, A.M.; Quigley, E.M.; Cryan, J.F.; Dinan, T.G. Early life stress alters behavior, immunity, and microbiota in rats: Implications for irritable bowel syndrome and psychiatric illnesses. *Biol. Psychiatry* **2009**, *65*, 263–267. [CrossRef] [PubMed]
95. Jasarevic, E.; Rodgers, A.B.; Bale, T.L. A novel role for maternal stress and microbial transmission in early life programming and neurodevelopment. *Neurobiol. Stress* **2015**, *1*, 81–88. [CrossRef] [PubMed]
96. Desbonnet, L.; Garrett, L.; Clarke, G.; Kiely, B.; Cryan, J.F.; Dinan, T.G. Effects of the probiotic Bifidobacterium infantis in the maternal separation model of depression. *Neuroscience* **2010**, *170*, 1179–1188. [CrossRef] [PubMed]
97. Eutamene, H.; Bueno, L. Role of probiotics in correcting abnormalities of colonic flora induced by stress. *Gut* **2007**, *56*, 1495–1497. [CrossRef] [PubMed]
98. Gareau, M.G.; Jury, J.; Macqueen, G.; Sherman, P.M.; Perdue, M.H. Probiotic treatment of rat pups normalises corticosterone release and ameliorates colonic dysfunction induced by maternal separation. *Gut* **2007**, *56*, 1522–1528. [CrossRef] [PubMed]

99. Sudo, N.; Chida, Y.; Aiba, Y.; Sonoda, J.; Oyama, N.; Yu, X.N.; Kubo, C.; Koga, Y. Postnatal microbial colonization programs the hypothalamic-pituitary-adrenal system for stress response in mice. *J. Physiol.* **2004**, *558*, 263–275. [CrossRef] [PubMed]
100. Neufeld, K.M.; Kang, N.; Bienenstock, J.; Foster, J.A. Reduced anxiety-like behavior and central neurochemical change in germ-free mice. *Neurogastroenterol. Motil.* **2011**, *23*, 255–264. [CrossRef] [PubMed]
101. Bravo, J.A.; Forsythe, P.; Chew, M.V.; Escaravage, E.; Savignac, H.M.; Dinan, T.G.; Bienenstock, J.; Cryan, J.F. Ingestion of Lactobacillus strain regulates emotional behavior and central GABA receptor expression in a mouse via the vagus nerve. *Proc. Natl. Acad. Sci. USA* **2011**, *108*, 16050–16055. [CrossRef] [PubMed]
102. Arseneault-Bréard, J.; Rondeau, I.; Gilbert, K.; Girard, S.A.; Tompkins, T.A.; Godbout, R.; Rousseau, G. Combination of Lactobacillus Helveticus R0052 and Bifidobacterium longum RO175 reduces post-myocardial infarction depression symptoms restores intestinal permeability in a rat model. *Br. J. Nutr.* **2012**, *107*, 1793–1799. [CrossRef] [PubMed]
103. Messaoudi, M.; Violle, N.; Bisson, J.; Desor, D.; Javelot, H.; Rougeot, C. Beneficial psychological effects of a probiotic formulation (*Lactobacillus helveticus* R0052 and *Bifidobacterium longum* R0175) in healthy human volunteers. *Gut Microbes* **2011**, *2*, 256–261. [CrossRef] [PubMed]
104. Huang, R.; Wang, K.; Hu, J. Effect of Probiotics on Depression: A Systematic Review and Meta-Analysis of Randomized Controlled Trials. *Nutrients* **2016**, *8*, 483. [CrossRef] [PubMed]
105. McNabney, S.M.; Henagan, T.M. Short Chain Fatty Acids in the Colon and Peripheral Tissues: A focus on Butyrate, Colon Cancer, Obesity and Insulin Resiatance. *Nutrients* **2017**, *9*, 1348. [CrossRef] [PubMed]
106. Duca, F.A.; Swartz, T.D.; Sakar, Y.; Covasa, M. Increased oral detection, but decreased intestinal signaling for fats in mice lacking gut microbiota. *PLoS ONE* **2012**, *7*, e39748. [CrossRef] [PubMed]
107. Savignac, H.M.; Tramullas, M.; Kiely, B.; Dinan, T.G.; Cryan, J.F. Bifidobacteria modulate cognitive processes in an anxious mouse strain. *Behav. Brain Res.* **2015**, *287*, 59–72. [CrossRef] [PubMed]
108. Distrutti, E.; O'Reilly, J.A.; McDonald, C.; Cipriani, S.; Renga, B.; Lynch, M.A.; Fiorucci, S. Modulation of intestinal microbiota by the probiotic VSL#3 resets brain gene expression ameliorates the age-related deficit in LTP. *PLoS ONE* **2014**, *9*, e106503.
109. Di Mauro, A.; Neu, J.; Riezzo, G.; Raimondi, F.; Martinelli, D.; Francavilla, R.; Indrio, F. Gastrointestinal function development and microbiota. *Ital. J. Pediatr.* **2013**, *39*, 15. [CrossRef] [PubMed]
110. Sung, V. Infantile colic. *Aust. Prescr.* **2018**, *41*, 105–110. [PubMed]
111. Zeevenhooven, J.; Koppen, I.J.; Benninga, M.A. The New Rome IV Criteria for Functional Gastrointestinal Disorders in Infants and Toddlers. *Pediatr. Gastroenterol. Hepatol. Nutr.* **2017**, *20*, 1–13. [CrossRef] [PubMed]
112. Shamir, R.; St James-Roberts, I.; Di Lorenzo, C.; Burns, A.J.; Thapar, N.; Indrio, F.; Riezzo, G.; Raimondi, F.; Di Mauro, A.; Francavilla, R.; et al. Infant crying, colic, and gastrointestinal discomfort in early childhood: A review of the evidence and most plausible mechanisms. *J. Pediatr. Gastroenterol. Nutr.* **2013**, *57* (Suppl. 1), S1–S45. [CrossRef] [PubMed]
113. Dryl, R.; Szajewska, H. Probiotics for management of infantile colic: A systematic review of randomized controlled trials. *Arch. Med. Sci.* **2018**, *14*, 1137–1143. [CrossRef] [PubMed]
114. Partty, A.; Kalliomaki, M.; Salminen, S.; Isolauri, E. Infant distress and development of functional gastrointestinal disorders in childhood: Is there a connection? *JAMA Pediatr.* **2013**, *167*, 977–978. [CrossRef] [PubMed]
115. Baldassarre, M.E.; Di Mauro, A.; Mastromarino, P.; Fanelli, M.; Martinelli, D.; Urbano, F.; Capobianco, D.; Laforgia, N. Administration of a Multi-Strain Probiotic Product to Women in the Perinatal Period Differentially Affects the Breast Milk Cytokine Profile and May Have Beneficial Effects on Neonatal Gastrointestinal Function Symptoms. A Randomized Clinical Trial. *Nutrients* **2016**, *8*, 677. [CrossRef] [PubMed]
116. Baldassarre, M.E.; Di Mauro, A.; Tafuri, S.; Rizzo, V.; Gallone, M.S.; Mastromarino, P.; Capobianco, D.; Laghi, L.; Zhu, C.; Capozza, M.; et al. Effectiveness and Safety of a Probiotic-Mixture for the Treatment of Infantile Colic: A Double-Blind, Randomized, Placebo-Controlled Clinical Trial with Fecal Real-Time PCR and NMR-Based Metabolomics Analysis. *Nutrients* **2018**, *10*, 195. [CrossRef] [PubMed]
117. Gutiérrez-Castrellón, P.; Indrio, F.; Bolio-Galvis, A.; Jiménez-Gutiérrez, C.; Jimenez-Escobar, I.; López-Velázquez, G. Efficacy of Lactobacillus reuteri DSM17938 for infantile colic: Systematic review with network meta-analysis. *Medicine* **2017**, *96*, e9375. [CrossRef] [PubMed]

118. Indrio, F.; Di Mauro, A.; Riezzo, G.; Civardi, E.; Intini, C.; Corvaglia, L.; Ballardini, E.; Bisceglia, M.; Cinquetti, M.; Brazzoduro, E.; et al. Prophylactic use of a probiotic in the prevention of colic, regurgitation, and functional constipation: A randomized clinical trial. *JAMA Pediatr.* **2014**, *168*, 228–233. [CrossRef] [PubMed]
119. Sung, V.; D'Amico, F.; Cabana, M.D.; Chau, K.; Koren, G.; Savino, F.; Szajewska, H.; Deshpande, G.; Dupont, C.; Indrio, F.; et al. Lactobacillus reuteri to Treat Infant Colic: A Meta-analysis. *Pediatrics* **2018**, *141*, e20171811. [CrossRef] [PubMed]
120. Boyle, R.J.; Robins-Browne, R.M.; Tang, M.L. Probiotic use in clinical practice: What are the risks? *Am. J. Clin. Nutr.* **2006**, *83*, 1256–1264. [CrossRef] [PubMed]
121. Besselink, M.G.; van Santvoort, H.C.; Buskens, E.; Boermeester, M.A.; van Goor, H.; Timmerman, H.M.; Nieuwenhuijs, V.B.; Bollen, T.L.; van Ramshorst, B.; Witteman, B.J.; et al. Probiotic prophylaxis in predicted severe acute pancreatitis: A randomised, double-blind, placebo-controlled trial. *Lancet* **2008**, *371*, 651–659. [CrossRef]
122. Allen, S.J.; Jordan, S.; Storey, M.; Thornton, C.A.; Gravenor, M.; Garaiova, I.; Plummer, S.F.; Wang, D.; Morgan, G. Dietary supplementation with lactobacilli and bifidobacteria is well tolerated and not associated with adverse events during late pregnancy and early infancy. *J. Nutr.* **2010**, *140*, 483–488. [CrossRef] [PubMed]
123. Luoto, R.; Laitinen, K.; Nermes, M.; Isolauri, E. Impact of maternal probiotic-supplemented dietary counselling on pregnancy outcome and prenatal and postnatal growth: A double-blind, placebo-controlled study. *Br. J. Nutr.* **2010**, *103*, 1792–1799. [CrossRef] [PubMed]
124. Kuitunen, M.; Kukkonen, K.; Savilahti, E. Pro- and prebiotic supplementation induces a transient reduction in hemoglobin concentration in infants. *J. Pediatr. Gastroenterol. Nutr.* **2009**, *49*, 626–630. [CrossRef] [PubMed]
125. Hooper, L.V.; Littman, D.R.; Macpherson, A.J. Interactions between the microbiota and the immune system. *Science* **2012**, *336*, 1268–1273. [CrossRef] [PubMed]
126. Rudensky, A.Y.; Chervonsky, A.V. A narrow circle of mutual friends. *Immunity* **2011**, *27*, 697–699. [CrossRef] [PubMed]
127. Baldassarre, M.E. Probiotic Genera/Species Identification Is Insufficient for Evidence-Based Medicine. *Am. J. Gastroenterol.* **2018**, *113*, 1561. [CrossRef] [PubMed]
128. Kolacek, S.; Hojsak, I.; Canani, R.B.; Guarino, A.; Indrio, F.; Pot, B.; Shamir, R.; Szajewska, H.; Vandenplas, Y.; van Goudoever, J.; et al. Commercial probiotic products: A call for improved quality control. A Position Paper by the ESPGHAN Working Group for Probiotics and Prebiotics. *J. Pediatr. Gastroenterol. Nutr.* **2017**, *65*, 117–124. [CrossRef] [PubMed]

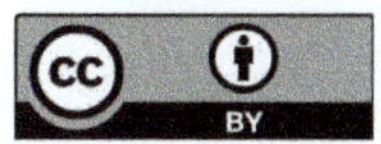

© 2018 by the authors. Licensee MDPI, Basel, Switzerland. This article is an open access article distributed under the terms and conditions of the Creative Commons Attribution (CC BY) license (http://creativecommons.org/licenses/by/4.0/).

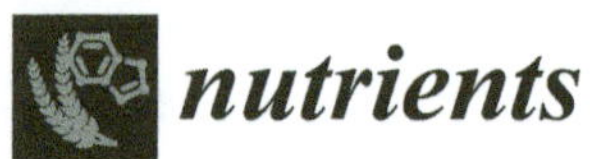 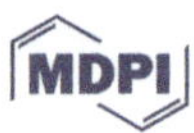

Review

Therapeutic Microbiology: The Role of *Bifidobacterium breve* as Food Supplement for the Prevention/Treatment of Paediatric Diseases

Nicole Bozzi Cionci, Loredana Baffoni, Francesca Gaggìa and Diana Di Gioia *

Department of Agricultural and Food Sciences (DISTAL), *Alma Mater Studiorum*—Università di Bologna, Viale Fanin 42, 40127 Bologna, Italy; nicole.bozzicionci@unibo.it (N.B.C.); loredana.baffoni@unibo.it (L.B.); francesca.gaggia@unibo.it (F.G.)

* Correspondence: diana.digioia@unibo.it; Tel.: +39-051-209-6269

Received: 15 October 2018; Accepted: 8 November 2018; Published: 10 November 2018 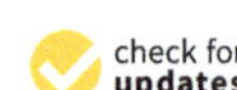

Abstract: The human intestinal microbiota, establishing a symbiotic relationship with the host, plays a significant role for human health. It is also well known that a disease status is frequently characterized by a dysbiotic condition of the gut microbiota. A probiotic treatment can represent an alternative therapy for enteric disorders and human pathologies not apparently linked to the gastrointestinal tract. Among bifidobacteria, strains of the species *Bifidobacterium breve* are widely used in paediatrics. *B. breve* is the dominant species in the gut of breast-fed infants and it has also been isolated from human milk. It has antimicrobial activity against human pathogens, it does not possess transmissible antibiotic resistance traits, it is not cytotoxic and it has immuno-stimulating abilities. This review describes the applications of *B. breve* strains mainly for the prevention/treatment of paediatric pathologies. The target pathologies range from widespread gut diseases, including diarrhoea and infant colics, to celiac disease, obesity, allergic and neurological disorders. Moreover, *B. breve* strains are used for the prevention of side infections in preterm newborns and during antibiotic treatments or chemotherapy. With this documentation, we hope to increase knowledge on this species to boost the interest in the emerging discipline known as "therapeutic microbiology".

Keywords: *Bifidobacterium breve*; probiotics; paediatrics; therapeutic microbiology

1. Introduction

The use of microorganisms to treat or prevent targeted diseases was conceived at the end of the last millennium. This concept has rapidly evolved giving rise to a new branch of applied microbiology known as "therapeutic microbiology" [1]. Since human organisms and gut microbiota establish an intimate symbiotic relationship that is fundamental for the maintenance of the host's health, the administration of beneficial microorganisms may represent a key determinant of the general health status and diseases susceptibility. The choice for the most suitable species for a certain pathology requires extensive studies, both *in vitro* and *in vivo*. Moreover, it is known that strains belonging to the same species may express different functions *in vivo* [2]. It has also been demonstrated that blending different microbial strains, species or even genera, may lead to a final effect that is not predicted by results from using each single microorganism. Several *Bifidobacterium* species are largely used as probiotics for their capability of reaching and colonizing the gastrointestinal tract and their documented history of safety. Among them, *Bifidobacterium breve*, originally isolated from infant faeces, represents one of the most used probiotics in infants. The multiple studies in which *B. breve* strains have been successfully used in diseased humans, especially children and newborns, witness the potentiality of strains belonging to this species for the prevention or treatment of human diseases. The aim of this review is to show the various applications of *B. breve* for preventing and treating paediatric diseases starting from *in vitro* and mice model assessment of efficacy to the clinical use. To the best of our knowledge, this work represents the first collection of works focused on the application in paediatrics of strains belonging to the *B. breve* species and is aimed to shed light on the role of this *Bifidobacterium* species in the scenario of "therapeutic microbiology." Moreover, this paper explores the effectiveness of *B. breve* used both as a single strain and combined with other microorganisms with a final short outcome of its application in adulthood.

2. The Human Intestinal Microbiota

The human intestinal microbiota is a complex ecosystem that includes not only bacteria but also fungi, Archaea, viruses and protozoans; bacteria concentration increases from the stomach and duodenum throughout the intestinal tract and in the large intestine it rises to 10^{11}–10^{12} CFU/g of lumen content [3]. It has been estimated that at least 1800 genera and a range of 15,000–36,000 bacterial species, depending on whether species are conservatively (97% OTUs) or liberally (99% OTUs) classified, can be found in the large intestine [4].

The symbiotic mutualistic relationship that the gut microbiota establishes with the host exerts several beneficial roles, the main of which are the maintenance of the gut epithelial barrier, the inhibition of pathogen adhesion to intestinal surfaces, the modulation and proper maturation of the immune system, the degradation of otherwise non-digestible carbon sources such as plant polysaccharides and the production of different metabolites including vitamins and short chain fatty acids (SCFAs) [5]. Furthermore, intestinal microorganisms seem to be responsible for a bidirectional interaction between the gut and the Central Nervous System (CNS) via the gut-brain axis [6]. Dysfunction in this interaction may be implicated in the development and prognosis of some neurological diseases, including autism [7], multiple sclerosis [8] or Parkinson disease [9]. Because of this symbiotic relationship, the human organism can be seen as a "superorganism," which consist of not only the microbial cells but also their genomes, that is, the microbiome and the related microproteome and micrometabolome [10]. The microbiome represents more than 100 times the human genome (1,000,000 genes vs. 23,000 genes) [10]. Indeed, the gut microbiome is influenced by external factors, such as diet, health status and xeno-metabolome. These factors shape the individual intestinal microbiota that can be considered as a "fingerprint" of the hosting organism.

Recently, the realization of global-collaborative projects has enriched the knowledge about the gut microbiota, such as the MetaHit project [11], the Human Microbiome project [12] and the MyNewGut project [13]. Moreover, the large amount of data from high throughput gene sequencing technology has allowed us to gain deeper insights in the composition of the "typical" human gut microbiota. The two principal bacterial phyla are *Firmicutes* and *Bacteroidetes*, followed by *Actinobacteria*, *Proteobacteria* and *Verrucomicrobia*. Fungi and Archaea constitute approximately 1% of the species of the intestinal microbiota [14,15]. The predominant fungal phyla are *Ascomycota* and *Basydiomicota*; some of the most abundant genera, that is, *Saccharomyces*, *Debaryomyces* and *Kluyveromyces*, are found in food, confirming the influence of diet habits also on the fungal intestinal population [16]. From the 80s some archaeal species belonging to *Methanobrevibacter* genus have been identified. *Methanobrevibacter* is the only genus detected in the gut probably due to the use of 16S primers not having sufficient resolution for Archaea. Within this genus, the species' composition depends on diet and host's health status, as for the entire microbiota [17,18].

Microbiologists' attention has been also focused on bacteriophages, which, living at bacteria expense and being vehicles of genetic transfer, could have an important role in shaping the biodiversity of the gut ecosystem. The first metagenomic analysis of an uncultured viral community from human faeces using partial shotgun sequencing suggested a large diversity of phages in gut microbiota [19]. The same authors investigated the viral community in the infant intestine using metagenomic sequencing: 72% of the detected viral community resulted to be siphoviruses and prophages and over 25% resulted to be phages that infect lactic acid bacteria; faecal viral sequences were not identified in breast milk, suggesting a non-dietary initial source of viruses [20]. The entire viral community composition changed dramatically between the first and the second week of age [20], remaining then stable during host's life [21].

Gut colonization begins at birth, although recent evidences suggest the existence of an intrauterine transmission of maternal bacteria to the foetus [22]. The first colonizer are facultative anaerobes (*Staphylococcus* spp., *Enterobacteriaceae* and *Streptococcus* spp.), followed by strict anaerobes, such as members of *Bifidobacterium*, *Bacteroides* and *Clostridium* genera [23,24]. The mode of delivery exerts a strong influence on the first microbial colonization of newborns' gut. Children born by natural delivery have an intestinal microbiota profile similar to their mother's vaginal one, characterized by *Lactobacillus* and *Prevotella* spp., while children born by caesarean section develop a microbiota similar to that of mother's skin (*Streptococcus*, *Corynebacterium* and *Propionibacterium* spp.) [25]. In addition, the type of feeding has a crucial role on the colonization of microbial groups in the gut. Indeed, the gut microbiota of formula-fed infants contains a higher amount of *Escherichia*, *Veillonella*, *Enterococcus* and *Enterobacter* members and the concentration of *Lactobacillus* and *Bifidobacterium* is lower with respect to in breast-fed infants [26]. The abundance of these genera can be due to a more acidic pH in the colon of breast-fed infants [27]. The prevalence of bifidobacteria in breast-fed infants is also due to their capability of fermenting oligosaccharides (referred to as human milk oligosaccharides, HMO) [28]. Diet continues to exert a crucial influence in the gut microbiota composition also in adulthood: De Filippis et al. [29] showed an association between plant-based diet and a prevalence of *Lachnospira* and *Prevotella* and a positive correlation between *Ruminococcus* and omnivore diet. Animal-based diets increase the abundance of bile-tolerant microorganism (*Alistipes*, *Bilophila* and *Bacteroides*) and decreases the levels of *Firmicutes* [30].

The use of antibiotics influences the gut microbiota composition, determining a significant decrease of the microbial diversity in the digestive tract [31,32]. However, the microbiota is a resilient system and tends to return to the pre-treatment state within 1 to 2 months after the end of the administration [33]. Moreover, the use of perinatal antibiotics, such as in the intrapartum prophylaxis, influences the establishment of a normal gut microbial composition and function, in particular reducing the levels of bifidobacteria and increasing potential pathogens [34–36].

It is well established that a functional and balanced microbiota reflects a healthy condition of the host; on the other hand, an unhealthy status may be associated with a compromised gut microbiota displaying a decrease of beneficial bacteria and increase of harmful ones.

3. Probiotics with a Special Emphasis on *Bifidobacterium breve*

"Probiotic" means "for life" and it is currently used to name bacteria associated with beneficial effects for humans and animals. In 2001 the Food and Agriculture Organization of the United Nations (FAO)/World Health Organization (WHO) defined them as "live microorganism which, when administered in adequate amounts confer a health benefit on the host" [37]. This definition has been revised in 2014 by the International Scientific Association for Probiotics and Prebiotics, including in the term probiotic "microorganism for which there are scientific evidence of safety and efficacy" and excluding "live cultures associated with fermented foods for which there is no evidence of a health benefit" [38].

Probiotics that have been largely studied in humans include species of the *Lactobacillus* and *Bifidobacterium* genera. Probiotic administration in the first stage of life results to be more effective in prevention and treatment of disorders, leading to a correct microbial colonization when the gut microbiota is still in a period of establishment. Several studies have shown the beneficial effects of *Lactobacillus reuteri*, one of the most used probiotics in infants, for the prevention and treatment of infant gastrointestinal disorders, including colics, regurgitation, vomit, constipation [39–41]. This species has been demonstrated to improve symptoms and reduce the number of anaerobic Gram negative bacteria, *Enterobacteriaceae* and enterococci in colicky infants [42,43]. Furthermore, *L. reuteri* ATCC 55730 was effective in children with distal active ulcerative colitis (UC) improving mucosal inflammation and modulating mucosal expression levels of some cytokines involved in the bowel inflammation [44]. *Lactobacillus* and *Saccharomyces* strains (*L. casei* CG, *L. reuteri* ATCC 55730 and a strain of *S. boulardii*) exerted positive effects as supplement for rehydration therapy for infectious diarrhoea in children by reducing the duration and stool frequency [45].

Several data are available for the use of bifidobacteria as probiotics for therapeutic purposes in infants [46]. As an example, *Bifidobacterium* strains belonging to the *animalis* (BB-12 strain) and *longum* species proved their efficacy against acute rotavirus diarrhoea in hospitalized children, particularly by increasing the immune response and decreasing duration of disease [47–49]. In addition, administration of *Bifidobacterium bifidum* and *B. animalis* strains in preterm and low birth weight infants demonstrated clinical positive effects for treatment of necrotizing enterocolitis (NEC) [50–52].

Among the different species belonging to the *Bifidobacterium* genus, *Bifidobacterium breve*, is the dominant one in breast-fed newborns [53] and one of the most used in infants. The species *B. breve* was firstly described by Reuter [54], who isolated from breast-fed infant faeces and named seven species of *Bifidobacterium*, including *B. parvulorum* and *B. breve*. The two species were then combined under the name of *B. breve* [55]. *B. breve* strains are also found in the vagina of healthy women [54]. Their presence in extra-body environments is a consequence of faecal contamination and the species is a useful indicator of human and animal faecal pollution [56]. *B. breve*, like other *Bifidobacterium* species, possess an array of enzymes for the utilization of different carbohydrates. These enzymes, useful to adapt and compete in an environment with changing nutritional conditions, are inducible in the presence of specific substrates. Amongst them, glycosidases, neuraminidases, glucosidases, galactosidase are included as well as extracellular glycosidases that degrade intestinal mucin oligosaccharides and glycosphingolipids [57]. *B. breve* also possess a glucosidase with a β-D-fucosidase activity, useful for the utilization of fucosilated HMO [58]. *B. breve* is included in the list of Qualified Presumption of Safety (QPS) biological agents [59]. Furthermore, recent studies have shown that human milk, traditionally considered as sterile, contains commensal, mutualistic and/or potentially probiotic bacteria for the infant gut. Among the different *Bifidobacterium* species found in human milk, *B. breve* strains have been detected with DNA-based techniques and also isolated and characterized [60]. These bacteria from human milk rapidly colonize the newborn's gut, protect the infant against infections and contribute to the maturation of the immune system [60].

Early studies by Akiyama et al. [61] showed that *B. breve* administration soon after birth was effective in developing a normal intestinal microbiota and, furthermore, *B. breve* showed a stronger affinity for immature bowel than other species, such as *B. longum*, evidencing its strong capabilities as probiotic. These achievements stimulated the development of further studies that gave new insights to the importance of this species as probiotic in infants.

Aloisio et al. [62] screened 46 *Bifidobacterium* strains for their capability of inhibiting the growth of gut pathogens including coliforms isolated from colicky infants. The most interesting strains belonged to the *B. breve* species, namely B632 strain (DSM 24706), B2274 strain (DSM 24707) and B7840 strain (DSM 24708). In addition to the antimicrobial activity against coliforms and other pathogenic bacteria, the strains did not possess transmissible antibiotic resistance traits and were not cytotoxic for gut epithelium, which are important pre-requisites for their use as probiotics. *B. breve* B632 was also able to stimulate the activity of mitochondrial dehydrogenases of macrophages and the production of IL-6, linked to a considerable activation of macrophages and endothelial cells in inflammatory condition. The potential of *B. breve* B632 as probiotic was also evidenced by Simone et al. [63]: it was able to inhibit the growth of *Enterobacteriaceae* in an *in vitro* gut model system stimulating the intestinal microbiota of a 2-month colicky infant, supporting the possibility to move to an *in vivo* study. Another strain of *B. breve*, BR03 (DSM 16604), revealed to be effective, as well as B632, in inhibiting the growth of 4 *E. coli* biotypes [64]. Mogna et al. [65] also underlined the validity of these two *B. breve* strains (B632 and BR03) in an *in vivo* study. The administration of both strains for 21 consecutive days as an oily suspension (daily dose of 100 million live cells of each strain) to healthy children was effective in obtaining gut colonization and in decreasing total faecal coliforms.

A biotechnological approach could improve the gastric transit survival, gastrointestinal persistence and therapeutic efficacy of the strain *B. breve* UCC2003, isolated from infant stool, via the heterologous expression of the listerial betaine uptake system gene, BetL [66]. In addition to the improved capability of colonizing the intestine of inoculated mice, the strain was also able to reduce *Listeria* proliferation in the organs of the infected mice. Although the introduction of genes from pathogens into probiotic cultures is unlikely to meet approval from regulatory authorities, this study underlined that probiotic characteristics can be susceptible to improvements. Future perspectives include the obtainment of BetL homologues from Generally Recognized as Safe (GRAS) organisms and natural selection of probiotic cultures with elevated expression of such homologues.

B. breve strain Yakult (BBG-01) is another widely used probiotic strain. It was one of the first *B. breve* strain shown to possess the ability to modulate the intestinal microbiota by reducing the count of several pathogenic bacteria, such as *Campylobacter*, *Candida* and *Enterococcus* spp., after oral administration [67,68]. This strain has also displayed an anti-infective activity against Shiga-toxin-producing *E. coli* (STEC) O157:H7 in infected mice [69].

For its valid properties as probiotic, *B. breve* has also found a notable place in food technology in the fermentation of milk. In this regard, the positive effects associated to *B. breve*-fermented soymilk has been reported in several studies, demonstrating to improve lipid metabolism, alcohol metabolism and mammary carcinogenesis in mice models [70–72].

Moreover, a strain of *B. breve* has been included in a widespread of commercial high concentrated probiotic preparation, known as VSL#3, which contains 10^{11}–10^{12} viable lyophilized cells of different bacterial species that are usual component of human gut microbiota. Specifically, the formulation contains four strains of *Lactobacillus* (*L. paracasei*, *L. plantarum*. *L. acidophilus* and *L. delbrueckii* subsp. *bulgaricus*), three strains of *Bifidobacterium* (*B. longum*, *B. breve* and *B. infantis*) and one strain of *Streptococcus salivarius* subsp. *thermophilus*. VSL#3 exhibited an immunomodulatory capacity in *in vitro* studies by increasing the production of anti-inflammatory cytokines and inhibiting the production of pro-inflammatory cytokines [73].

4. *B. breve* Effectiveness in Mice Models

The strong evidence of the immune modulating capability of *B. breve* strains has been consolidated and well documented in a large number of animal models studies, which are the basis for human clinical trials.

The oral administration of *B. breve* YIT4064 strain, isolated from faeces of a healthy breast-fed infant, in mice immunized orally with an influenza virus was able to increase anti-influenza virus IgG levels in serum, thus protecting mice against infection. The authors concluded that the oral administration of this strain may enhance antigen-specific IgG against various pathogenic antigens taken orally and induce protection against various viral infections [74]. This conclusion was also supported by the study of Yasui et al. [75] that proved that the same strain stimulated anti-influenza virus hemagglutinin IgA by Peyer's patch cells in response to addition of hemagglutinins. These antibodies may reach the mucosal tissue and prevent influenza virus infection.

B. breve UCC2003 possessed a cell surface exopolysaccharide (EPS) able to play an important role in immunomodulation in B cell response. Administration for 3 consecutive days of EPS^{+} *B. breve* strains in mice infected with *Citrobacter rodentium*, a diarrheagenic pathogen related to human *E. coli*, is effective in reducing the pathogen colonization, differently from mice fed with EPS^{-} *B. breve* [76]. EPS was involved in the production of a biofilm on the gut epithelium [77] preventing the attachment of *C. rodentium*.

Natividad et al. [78] illustrated the relationship between *B. breve* NCC2950 and regenerating (REG) III proteins, molecules belonging to the family of C-type lectins, which are expressed in the intestine and involved in maintaining gut homeostasis. The group REGIII-γ was measured in the ileum and colon of germ-free (GF) mice, mice colonized with specific pathogen free (SPF) microbiota and with a low diversity microbiota (altered Schaedler flora–ASF). Monocolonization with the probiotic *B. breve* NCC2950 but not with the commensal *E. coli* JM83, significantly induced REGIII-γ expression.

B. breve MRx0004, isolated from faeces of healthy humans, possessed a protective action in a severe asthma condition [79]. The study remarked an important decrease of neutrophil and eosinophil infiltration in lung bronchoalveolar lavage fluid in a mouse model of severe asthma after the probiotic treatment. This result, together with the demonstrated reduction of pro-inflammatory cytokines and chemokines involved in neutrophil migration, showed that *B. breve* MRx0004 effectiveness in reducing the above-mentioned inflammation condition paves the way for next-generation drug for management of severe asthma.

Many *B. breve* strains played an important role in prevention and treatment of various allergy conditions. Oral administration of *B. breve* M-16V, isolated from faecal sample of a healthy infant, in ovalbumin (OVA)-immunized mice significantly reduced the serum levels of total IgE, OVA-specific IgE and OVA-specific IgG1 and *ex vivo* production of IL-4 by the splenocytes [80]. Schouten et al. [81] showed that an intervention with a synbiotic formulation, comprising *B. breve* M-16V and a GOS/FOS mixture, was protective against the development of symptoms in mice orally sensitized with whey. The promising effect was confirmed by Kostadinova et al. [82] demonstrating the partially prevention of skin reaction due to cow's milk allergy, following the probiotic administration in combination with specific β-lactoglobulin—derived peptides and a specific blend of short- and long-chain fructo-oligosaccharides in mice. Particularly, the treatment, besides increasing the cecal content of propionic and butyric acid, determined an increase of IL-22 expression, which plays an antimicrobial role in the innate immunity response and of the anti-inflammatory cytokine IL-10 in the Peyer's patches. This outcome agrees with Jeon et al. [83], who demonstrated that the administration of the *B. breve* Yakult strain increased the number of IL-10-producing $CD4^+$ T cells in the large intestine of murine models and an increased production of acetic acid [69].

B. breve was also involved in protective mechanisms against obesity; the orally administration of *B. breve* B-3 in a mouse model with diet-induced obesity could suppress the increase of body weight and epididymal fat, with improved serum levels of total cholesterol, fasting glucose and insulin and act by regulating gene expression pathways involved in lipid metabolism and response to stress in the liver [84,85].

Increasing evidence suggests that a brain–gut–microbiome axis exists, although its role in cognition remains relatively unexplored [6,86]. Bifidobacteria were found to improve the behavioural deficits and to possess a potential action on stress-related disorders in model mice [87]. *B. breve* strains potential has also been investigated for the capability of conferring beneficial effects on neurological diseases. Savignac et al. [88] showed that 6 weeks feeding of *B. breve* 1205 strain resulted in positive effects on compulsive behaviour in marble burying test, anxiolytic effects in the elevated plus maze and reduced body weight gain in model mice, contributing to a general amelioration of anxiety and metabolism. Kobayashi et al. [89] showed that oral administration of *B. breve* A1, isolated from faeces of human infants, prevented cognitive decline in Alzheimer disease (AD) model mice, with a reduction of neural inflammation; they observed that the probiotic provided ameliorations in both working memory and long-term memory. Furthermore, they found an increase of plasma acetate levels after the probiotic treatment and the neural inflammation reduction can be considered as a consequence of this increase due to *B. breve* administration, since SCFAs have been shown to have immune modulatory functions in model mice [90]. This evidence suggests that *B. breve* A1 has therapeutic potential for preventing cognitive impairment in Alzheimer disease and the necessity to move to a clinical intervention to evaluate the effects on diseased humans.

B. breve supplementation can affect the metabolism of fatty acids. Among them, eicosapentaenoic acid (EPA), which derives from α-linolenic acid metabolization, is an essential constituent of the cell membrane, plays an important role in brain and nervous system development and in inflammatory response [91]; docosahexanoic acid (DHA), which derives from EPA metabolization, is one of the major n-3 polyunsaturated fatty acids (PUFA) in the brain and is essential for a correct development of foetal encephalon [92]. Some studies revealed that human commensal microorganisms are able to synthetize bioactive isomers of conjugated linoleic acids (CLA) from free linoleic acid [93]; CLA was proven to possess antiatherosclerotic, antidiabetic and immunomodulatory properties [94,95]. Wall et al. [96] demonstrated that oral administration for 8 weeks to different animals (pigs and mice) of *B. breve* NCIMB 702258, a CLA producer strain, in combination with linoleic acid as substrate, increased the concentration of the predominant CLA isomer found in nature (*c*9, *t*11) in the liver. Furthermore, this supplementation in mice increased EPA and DHA levels in the adipose tissue and reduced proinflammatory cytokines tumour necrosis factor-α (TNF-α) and interferon-γ (IFN-γ) levels. The same authors demonstrated that a 8 weeks administration with the same *B. breve* strain and α-linolenic acid, the precursor of EPA, resulted in an increase in the liver EPA and brain DHA concentrations in mice. These results outline that the *B. breve* strain is a notable candidate for the treatment of inflammatory and neurodegenerative being able to modulate the hippocampal expression of brain-derived neutrophic factor (BDNF), a neurotrophin involved in development of the nervous system [97,98]. Particularly, the probiotic treatment reduced the expression of BDNF exon IV, which has been described as being highly responsive and increased by stress [99].

5. *B. breve* Application in Clinical Trials in Paediatrics

The use of *B. breve* strains for treatment and prevention of human diseases have been increasingly expanding in the last decade. Being bifidobacteria the most abundant bacterial group in infant gut, most of the studies are focused on paediatric subjects. Figure 1 summarizes the main applications of *B. breve* in paediatric diseases.

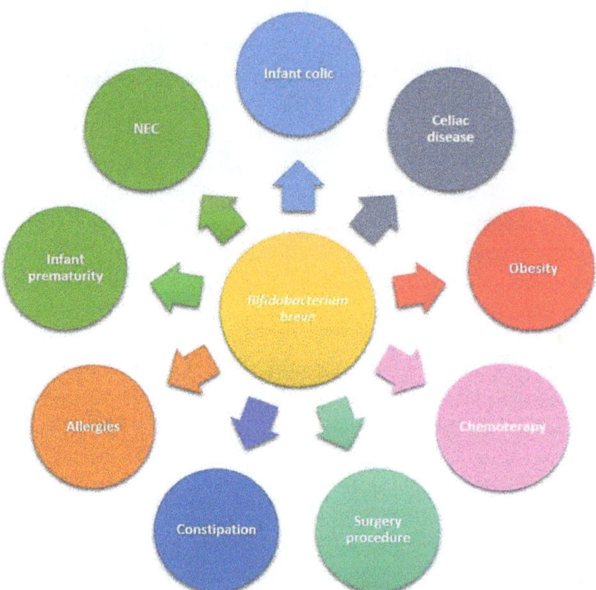

Figure 1. Paediatric diseases in which an amelioration of symptoms has been obtained upon *B. breve* strains administration.

Therapeutic and protective role for human health of *B. breve* strains both as single strain or as a mixture of two strains of the same species has been demonstrated. As already mentioned, several researchers account for the improved efficacy of multi-species and multi-strain formulations that acting with a synergic effect, may enhance the effectiveness of each single strain [100,101].

5.1. Preterm Infants and Necrotising Enterocolitis (NEC)

A consistent number of preterm infants, especially those of very low birth weight, are subjected to episodes of systemic infection caused by antibiotic resistant bacteria and fungi that can lead to chronic diseases and brain injuries [102,103]. These episodes can result from a combination of factors, including immature gastrointestinal tract mucosal barrier and undeveloped gastrointestinal tract immune system, which may predispose premature infants to bacterial translocation, causing systemic infection and necrotising enterocolitis (NEC) [104,105]. In addition, preterm infants have revealed an altered microbiota composition, resulting in almost undetectable bifidobacteria counts during the first and second week of life, differently for those at term [106–108]. This observation has allowed the formulation of the hypothesis that a bifidobacteria treatment could lead to a reintegration of beneficial bacteria in the intestinal environment and a reduction of bacterial translocation to other districts, stimulating researches in this sector. One of the first study that investigated the effects of a *B. breve* supplementation in preterm neonates reported that the strain YIT4010, administered as a suspension of distilled water containing 0.5×10^9 bacterial cells for 28 days, was able to colonize efficiently the intestinal tract, to reduce abnormal abdominal symptoms and to improve the weight gain [109]. A later study compared the effects of the administration of a *B. breve* strain a few hours after birth and 24 h after birth; the supplement was prepared by dissolving 1.6×10^8 cells in 0.5 mL of 5% glucose solution and administered twice a day for all the duration of hospitalization [110]. In newborns administered with the probiotic soon after birth, bifidobacteria were detected significantly earlier and the number of *Enterobacteriaceae* at 2 weeks after birth was significantly lower, compared to the infants treated 24 h after birth demonstrating that a very early probiotic intervention may contribute to the establishment of a beneficial gut microbiota and the prevention of infectious diseases [110].

A more recent work proved the suitability of *B. breve* M-16V administration for routine use in preterm infants in order to control the gut microbiota colonization and shift it towards a healthy profile [111]. Moreover, a retrospective cohort study was performed with the purpose of evaluating whether the supplementation with the same probiotic to preterm neonates would reduce the risk of NEC [112]. NEC represents the most life-threatening pathology of preterm neonates with incidence and mortality of 10–12% and 40–45%, respectively. It is characterized by gastrointestinal dysfunction progressing to pneumatosis intestinalis, systemic shock and rapid death in severe cases [113,114]. NEC is categorized into 3 different stages based on the severity of the disease, from stage I, a suspicion for disease, to stage III, corresponding to a severe progression of the disease [115]. Although the pathogenesis of this condition remains obscure, some important prevention strategies have been adopted, such as the use of antenatal glucocorticoids, early preferential feeding with breast-milk, prevention and treatment of infections [116]. Since preterm infants have shown an intestinal reduction of total bifidobacteria and a predominance of facultative anaerobes, some of which potentially pathogens, until the 20th day of life, it has been suggested that a major etiological factor for NEC could be an altered microbiota composition [117]. Therefore, a probiotic treatment can be an additional strategy for NEC prevention. A 3-week *B. breve* M-16V supplementation (3×10^9 CFU/day) has been associated with a lower incidence of NEC ($\geq$stage II) in very low birth weight infants born before 34 weeks; the incidence in those born before 28 weeks resulted lower but not statistically significant [112]. Satoh et al. [118] had already demonstrated the efficacy of *B. breve* M-16V administration in preventing NEC in extremely low and very low birth weight infants: the probiotic was daily supplemented at a dose of 1×10^9 CFU dissolved in breast milk or breast-mixed with formula milk several hours after birth and continued until discharge from hospital (achievement of body weight 2300 g or gestational age of 37 weeks); the treatment led to a significant reduction of infection and mortality rate.

Various studies suggested that an overproduction of SCFAs in the intestinal environment can lead to mucosal injuries, which may evolve in NEC in premature infants [119,120]. Wang et al. [121] demonstrated that a 4 weeks *B. breve* M-16V supplementation (1.6×10^8 cells suspended in 0.5% glucose solution) was associated with a reduction of butyric acid levels in very and extremely low birth weight newborns. Since butyric acid increases the IL-8 secretion in enterocytes, condition that may lead to neutrophil invasion, a known hallmark of NEC, *B. breve* administration can be considered protective against NEC onset.

Immediately after delivery, some physiological changes, especially in the immunologic system, occur in newborns in order to adapt themselves to the new environment. *B. breve* M-16V, administered at 10^9 cells in 0.5 mL of 5% glucose solution starting several hours after birth, can increase the transforming growth factor β1 (TGF-β1) signals in preterm infants [122]. This increase has a relevant importance as it is known to induce oral tolerance, exert anti-inflammatory effects, express mucosal IgA and promote epithelial cell proliferation and differentiation [123]. A further study investigated the preventive effects of the same *B. breve* strain against infections and sepsis in extremely and very low birth weight newborns. The probiotic consisted on a freeze-dried preparation with a dose of 10^9 CFU dissolved in breast- or formula-milk; the development of infection and sepsis resulted significantly lower in the supplemented group compared with the non-supplemented one [124], highlighting once more the efficacy of a *B. breve* treatment in the prevention of developing infections, sepsis and NEC.

According to Braga et al. [125] the combined use of *B. breve* Yakult and *L. casei* was able to reduce the occurrence of NEC and was associated with an improvement in intestinal motility in newborns. The intervention started at the second day of life and continued for 30 days, provided *L. casei* and *B. breve* mixed to human milk in a daily dosage of 3.5×10^7 and 3.5×10^9 CFU, respectively. The number of NEC confirmed cases (≥stage II) was reduced upon probiotic treatment.

5.2. Gastrointestinal Disorders

A disorder that affects up to 30% of newborns in the first months of life is infant colic. It is characterized by paroxysmal, excessive and incontrollable crying without identifiable causes [126] representing a serious problem for the family and, in many cases, it can cause disorders later in life [127,128]. The aetiology remains obscure but an unbalanced intestinal microbiota has been suggested to play a role in the disease pathogenesis. Several studies support the use of probiotics as therapeutic or preventive agent against colics but very few clinical trials have been performed on bifidobacteria application. A mixture of *B. breve* strains (BR03 and B632), whose probiotic potential, as already highlighted in Section 3, has been extensively demonstrated *in vitro*, was prepared as oily suspension and administered at a daily dosage of 5 drops containing 10^8 CFU of each strain to 83 infants, involving both breast and bottle-fed subjects [129]. Preliminary results showed that administration was effective in reducing minutes of daily crying. The clinical trial was then completed (155 infants, 130 breast- and 25 bottle-fed), as described in Aloisio et al. [130]; the *B. breve* mixture was able to prevent gastrointestinal disorders in healthy breast-fed infants, principally by reducing 56% of daily vomit frequency, decreasing 46.5% of daily evacuation over time and improving stool consistency. The strength of this study is the interrelation among a prolonged probiotic treatment, several clinical and anthropometric parameters (e.g., crying time, stool frequency, colour and consistency, regurgitation, vomits, weight, length, head circumference of newborn, delivery mode, type of feeding, gestational age) and main gut microbial groups. Epidemiological data have shown the predisposition of neonates born by caesarean section to develop obesity later in life [131,132]. However, the *B. breve* supplementation in infants born by caesarean section [130] resulted in a lower catch-up growth in weight, thus allowing the authors to speculate a protective effect of the probiotic strains against the risk to develop metabolic disturbance later in life.

Another common disease in childhood related to the intestinal tract is functional constipation, a chronic condition characterized by infrequent defecation (less than three times per week) and more than two episodes of faecal incontinence per week [133]; the pathogenesis, undoubtedly multifactorial, has not a well-defined aetiology. It has been shown that, despite intensive medical and behavioural therapy, 25% of patients developing constipation before the age of 5 years continue to have constipation upsets beyond puberty [134]. A pilot study showed the beneficial effects of 4 weeks treatment with *B. breve* Yakult (BBG-01) in constipated children: daily administration of 10^8–10^9 CFU led to a significantly increase in defecation frequency and amelioration of stool consistency, frequency of episodes of faecal incontinence and abdominal pain [135]. There is a debate of whether it is more effective the use of single strains or an association of them for constipation treatment; however, the mentioned study demonstrated that the intake of only one *B. breve* strain is even effective. Giannetti et al. [136] investigated the effects deriving from the administration of a mixture of 3 bifidobacteria, namely *B. infantis* M-63, *B. breve* M-16V and *B. longum* BB536, in children suffering from irritable bowel syndrome (IBS). IBS is a functional bowel disorder characterized by chronic abdominal pain, discomfort, bloating and altered bowel habits including diarrhoea or constipation [137]. The daily dose was about 10^9 cells for each strain administered as bacterial powder and the treatment lasted 6 weeks. The bifidobacteria mixture intake resulted in a significant decrease in prevalence and frequency of abdominal pain and an improvement of the quality of life, assessed by an interview-administered validated questionnaire.

The commercial formulation VSL#3, already described in Section 3, was used in several clinical studies targeted to different diseases in paediatrics resulting in an amelioration of the health status of children suffering from IBS [138]. In this randomized, double-blind, placebo-controlled, multicentre trial, patients were treated with one sachet (twice in those 12–18 years old) of probiotic mixture containing 4.5×10^{12} bacteria for 6 weeks. The preparation was effective in improving the overall perception of symptoms, the severity and frequency of abdominal pain, abdominal bloating and family assessment of life disruption, leading to a general improving of quality of life in children suffering from IBS.

Miele et al. [139] carried out the first paediatric, randomized, placebo-controlled trial using VSL#3 for the treating of ulcerative colitis (UC). This disorder belongs to the chronic inflammatory bowel disease (IBD) category, has a prevalence of about 100 cases per 100,000 children [140] and occurs as diffuse mucosal inflammation in the colon; it is characterized by periods of remission and relapse episodes, not all the patients tolerate the existing treatment to induce remission for their adverse effects and in 20–30% of paediatric patients failure of the treatment occurs [141]. Since the pathogenesis, beside genetic susceptibility, is linked to compromised immune response and alteration in gut microbiota composition, the idea beyond the study was that 1 year of VSL#3 administration might improve the health status of patients. Subjects with an average age of 10 were supplemented with a weight-base dose of probiotic (4.5×10^{11}–1.8×10^{12} bacteria per day); treated patients showed a significantly higher rate of remission compared to placebo and a significantly lower incidence of relapse within 1 year of follow-up. According to the authors, this success may be related to the use of a mixture of various probiotics, which might have a strong synergic action and to the high bacterial concentration of viable cells contained in the mixture. Furthermore, the probiotic preparation showed to be safe and well tolerable by children with a diagnosis of UC.

The efficacy of VSL#3 in paediatric diseases was also evaluated by Dubey et al. [142], who conducted a double-blind, randomized, placebo-controlled trial treating acute rotavirus diarrhoea in children. VSL#3, containing a total of 9×10^9 bacteria/dose and administered for 4 days, significantly reduced, already on day 2, mean stool frequency and improved stool consistency; these results were also reflected in the lower volume of oral rehydration salts administered in children who received the probiotic. The functional role of VSL#3 was investigated by Sinha et al. [143], who focused on the prevention of neonatal sepsis in low birth weight infants, one of the infections which evolves more rapidly in this paediatric category. The mixture, containing 10^9 bacteria/dose, was administered for 30 days. VSL#3 intake in low birth weight was associated with a non-significant 21% reduction in the risk of suspected sepsis; nevertheless, in the sub-group of infants weighing 1.5–1.99 kg, the reduction of the risk of suspected sepsis was statistically significant, differently from newborns weighing 2.0–2.49 kg. The results of the study allowed to conclude that the intervention may be useful for the most vulnerable subjects of low birth weight.

As infant feeding has a crucial role in developing infant gut microbiota and consequently intestinal immunity, fermented formula milk containing probiotics or prebiotics has been developed. This approach is aimed at protecting infants from various gastrointestinal disorders by modulating gut microbial composition. The first study that evaluated the effects of a fermented formula milk with *B. breve* C50 and *Streptococcus thermophilus* 065 on the incidence of acute diarrhoea in healthy infants was a randomized, double-blind, placebo-controlled multicentre study, which involved 971 subjects belonging to three different areas of France [144]. The trial was planned to occur in a high risk predicted period for diarrhoea incidence in France (from October to January) and the supplementation lasted 5 months. Although no reduction in the incidence and duration of diarrhoea episodes were observed after the intervention, a lower number of dehydration cases, a lower number of medical consultation cases with fewer oral rehydration solution prescriptions and changes of formula were registered. These outcomes can be considered as indicators of probiotic positive effects on the severity of the disease. According to the authors, these results may be related to the bifidogenic and immunomodulatory properties of fermentation products contained in formula-milk.

5.3. Celiac Disease

The efficacy of the probiotic mixture containing *B. breve* B632 and *B. breve* BR03 was also shown in children affected by celiac disease. In this case, the strains were administered as lyophilized powder at a daily dosage of 10^9 CFU of each strain for 3 months in celiac children on a gluten free diet (GFD). A preliminary important outcome obtained from the intervention was the reduction of pro-inflammatory cytokine TNF-α in blood samples of celiac children on GFD [145]. The gut microbiota composition was also studied with Next Generation Sequencing (NGS) technology. Unexpectedly, the intervention did not cause changes at the level of the genus or phylum to which the administered probiotics belong but the probiotic acted as a "trigger" element for the increase of *Firmicutes* and the restoration of the physiological *Firmicutes/Bacteroides* ratio that was altered in celiacs with respect to healthy subjects. Moreover, the intervention restored the normal amount of *Lactobacillaceae* members, reaching almost the same values of healthy subjects [146]. Besides modulating inflammatory condition and gut microbiota composition of celiac children, *B. breve* supplementation influenced the SCFAs profile; acetic acid had a negative correlation with *Verrucomicrobia*, *Euryarcheota* and particularly *Synergisestes* [147]. Although *Synergisestes* is a minor phylum in human faeces (abundance of 0.01%) of healthy subjects, it was found to have a considerable role for human health because of its negative correlation with TNF-α that may indicate an anti-inflammatory role [148,149]. In the study of Primec et al. [147], the *Synergisestes* phylum clearly confirmed its anti-inflammatory role negatively correlating with pro-inflammatory acetic acid after three months of probiotic treatment.

5.4. Paediatric Obesity

Another pathology in which the gut microbiota may play a notable role is obesity. Although it is accepted that obesity results from disequilibrium between energy intake and expenditure, it is a complex disease and not completely understood. Nowadays, obesity prevalence is spreading especially among children and adolescents and it can be considered a worldwide epidemic. Obesity has been associated with a chronic inflammation that may conduct to insulin resistance [150,151]. Recently, obesity has been associated with a specific profile of the gut microbiota characterized by lower levels of bacteria belonging to *Bacteroides* and *Bifidobacterium* genera compared to that of lean individuals [152]. In addition, bifidobacteria were shown to be higher in children maintaining normal weight at 7 years old than in children developing overweight and their administration was able to reduce serum and liver triglyceride levels and to decrease hepatic adiposity [153,154]. The mixture of *B. breve* already mentioned (BR03 and B632) was used in a cross-over double-blind randomized controlled trial in order to re-establish metabolic homeostasis and reduce chronic inflammation in obese children [155]. Although the study is still on-going, preliminary results related to the part previous the cross-over demonstrated that a *B. breve* administration in obese children is promising: 8 weeks treatment seems to ameliorate glucose metabolism and could help in weight management by reducing BMI, waist to height ratio and waist circumference [155].

5.5. Allergies

There are increasing evidences that the intestinal microbiota plays an important role in the development of allergic diseases, in particular, low bifidobacteria levels appear to be associated with atopic dermatitis [156]; in the previous section, the potential of *B. breve* in preventing and treating allergy conditions was reported and this impressive role has been confirmed in clinical studies. *B. breve* M-16V revealed to be effective in the treatment of cow's milk hypersensitivity infants with atopic dermatitis [157]. *B. breve*, added to the casein-hydrolysed milk formula at the dosage of 5×10^9 CFU or 15×10^9 CFU per day, increased the proportion of bifidobacteria in the gut microbial composition and ameliorated allergic symptoms by interacting with the immune system and no remarkable dose dependent differences were detected [157]. The synergetic combination of probiotics and prebiotics, known as synbiotic, seems also to be promising in atopic dermatitis treatment. In this regard, Van der Aa et al. [158] studied the effects of a synbiotic mixture on atopic dermatitis in formula-fed infants; the formulation consisted of *B. breve* M-16V at a dose of 1.3×10^9 CFU/100 mL and a mixture of 90% short-chain galactooligosaccharides (scGOS) and 10% long-chain fructooligosaccharides (IcFOS), 0.8 g/100 mL added to formula milk. Although the formulation, administered for 12 weeks, had no effect on atopic dermatitis severity, it significantly modulated the composition and the metabolic activity of gut microbiota, leading to a decrease of pH, high lactate and low butyric levels resembling the metabolic profile of breast-fed infants [159]. The same synbiotic mixture has demonstrated to reduce the prevalence of asthma-like symptoms and the prevalence of asthma medications use after the fulfilment of a 1-year follow-up [160].

The effects of a formulation containing *B. breve* M-16V and *B. longum* BB536 for the prevention of allergies in infants enrolling both mothers and newborns was studied [161]. The formulation was provided as powder daily doses containing 5×10^9 CFU/g of each strain. Pregnant women begun the supplementation 4 weeks before the expected date of delivery and the newborns received the probiotic mixed to water, breast- or formula-milk starting 1 week after birth and continuing for 6 months. The study revealed that prenatal and postnatal supplementation with a bifidobacteria mixture reduced the risk of developing eczema and atopic dermatitis in infants. NGS analyses of newborns' faecal samples showed significant differences of the major intestinal microbial phyla (*Actinobacteria, Bacteroidetes, Proteobacteria*) of allergic and non-allergic infants at 4 months of age. However, these differences were lost at 10 months of age, highlighting that the microbiota of early stages is particularly important in regulating allergies upset in infants.

5.6. Surgical Procedures

Surgical procedures can also alter gut microbiota composition and functions and disrupt intestinal barrier function, inducing the patient in a condition at risk for infection [162]. A probiotic therapy may be functional for patients improving the immunological function of the intestine and competing against harmful bacteria infection. A pilot study demonstrated that daily administration of *B. breve* Yakult BBG-01 (10^9 freeze-dried cells per day) to children younger than 15 years 7 days before surgery until discharge from hospital, simultaneously to intravenous antibiotics postoperatively treatment, reduced the incidence of bacteria in blood samples. Moreover, the intestinal microbial composition was improved by increasing *Bifidobacterium* spp. and reducing potential pathogens such as *Clostridium difficile, Pseudomonas* and *Enterobacteriaceae*. Higher concentrations of faecal acetate and lower faecal pH levels were detected in children who received the probiotic 2 weeks after surgery [163]. Improvement of intestinal environment resulting from a perioperative supplementation with the same strain was also observed in neonates undergoing surgery for congenital heart disease [164]. Daily dosage of 3×10^9 CFU of *B. breve* Yakult (BBG-01) was administered starting 1 week before surgery and ending 1 week after the operation; infants who received the probiotic supplement showed significantly higher bifidobacteria levels and lower *Enterobacteriaceae, Staphylococcus* and *Pseudomonas* levels in faecal microbiota compared to infants not receiving the supplement. Moreover, probiotic treated infants exhibited significantly higher concentration of total organic acids levels compared to non-treated ones, in particular acetic acid increased immediately and 1 week after surgery; furthermore, the faecal pH tended to decrease with the probiotic intervention.

Kanamori et al. [165] documented in a case-report the efficacy of a synbiotic therapy, consisting in a combination of *B. breve* Yakult (BBG-01), *L. casei* Shirota and galactoolicosaccharides as prebiotic components, in a newborn with short bowel syndrome resulting from a consistent bowel resection performed soon after delivery. Patients affected from this pathology are subjected to an intestinal bacteria overgrowth due to their dilated intestine [166]; this condition can lead to a bacteria translocation in other districts inducing catheter sepsis, compromised carbohydrates fermentation resulting in high level of lactate, with consequent acidosis [167] and a possible incontrollable growth of intestinal pathogens. One year of synbiotic therapy, consisting in 3 g of bacteria (1×10^9 bacteria/g per each strain) and 3 g of prebiotic per day, improved the nutritional state, prior compromised, by increasing the intestinal motility and suppressed the intestinal pathogen overgrowth, in particular *E. coli* and *Candida* spp.

The same synbiotic combination was used as a therapy for refractory and repetitive enterocolitis [168]; this disorder often occurs in paediatric surgery patients and the severe type may be fatal. The 7 recruited patients, having short bowels as a result of surgical resection and suffering from repetitive enterocolitis, were administered with 1 g of probiotic (10^9 bacteria/g) 3 times daily for 36 months. All patients had an altered gut microbial composition prior to the therapy characterized by low levels of anaerobic bacteria and high levels of resident pathogenic bacteria. In spite of the frequent antibiotic treatments to which patients were exposed, the long synbiotic administration was effective in highly increasing bifdobacteria and lactobacilli levels, which were almost undetectable before the supplementation and incrementing faecal SCFAs, inducing a more normal ecosystem profile in the intestine. Moreover, most of patients accelerated their body weight gain and showed increased serum rapid turnover, with a general amelioration of their health status.

With the developing of therapies and surgeries in the field of perinatal and foetal cares, neonate survival outcomes have extraordinary increased; newborns that are subjected to these interventions need prolonged intensive care periods, which include use of antibiotics, respiratory care and restriction of enteral feeding. All these factors may affect the normal microbial gut colonization leading to severe infection and malnutrition [169]. A synbiotic therapy, including *B. breve*, as already observed, could be effective in preventing or correcting an abnormal microbial colonization in intensive care newborns. The same synbiotic therapy, largely and positively tested, including *B. breve* Yakult, *L. casei* Shirota and galactooligosaccharides, was applied to newborns with diagnosis of severe congenital anomalies [169]. The product contained 10^9–10^{10} bacteria/g and was administered immediately after birth via a nasogastric tube, as soon as intestinal feeding was possible, first at a dose of 0.12 g per day in four equal dose and then, when the amount of milk increased, at 3 g per day in three equal doses. As results of the therapy, none of patients manifested enterocolitis, they showed an improvement in their clinical course and reached a body weight gain equivalent to that of normal infants. This last outcome has been hypothesized to be linked to the potential metabolic activity of the administered probiotics to promote liver lipogenesis and fat storage in the peripheral fat tissue contributing to the growth observed in these infants despite the congenital disorders [170].

5.7. Coadjuvant in Chemotherapic Treatment

A condition in which the use of probiotics may have a reliving effect is chemotherapy. The cancer itself and the drug-therapy inducing bone marrow suppression lead to an immunocompromising state in which an infectious could be fatal. Since the main source of infection is endogenous intestinal harmful bacteria [171], a probiotic treatment can certainly benefit the patient's state by not only competing against pathogens for nutrients and attachments sites but also by stimulating gut immunity, producing organic acids and improving transepithelial resistance [172]. A study conducted in 2009 evaluated the effect of *B. breve* Yakult (BBG-01) strain in cancer paediatric subjects, administered with 10^9 freeze-dried cells, corn starch and hydroxipropyl cellulose in 1 g of formulation. The administration was found to be effective in reducing febrile episodes, which may be the only sign of infection and the use of intravenous antibiotics by stabilizing the intestinal microbial composition [173].

An overview in chronological order of *B. breve* applications as a single strain and as a component of a multi-strain/multi-species formulation is reported in Tables 1 and 2, respectively.

Table 1. Overview of *B. breve* strains applications in *in vitro* studies, mice model and paediatric trials.

B. breve Strains	Reported Effect(s)	References
B. breve B632	Strong antimicrobial activity against pathogens, stimulation of mitochondrial dehydrogenase activity of macrophages, stimulation of proinflammatory cytokines production in *in vitro* study	[62]
B. breve BR03	Inhibition of the growth of 4 *E. coli* biotypes in *in vitro* study	[64]
B. breve B632 + *B. breve* BR03	Reduction of total faecal coliforms in healthy children	[65]
	Reduction of pro-inflammatory TNF-α in blood samples of celiac children	[145]
	Reduction of minutes of daily crying in healthy infants	[129]
	Restoration of the healthy percentage of main gut microbial components in celiac children	[146]
	Improvement of glucose metabolism and weight management in obese children	[155]
	Reduction of daily vomit frequency, daily evacuation, improved stool consistency, protection against developing metabolic disturbance in healthy infants	[130]
	Modulation of faecal SCFAs profile in celiac children	[147]
B. breve Yakult (BBG-01)	Anti-infective activity against Shiga-toxin-producing *E. coli* in mice model	[69]
	Reduction of febrile episodes and use of intravenous antibiotics in cancer paediatric subjects	[173]
	Improvement of composition and metabolic activity of gut microbiota and reduction of incidence of bacteria in blood in paediatric surgery subjects	[163]
	Increased defecation frequency, improvement of stool consistency, frequency episodes of faecal incontinence and abdominal pain in constipated children	[133]
	Stimulation of anti-inflammatory IL-10-producing CD4+T cells in mice model	[83]
	Improvement of composition and metabolic activity of gut microbiota in paediatric surgery infants with congenital heart disease	[164]
B. breve YIT4064	Stimulation of anti-influenza virus hemagglutinin IgA production by Peyer's patch cells in mice model	[75]
	Stimulation of antigen-specific IgG production against pathogenic antigens in mice model	[74]
B. breve UCC2003	Reduction of *Citrobacter rodentium* gut colonization in mice model	[76]
B. breve NCC2950	Induction of REGIII-γ expression in mice model and REGIII-α in *in vitro* study	[78]
B. breve MRx0004	Reduction of pro-inflammatory cytokines and lung neutrophil and eosinophil infiltration in severe asthma mice model	[79]
B. breve M-16V	Improvement of allergic symptoms associated to cow's milk hypersensitivity in infants	[157]
	Immunomodulation activity by increasing TGF-β1 in preterm infants	[122]
	Reduction of infections and mortality for NEC in extremely and very low birth weight infants	[118]
	Reduction of faecal butyric acid in extremely and very low birth weight infants	[121]
	Reduction of total IgE, OVA-specific IgE and OVA-specific IgG in mice model	[80]
	Protection against developing of whey allergy symptoms in model mice	[81]
	Reduction of infections and sepsis incidence in extremely and very low birth weight infants	[124]
	Improvement of composition and metabolic activity of gut microbiota in infants with atopic dermatitis	[158]
	Reduction of asthma-like symptoms prevalence and asthma medication use prevalence in infants with atopic dermatitis	[160]
	Shifted gut microbiota towards a healthy profile in preterm infants	[111]
	Low incidence of NEC (≥stage II) in very low birth weight infants	[112]
	Partially protection against developing skin reaction due to cow's milk allergy, increased cecal content of butyrate and propionate and increased antimicrobial IL-22 expression in mice model	[82]

Table 1. *Cont.*

B. breve Strains	Reported Effect(s)	References
B. breve B-3	Suppression of epididymal fat and body weight gain in mice model with diet-induced obesity	[84,85]
B. breve 1205	Amelioration of anxiety condition and general metabolism in mice model	[88]
B. breve A1	Prevention of cognitive decline in Alzheimer disease and reduction of neural inflammation in mice model	[89]
B. breve NCIMB 702258	Increased CLA isomer (*c*9, *t*11), EPA and DHA in adipose tissue and reduced proinflammatory cytokines in mice model	[96]
B. breve YIT4010	Reduced abdominal symptoms and improved weight gain in preterm infants	[109]
	Establishment of beneficial gut microbiota and prevention of infections in preterm infant	[110]

Table 2. Overview of applications of *B. breve* strains combined to other bacterial strains in paediatric trials.

B. breve Strains	Probiotic Mixture	Reported Effect(s)	References
B. breve M-16V	*B. breve* M-16V *B. longum* BB536	Reduction of developing eczema and atopic dermatitis in infants	[161]
	B. breve M-16V *B. infantis* M-63 *B. longum* BB536	Reduction of abdominal pain prevalence and frequency, improvement of quality of life in IBS children	[134]
B. breve Yakult (BBG-01)	*B. breve* Yakult *L. casei* Shirota	Improvement of composition and metabolic activity of gut microbiota and of overall health status in infants with short bowel syndrome	[165,168]
		Prevention of enterocolitis, improvement of body weight and clinical course in infants with congenital disorders	[169]
	B. breve Yakult *L. casei*	Reduction of NEC incidence and improvement of intestinal motility in infants	[125]
B. breve C50	*B. breve* C50 *S. thermophilus* 065	Reduction of number of dehydration cases and medical consultation cases in children exposed to risk of developing acute diarrhoea	[144]
B. breve DSM 24732	VSL#3	Reduction of stool frequency and improving of stool consistency in children with acute rotavirus diarrhoea	[142]
		Manifestation of high rate of remission and low incidence of relapse in UC children	[139]
		Improvement of symptoms, severity and frequency of abdominal pain and bloating and family assessment of life disruption in IBS children	[138]
		Reduction of the risk of suspected sepsis in most vulnerable very low birth weight infants	[144]

6. *B. breve* Administration in Adults: A Short Outcome

The use of *B. breve* has been largely investigated in paediatric scenery and its therapeutic role has been strongly supported by significant and solid outcomes; its use is not limited to paediatric supplementation but it is also involved in improving health condition in briefly outlined.

Minami et al. [174] investigated the use of *B. breve* B-3 at a daily dosage of 5×10^{10} CFU/capsule for 12 weeks in adults with a tendency for obesity. A significant decrease of the fat mass and an amelioration of blood parameters were observed, in particular a significant reduction of γ-glutamyltranspeptidase (γ-GTP), a marker used to evaluate liver injury and high-sensitivity protein C-reactive (hCRP), a marker used to evaluate the inflammatory reaction, were detected. Interestingly, a significant negative correlation between the value of fat mass and 1,5-anhydroglucitol, a marker that closely reflect short-term glucose status and glycaemic variability, was recorded suggesting the potential role of *B. breve* in the improvement of diabetes.

Ishikawa et al. [175] showed the effects of one year of *B. breve* Yakult treatment, in association with galactooligosaccharides as prebiotic, in patients diagnosed with UC. The probiotic, containing 10^9 CFU/dose of freeze-dried powder, was administered immediately after every meal 3 times a day and the prebiotic, at a dosage of 5.5 g, was administered once a day. The synbiotic intervention improved the endoscopic score by decreasing the values of severity mucosa damage [176] and reduced the level of myeloperoxidase, which is secreted by neutrophils and macrophages accumulated in the inflamed lesions and positively correlated with the disease severity [177]. Regarding gut environment results, the synbiotic treatment significantly reduced *Bacteroidaceae* counts and faecal pH, which may be connected to an increment of faecal SCFAs.

An interesting relationship was evaluated by Kano et al. [178]: since a Japanese 2007 survey evidenced that women who suffer from abnormal bowel movements also showed skin disorders, they conducted a double-blind, placebo-controlled, randomized trial to investigate the effects of probiotic and prebiotic fermented milk on skin of healthy adult women. The fermented milk contained galactooligosaccharides, polydextrose, *B. breve* Yakult, *Lactococcus lactis* and *S. thermophilus* at a daily dose of 6×10^{10}, 5×10^{10}, 5×10^{10} CFU/100 mL of milk, respectively. The synbiotic intake, which lasted 4 weeks, resulted to prevent hydration level decreases in the stratum corneum. The intervention increased cathepsin L-like protease activity, which can be considered as an indicator of keratocyte differentiation, as proteolysis of cathepsin L activates transglutaminase 3, which plays an important role in the *stratum corneum* formation [179]. Moreover, the administration reduced phenol levels in serum and urine and since the production of phenols is inhibited at low intestinal pH, an increase of intestinal organic acid levels might be occurred after the treatment.

The probiotic preparation VSL#3 has been extensively used for the treatment of IBD in adulthood. Brigidi et al. [180] investigated the effects of 20 days VSL#3 administration in patients with diarrhoea predominant-IBS or functional diarrhoea; the probiotic intake caused changes in gut microbiota composition with a significantly increase of total lactobacilli, total bifidobacteria and *S. thermophilus*, which are component of VSL#3. The treatment led also to an improvement of some enzymes functions, whose actions are compromised in IBD, by reducing urease activity, whose products usually allow pathogenic bacteria to survive in the gastrointestinal tract and contribute to mucosal tissue damages [181] and by increasing β-galactosidase activity, which is involved in the metabolism of unabsorbed carbohydrates. Pronio et al. [182] confirmed the positive role of VSL#3 upon treatment of patients undergoing ileal pouch anal anastomosis for ulcerative colitis. The probiotic intervention reduced signs and symptoms of inflammation inducing a significant expansion of cells associated to an improvement of the inflammatory condition of the pouch mucosa. An interesting microbial outcome was evidenced by Kühbacher et al. [183]: the UC remission maintained by VSL#3 administration was accompanied by a higher bacterial diversity actually not related to the probiotic intake. However, the increase of bacterial diversity may represent a therapeutic mechanism that supports the VSL#3 activity in maintaining UC remission. Bibiloni et al. [184] showed that 6 weeks administration with the probiotic mixture improved UC remission and response in patients not responding to traditional therapy. Since VSL#3 has been demonstrated to maintain remission in UC patients intolerant or allergic to 5-aminosalicylic acid (5-ASA), known also as mesalazine [185], Tursi et al. [186] demonstrated the efficacy on UC of another therapeutic combination: VSL#3, in association with balsalazide, 5-ASA prodrug, was shown to be significantly superior to balsalazide alone and to mesalazide in the treatment of active mild-to-moderate UC. One of the key points of the study is the low dosage of balsalazide used (2.25 g/day), usually not effective in reducing UC symptoms and inducing remission. Therefore, the low dosage appeared to be effective only in combination with VSL#3. In this regard, a more recent study, involving a larger number of patients, highlighted the superior ability of VSL#3 to improve relapsing mild-to-moderate UC when added to standard UC treatment with respect to patients on standard treatment only, confirming the potential synergic action exerted by standard UC pharmacological treatments and VSL#3 [187]. The reason for this synergic action may be a combined effect of the chemotherapic on the disease and of the probiotic on the general well-being of the host. Clinical studies proved that this probiotic mixture was particularly effective in the treatment of IBD, improving abdominal pain duration and distention severity score in patients suffering from IBS [188]. Moreover, it was effective in clinical condition of diarrhoea-predominant IBS subjects [189,190].

7. Conclusions

This review has outlined the large number of cases in which *B. breve* strains, mainly as single strains but also in combination with other *Bifidobacterium* species or *Lactobacillus* strains, are used for therapeutic and prevention purposes and/or to prevent further complications of the disease in the paediatric sector. The analysis of the outlined results allows to conclude that, whereas *in vitro* or animal-model study are performed with a large number of different *B. breve* strains, clinical studies are performed with a restricted number of strains (mainly *B. breve* YIT4010, M-16V, the associations B632/BR03 and Yakult BBG-01). Therefore, there is the opportunity of expanding the potentialities of the strains used in clinical studies on the basis of the positive results obtained in pre-clinical studies and, therefore, more opportunities for a further development of "therapeutic microbiology." A second interesting aspect outlined in this review is the frequent association of the *B. breve* administration with traditional chemotherapeutic treatment. This is particularly important in the treatment of very serious diseases in which stopping the traditional therapies may be considered risky for the patient. The probiotic can act as a supplement to prevent complication and improve the general health status of the patient. We are all confident that the improvement in the "therapeutic microbiology" sector will be a great aid to medical approach in the near future.

Author Contributions: All the authors designed the outline of the review; N.B.C. wrote the main sections of the manuscript, L.B. contributed to the general description of *B. breve* species, F.G. contributed to the studies on adults, D.D.G. supervised the work and critically revised the paper.

Funding: This research received no external funding.

Acknowledgments: The authors would like to acknowledge the EU project FOODstars (Innovative Food Product Development Cycle: Frame for Stepping Up Research Excellence of FINS, GA 692276) for the grant supplied to N.B.C.

Conflicts of Interest: The authors declare no conflict of interest.

References

1. Spinler, J.K.; Versalovic, J. Probiotics in Human Medicine: Overview. In *Therapeutic Microbiology: Probiotics and Related Strategies*, 1st ed.; Versalovic, J., Wilson, M., Eds.; ASM Press: Washington, DC, USA, 2008; pp. 225–229.
2. Maassen, C.B.M.; Van Holten-Neelen, C.; Balk, F.; Heijne Den Bak-Glashouwer, M.J.; Leer, R.J.; Laman, J.D.; Boersma, W.J.A.; Claassen, E. Strain-dependent induction of cytokine profiles in the gut by orally administered Lactobacillus strains. *Vaccine* **2000**, *18*, 2613–2623. [CrossRef]
3. O'Hara, A.M.; Shanahan, F. The gut flora as a forgotten organ. *EMBO Rep.* **2006**, *7*, 688–693. [CrossRef] [PubMed]
4. Frank, D.N.; St. Amand, A.L.; Feldman, R.A.; Boedeker, E.C.; Harpaz, N.; Pace, N.R. Molecular-phylogenetic characterization of microbial community imbalances in human inflammatory bowel diseases. *Proc. Natl. Acad. Sci. USA* **2007**, *104*, 13780–13785. [CrossRef] [PubMed]
5. Sánchez, B.; Delgado, S.; Blanco-Míguez, A.; Lourenço, A.; Gueimonde, M.; Margolles, A. Probiotics, gut microbiota, and their influence on host health and disease. *Mol. Nutr. Food Res.* **2016**, *61*, 1600240. [CrossRef] [PubMed]
6. Cryan, J.F.; O'Mahony, S.M. The microbiome-gut-brain axis: From bowel to behavior. *Neurogastroenterol. Motil.* **2011**, *23*, 187–192. [CrossRef] [PubMed]

7. De Theije, C.G.M.; Wu, J.; Da Silva, S.L.; Kamphuis, P.J.; Garssen, J.; Korte, S.M.; Kraneveld, A.D. Pathways underlying the gut-to-brain connection in autism spectrum disorders as future targets for disease management. *Eur. J. Pharmacol.* **2011**, *668*, 70–80. [CrossRef] [PubMed]
8. Berer, K.; Gerdes, L.A.; Cekanaviciute, E.; Jia, X.; Xiao, L.; Xia, Z.; Liu, C.; Klotz, L.; Stauffer, U.; Baranzini, S.E.; et al. Gut microbiota from multiple sclerosis patients enables spontaneous autoimmune encephalomyelitis in mice. *Proc. Natl. Acad. Sci. USA* **2017**, *114*, 10719–10724. [CrossRef] [PubMed]
9. Scheperjans, F.; Aho, V.; Pereira, P.A.B.; Koskinen, K.; Paulin, L.; Pekkonen, E.; Haapaniemi, E.; Kaakkola, S.; Eerola-Rautio, J.; Pohja, M.; et al. Gut microbiota are related to Parkinson's disease and clinical phenotype. *Mov. Disord.* **2015**, *30*, 350–358. [CrossRef] [PubMed]
10. Del Chierico, F.; Vernocchi, P.; Bonizzi, L.; Carsetti, R.; Castellazzi, A.M.; Dallapiccola, B.; de Vos, W.; Guerzoni, M.E.; Manco, M.; Marseglia, G.L.; et al. Early-life gut microbiota under physiological and pathological conditions: The central role of combined meta-omics-based approaches. *J. Proteomics* **2012**, *75*, 4580–4587. [CrossRef] [PubMed]
11. Metagenomics of the Human Intestinal Tract. Available online: http://www.metahit.eu/ (accessed on 24 August 2018).
12. NIH Human Microbiome Project. Available online: https://hmpdacc.org/ (accessed on 24 August 2018).
13. My New Gut. Available online: http://www.mynewgut.eu/ (accessed on 24 August 2018).
14. Lynch, S.V.; Pedersen, O. The Human Intestinal Microbiome in Health and Disease. *N. Engl. J. Med.* **2016**, *375*, 2369–2379. [CrossRef] [PubMed]
15. Graf, D.; Di Cagno, R.; Fåk, F.; Flint, H.J.; Nyman, M.; Saarela, M.; Watzl, B. Contribution of diet to the composition of the human gut microbiota. *Microb. Ecol. Health Dis.* **2015**, *26*, 26164. [CrossRef] [PubMed]
16. Sokol, H.; Leducq, V.; Aschard, H.; Pham, H.-P.; Jegou, S.; Landman, C.; Cohen, D.; Liguori, G.; Bourrier, A.; Nion-Larmurier, I.; et al. Fungal microbiota dysbiosis in IBD. *Gut* **2017**, *66*, 1039–1048. [CrossRef] [PubMed]
17. Dridi, B.; Raoult, D.; Drancourt, M. Archaea as emerging organisms in complex human microbiomes. *Anaerobe* **2011**, *17*, 56–63. [CrossRef] [PubMed]
18. Ishaq, S.L.; Moses, P.L.; Wright, A.-D.G. The Pathology of Methanogenic Archaea in Human Gastrointestinal Tract Disease. In *The Gut Microbiome*; Mozsik, G., Ed.; IntechOpen: Rijeka, Croatia, 2016.
19. Breitbart, M.; Hewson, I.; Felts, B.; Mahaffy, J.M.; Nulton, J.; Salamon, P.; Rohwer, F. Metagenomic Analyses of an Uncultured Viral Community from Human Feces. *J. Bacteriol.* **2003**, *185*, 6220–6223. [CrossRef] [PubMed]
20. Breitbart, M.; Haynes, M.; Kelley, S.; Angly, F.; Edwards, R.A.; Felts, B.; Mahaffy, J.M.; Mueller, J.; Nulton, J.; Rayhawk, S.; et al. Viral diversity and dynamics in an infant gut. *Res. Microbiol.* **2008**, *159*, 367–373. [CrossRef] [PubMed]
21. Scarpellini, E.; Ianiro, G.; Attili, F.; Bassanelli, C.; De Santis, A.; Gasbarrini, A. The human gut microbiota and virome: Potential therapeutic implications. *Dig. Liver Dis.* **2015**, *47*, 1007–1012. [CrossRef] [PubMed]
22. Francino, M. Early Development of the Gut Microbiota and Immune Health. *Pathogens* **2014**, *3*, 769–790. [CrossRef] [PubMed]
23. Solís, G.; de los Reyes-Gavilan, C.G.; Fernández, N.; Margolles, A.; Gueimonde, M. Establishment and development of lactic acid bacteria and bifidobacteria microbiota in breast-milk and the infant gut. *Anaerobe* **2010**, *16*, 307–310. [CrossRef] [PubMed]
24. Sharon, I.; Morowitz, M.J.; Thomas, B.C.; Costello, E.K.; Relman, D.A.; Banfield, J.F. Time series community genomics analysis reveals rapid shifts in bacterial species, strains, and phage during infant gut colonization. *Genome Res.* **2013**, *23*, 111–120. [CrossRef] [PubMed]
25. Azad, M.B.; Konya, T.; Maughan, H.; Guttman, D.S.; Field, C.J.; Chari, R.S.; Sears, M.R.; Becker, A.B.; Scott, J.A.; Kozyrskyj, A.L. Gut microbiota of healthy Canadian infants: Profiles by mode of delivery and infant diet at 4 months. *Can. Med. Assoc. J.* **2013**, *185*, 385–394. [CrossRef] [PubMed]
26. Lee, S.A.; Lim, J.Y.; Kim, B.S.; Cho, S.J.; Kim, N.Y.; Kim, O.B.; Kim, Y. Comparison of the gut microbiota profile in breast-fed and formula-fed Korean infants using pyrosequencing. *Nutr. Res. Pract.* **2015**, *9*, 242–248. [CrossRef] [PubMed]
27. Tham, C.S.C.; Peh, K.K.; Bhat, R.; Liong, M.T. Probiotic properties of bifidobacteria and lactobacilli isolated from local dairy products. *Ann. Microbiol.* **2012**, *62*, 1079–1087. [CrossRef]
28. Liepke, C.; Adermann, K.; Raida, M.; Mägert, H.J.; Forssmann, W.G.; Zucht, H.D. Human milk provides peptides highly stimulating the growth of bifidobacteria. *Eur. J. Biochem.* **2002**, *269*, 712–718. [CrossRef] [PubMed]

29. De Filippis, F.; Pellegrini, N.; Vannini, L.; Jeffery, I.B.; La Storia, A.; Laghi, L.; Serrazanetti, D.I.; Di Cagno, R.; Ferrocino, I.; Lazzi, C.; et al. High-level adherence to a Mediterranean diet beneficially impacts the gut microbiota and associated metabolome. *Gut* **2016**, *65*, 1812–1821. [CrossRef] [PubMed]
30. David, L.A.; Maurice, C.F.; Carmody, R.N.; Gootenberg, D.B.; Button, J.E.; Wolfe, B.E.; Ling, A.V.; Devlin, A.S.; Varma, Y.; Fischbach, M.A.; et al. Diet rapidly and reproducibly alters the human gut microbiome. *Nature* **2014**, *505*, 559–563. [CrossRef] [PubMed]
31. Huse, S.M.; Dethlefsen, L.; Huber, J.A.; Welch, D.M.; Relman, D.A.; Sogin, M.L. Exploring microbial diversity and taxonomy using SSU rRNA hypervariable tag sequencing. *PLoS Genet.* **2008**, *4*, 1000255. [CrossRef]
32. Jernberg, C.; Löfmark, S.; Edlund, C.; Jansson, J.K. Long-term ecological impacts of antibiotic administration on the human intestinal microbiota. *ISME J.* **2007**, *1*, 56–66. [CrossRef] [PubMed]
33. De La Cochetière, M.F.; Durand, T.; Lepage, P.; Bourreille, A.; Galmiche, J.P.; Doré, J. Resilience of the Dominant Human Fecal Microbiota upon Short-Course Antibiotic Challenge. *J. Clin. Microbiol.* **2005**, *43*, 5588–5592. [CrossRef]
34. Arboleya, S.; Sánchez, B.; Solís, G.; Fernández, N.; Suárez, M.; Hernández-Barranco, A.M.; Milani, C.; Margolles, A.; De Los Reyes-Gavilán, C.G.; Ventura, M.; et al. Impact of prematurity and perinatal antibiotics on the developing intestinal microbiota: A functional inference study. *Int. J. Mol. Sci.* **2016**, *17*, 649. [CrossRef] [PubMed]
35. Aloisio, I.; Quagliariello, A.; De Fanti, S.; Luiselli, D.; De Filippo, C.; Albanese, D.; Corvaglia, L.T.; Faldella, G.; Di Gioia, D. Evaluation of the effects of intrapartum antibiotic prophylaxis on newborn intestinal microbiota using a sequencing approach targeted to multi hypervariable 16S rDNA regions. *Appl. Microbiol. Biotechnol.* **2016**, *100*, 5537–5546. [CrossRef] [PubMed]
36. Mazzola, G.; Murphy, K.; Ross, R.P.; Di Gioia, D.; Biavati, B.; Corvaglia, L.T.; Faldella, G.; Stanton, C. Early gut microbiota perturbations following intrapartum antibiotic prophylaxis to prevent group B streptococcal disease. *PLoS ONE* **2016**, *11*, e0157527. [CrossRef] [PubMed]
37. Joint FAO/WHO. *Expert consultation on evaluation of health and nutritional properties of probiotics in food including powder milk with live lactic acid bacteria.* Health and Nutritional Properties of Probiotics in Food including Powder Milk with Live Lactic Acid Bacteria: Cordoba, Argentina, 1–4 October 2001. Available online: http://isappscience.org/wp-content/uploads/2015/12/FAO-WHO-2001-Probiotics-Report.pdf (accessed on 28 August 2018).
38. Hill, C.; Guarner, F.; Reid, G.; Gibson, G.R.; Merenstein, D.J.; Pot, B.; Morelli, L.; Canani, R.B.; Flint, H.J.; Salminen, S.; et al. The International Scientific Association for Probiotics and Prebiotics consensus statement on the scope and appropriate use of the term probiotic. *Nat. Rev. Gastroenterol. Hepatol.* **2014**, *11*, 506–514. [CrossRef] [PubMed]
39. Indrio, F.; Di Mauro, A.; Riezzo, G.; Civardi, E.; Intini, C.; Corvaglia, L.; Ballardini, E.; Bisceglia, M.; Cinquetti, M.; Brazzoduro, E.; et al. Prophylactic use of a probiotic in the prevention of colic, regurgitation, and functional constipation a randomized clinical trial. *JAMA Pediatr.* **2014**, *168*, 228–233. [CrossRef] [PubMed]
40. Szajewska, H.; Gyrczuk, E.; Horvath, A. *Lactobacillus reuteri* DSM 17938 for the management of infantile colic in breastfed infants: A randomized, double-blind, placebo-controlled trial. *J. Pediatr.* **2013**, *162*, 257–262. [CrossRef] [PubMed]
41. Chau, K.; Lau, E.; Greenberg, S.; Jacobson, S.; Yazdani-Brojeni, P.; Verma, N.; Koren, G. Probiotics for infantile colic: A randomized, double-blind, placebo-controlled trial investigating *Lactobacillus reuteri* DSM 17938. *J. Pediatr.* **2015**, *166*, 74–78. [CrossRef] [PubMed]
42. Savino, F.; Cordisco, L.; Tarasco, V.; Palumeri, E.; Calabrese, R.; Oggero, R.; Roos, S.; Matteuzzi, D. *Lactobacillus reuteri* DSM 17938 in Infantile Colic: A Randomized, Double-Blind, Placebo-Controlled Trial. *Pediatrics* **2010**, *126*, e526–e533. [CrossRef] [PubMed]
43. Savino, F.; Fornasero, S.; Ceratto, S.; De Marco, A.; Mandras, N.; Roana, J.; Tullio, V.; Amisano, G. Probiotics and gut health in infants: A preliminary case-control observational study about early treatment with *Lactobacillus reuteri* DSM 17938. *Clin. Chim. Acta* **2015**, *451*, 82–87. [CrossRef] [PubMed]
44. Oliva, S.; Di Nardo, G.; Ferrari, F.; Mallardo, S.; Rossi, P.; Patrizi, G.; Cucchiara, S.; Stronati, L. Randomised clinical trial: The effectiveness of *Lactobacillus reuteri* ATCC 55730 rectal enema in children with active distal ulcerative colitis. *Aliment. Pharmacol. Ther.* **2012**, *35*, 327–334. [CrossRef] [PubMed]

45. Allen, S.J.; Martinez, E.G.; Gregorio, G.V.; Dans, L.F. Cochrane Review: Probiotics for treating acute infectious diarrhoea. *Evid.-Based Child Health Cochrane Rev. J.* **2011**, *6*, 1894–2021. [CrossRef]
46. Sanders, M.E.; Akkermans, L.M.A.; Haller, D.; Hammerman, C.; Heimbach, J.T.; Hörmannsperger, G.; Huys, G. Safety assessment of probiotics for human use. *Gut Microbes* **2010**, *1*, 164–185. [CrossRef] [PubMed]
47. Weizman, Z.; Asli, G.; Alsheikh, A. Effect of a Probiotic Infant Formula on Infections in Child Care Centers: Comparison of Two Probiotic Agents. *Pediatrics* **2005**, *115*, 5–9. [CrossRef] [PubMed]
48. Grandy, G.; Medina, M.; Soria, R.; Terán, C.G.; Araya, M. Probiotics in the treatment of acute rotavirus diarrhoea. A randomized, double-blind, controlled trial using two different probiotic preparations in Bolivian children. *BMC Infect. Dis.* **2010**, *10*, 253. [CrossRef] [PubMed]
49. Vandenplas, Y.; De Hert, S.G. Randomised clinical trial: The synbiotic food supplement Probiotical vs. placebo for acute gastroenteritis in children. *Aliment. Pharmacol. Ther.* **2011**, *34*, 862–867. [CrossRef] [PubMed]
50. Lin, H.; Hsu, C.; Chen, H.; Chung, M.; Hsu, J.; Lien, R.; Tsao, L.; Chen, C.; Su, B. Oral Probiotics Prevent Necrotizing Enterocolitis in Very Low Birth Weight Preterm Infants: A Multicenter, Randomized, Controlled Trial. *Pediatrics* **2008**, *122*, 693–700. [CrossRef] [PubMed]
51. Khailova, L.; Dvorak, K.; Arganbright, K.M.; Halpern, M.D.; Kinouchi, T.; Yajima, M.; Dvorak, B. *Bifidobacterium bifidum* improves intestinal integrity in a rat model of necrotizing enterocolitis. *AJP Gastrointest. Liver Physiol.* **2009**, *1297*, 940–949. [CrossRef] [PubMed]
52. Underwood, M.A.; Kananurak, A.; Coursodon, C.F.; Adkins-Reick, C.K.; Chu, H.; Bennett, S.H.; Wehkamp, J.; Castillo, P.A.; Leonard, B.C.; Tancredi, D.J.; et al. *Bifidobacterium bifidum* in a rat model of necrotizing enterocolitis: Antimicrobial peptide and protein responses. *Pediatr. Res.* **2012**, *71*, 546–551. [CrossRef] [PubMed]
53. Turroni, F.; Peano, C.; Pass, D.A.; Foroni, E.; Severgnini, M.; Claesson, M.J.; Kerr, C.; Hourihane, J.; Murray, D.; Fuligni, F.; et al. Diversity of bifidobacteria within the infant gut microbiota. *PLoS ONE* **2012**, *7*, e36957. [CrossRef] [PubMed]
54. Reuter, G. Vergleichende Untersuchungen uber die Bifidus-flora im Sauglings-und Erwachsenenstuhl. *Zentbl Bakteriol* **1963**, *191*, 486–507.
55. Rogosa, M. Genus III, *Bifidobacterium* Orla-Jensen. In *Bergley's Manual of Determinative Bacteriology*, 8th ed.; Buchanan, R.E., Gibbons, N.E., Eds.; Williams and Wilkins Co.: Baltimore, MD, USA, 1974; pp. 669–676.
56. Mara, D.D.; Oragui, J.I. Sorbitol-fermenting bifidobacteria as specific indicators of human faecal pollution. *J. Appl. Bacteriol.* **1983**, *55*, 349–357. [CrossRef] [PubMed]
57. Falk, P.; Hoskins, L.C.; Larson, G. Bacteria of the human intestinal microbiota produce glycosidases specific for lacto-series glycosphingolipids. *J. Biochem.* **1990**, *108*, 466–474. [CrossRef] [PubMed]
58. Asakuma, S.; Hatakeyama, E.; Urashima, T.; Yoshida, E.; Katayama, T.; Yamamoto, K.; Kumagai, H.; Ashida, H.; Hirose, J.; Kitaoka, M. Physiology of consumption of human milk oligosaccharides by infant gut-associated bifidobacteria. *J. Biol. Chem.* **2011**, *286*, 34583–34592. [CrossRef] [PubMed]
59. EFSA Panel on Biological Hazards (BIOHAZ). Scientific opinion on the maintenance of the list of QPS biological agents intentionally added to food and feed (2012 update). *EFSA J.* **2012**, *11*, 3449. [CrossRef]
60. Fernández, L.; Langa, S.; Martín, V.; Maldonado, A.; Jiménez, E.; Martín, R.; Rodríguez, J.M. The human milk microbiota: Origin and potential roles in health and disease. *Pharmacol. Res.* **2013**, *69*, 1–10. [CrossRef] [PubMed]
61. Akiyama, K.; Hosono, S.; Takahashi, E.; Ishizeki, S.; Takigawa, I.; Imura, S.; Yamauchi, K.; Yaeshima, T.; Hayasawa, H.; Shimamura, S. Effects of oral administration of *Bifidobacterium breve* on development of intestinal microflora in extremely premature infants. *Acta Neonatol. Jpn.* **1994**, *30*, 130–137.
62. Aloisio, I.; Santini, C.; Biavati, B.; Dinelli, G.; Cencič, A.; Chingwaru, W.; Mogna, L.; Di Gioia, D. Characterization of *Bifidobacterium* spp. strains for the treatment of enteric disorders in newborns. *Appl. Microbiol. Biotechnol.* **2012**, *96*, 1561–1576. [CrossRef] [PubMed]
63. Simone, M.; Gozzoli, C.; Quartieri, A.; Mazzola, G.; Di Gioia, D.; Amaretti, A.; Raimondi, S.; Rossi, M. The probiotic *Bifidobacterium breve* B632 inhibited the growth of enterobacteriaceae within colicky infant microbiota cultures. *BioMed Res. Int.* **2014**. [CrossRef] [PubMed]
64. Mogna, L.; Del Piano, M.; Deidda, F.; Nicola, S.; Soattini, L.; Debiaggi, R.; Sforza, F.; Strozzi, G.; Mogna, G. Assessment of the in vitro inhibitory activity of specific probiotic bacteria against different *Escherichia coli* strains. *J. Clin. Gastroenterol.* **2012**, *46*, S29–S32. [CrossRef] [PubMed]

65. Mogna, L.; Del Piano, M.; Mogna, G. Capability of the two microorganisms *Bifidobacterium breve* B632 and *Bifidobacterium breve* BR03 to colonize the intestinal microbiota of children. *J. Clin. Gastroenterol.* **2014**, *48*, S37–S39. [CrossRef] [PubMed]
66. Sheehan, V.M.; Sleator, R.D.; Hill, C.; Fitzgerald, G.F. Improving gastric transit, gastrointestinal persistence and therapeutic efficacy of the probiotic strain *Bifidobacterium breve* UCC2003. *Microbiology* **2007**, *153*, 3563–3571. [CrossRef] [PubMed]
67. Tojo, M.; Oikawa, T.; Morikawa, Y.; Yamashita, N.; Iwata, S.; Satoh, Y.; Hanada, J.; Tanaka, R. The Effects of *Bifidobacterium breve* Administration on *Campylobacter Enteritis*. *Pediatr. Int.* **1987**, *29*, 160–167. [CrossRef]
68. Hotta, M.; Sato, Y.; Iwata, S.; Yamashita, N.; Sunakawa, K.; Oikawa, T.; Tanaka, R.; Takayama, H.; Yajima, M.; Watanabe, K.; et al. Clinical Effects of *Bifidobacterium* Preparations on Pediatric Intractable Diarrhea. *Keio J. Med.* **1987**, *36*, 298–314. [CrossRef] [PubMed]
69. Asahara, T.; Shimizu, K.; Nomoto, K.; Hamabata, T.; Ozawa, A.; Takeda, Y. Probiotic Bifidobacteria Protect Mice from Lethal Infection with Shiga Toxin-Producing *Escherichia coli* O157:H7. *Society* **2004**, *72*, 2240–2247. [CrossRef]
70. Kikuchi-Hayakawa, H.; Onodera, N.; Matsubara, S.; Yasuda, E.; Shimakawa, Y.; Ishikawa, F. Effects of soya milk and *Bifidobacterium*-fermented soya milk on plasma and liver lipids, and faecal steroids in hamsters fed on a cholesterol-free or cholesterol-enriched diet. *Br. J. Nutr.* **1998**, *79*, 97–105. [CrossRef] [PubMed]
71. Kano, M.; Ishikawa, F.; Matsubara, S.; Kikuchi-Hayakawa, H.; Shimakawa, Y. Soymilk products affect ethanol absorption and metabolism in rats during acute and chronic ethanol intake. *J. Nutr.* **2002**, *132*, 238–244. [CrossRef] [PubMed]
72. Ohta, T.; Nakatsugi, S.; Watanabe, K.; Kawamori, T.; Ishikawa, F.; Morotomi, M.; Sugie, S.; Toda, T.; Sugimura, T.; Wakabayashi, K. Inhibitory effects of *Bifidobacterium*-fermented soy milk on 2-amino-1-methyl-6-phenylimidazo[4,5-b] pyridine-induced rat mammary carcinogenesis, with a partial contribution of its component isoflavones. *Carcinogenesis* **2000**, *21*, 937–941. [CrossRef] [PubMed]
73. Chapman, T.M.; Plosker, G.L.; Figgitt, D.P. VSL# 3 probiotic mixture. *Drugs* **2006**, *66*, 1371–1387. [PubMed]
74. Yasui, H.; Kiyoshima, J.; Hori, T.; Shida, K. Protection against influenza virus infection of mice fed *Bifidobacterium breve* YIT4064. *Clin. Diagn. Lab. Immunol.* **1999**, *6*, 186–192. [PubMed]
75. Yasui, H.; Ohwaki, M. Enhancement of Immune Response in Peyer's Patch Cells Cultured with *Bifidobacterium breve*. *J. Dairy Sci.* **1991**, *74*, 1187–1195. [CrossRef]
76. Fanning, S.; Hall, L.J.; van Sinderen, D. *Bifidobacterium breve* UCC2003 surface exopolysaccharide production is a beneficial trait mediating commensal-host interaction through immune modulation and pathogen protection. *Gut Microbes* **2012**, *3*, 420–425. [CrossRef] [PubMed]
77. Frederick, M.R.; Kuttler, C.; Hense, B.A.; Eberl, H.J. A mathematical model of quorum sensing regulated EPS production in biofilm communities. *Theor. Biol. Med. Model.* **2011**, *8*, 8. [CrossRef] [PubMed]
78. Natividad, J.M.M.; Hayes, C.L.; Motta, J.P.; Jury, J.; Galipeau, H.J.; Philip, V.; Garcia-Rodenas, C.L.; Kiyama, H.; Bercik, P.; Verdú, E.F. Differential induction of antimicrobial REGIII by the intestinal microbiota and *Bifidobacterium breve* NCC2950. *Appl. Environ. Microbiol.* **2013**, *79*, 7745–7754. [CrossRef] [PubMed]
79. Raftis, E.J.; Delday, M.I.; Cowie, P.; McCluskey, S.M.; Singh, M.D.; Ettorre, A.; Mulder, I.E. *Bifidobacterium breve* MRx0004 protects against airway inflammation in a severe asthma model by suppressing both neutrophil and eosinophil lung infiltration. *Sci. Rep.* **2018**, *8*, 12024. [CrossRef] [PubMed]
80. Inoue, Y.; Iwabuchi, N.; Xiao, J.; Yaeshima, T.; Iwatsuki, K. Suppressive Effects of *Bifidobacterium breve* Strain M-16V on T-Helper Type 2 Immune Responses in a Murine Model. *Biol. Pharm. Bull.* **2009**, *32*, 760–763. [CrossRef] [PubMed]
81. Schouten, B.; van Esch, B.C.A.M.; Hofman, G.A.; van Doorn, S.A.C.M.; Knol, J.; Nauta, A.J.; Garssen, J.; Willemsen, L.E.M.; Knippels, L.M.J. Cow Milk Allergy Symptoms Are Reduced in Mice Fed Dietary Synbiotics during Oral Sensitization with Whey. *J. Nutr.* **2009**, *139*, 1398–1403. [CrossRef] [PubMed]
82. Kostadinova, A.I.; Meulenbroek, L.A.; van Esch, B.C.; Hofman, G.A.; Garssen, J.; Willemsen, L.E.; Knippels, L.M. A Specific Mixture of Fructo-Oligosaccharides and *Bifidobacterium breve* M-16V Facilitates Partial Non-Responsiveness to Whey Protein in Mice Orally Exposed to β-Lactoglobulin-Derived Peptides. *Front. Immunol.* **2017**, *7*, 673. [CrossRef] [PubMed]
83. Jeon, S.G.; Kayama, H.; Ueda, Y.; Takahashi, T.; Asahara, T.; Tsuji, H.; Tsuji, N.M.; Kiyono, H.; Ma, J.S.; Kusu, T.; et al. Probiotic *Bifidobacterium breve* induces IL-10-producing Tr1 cells in the colon. *PLoS Pathog.* **2012**, *8*, 1002714. [CrossRef] [PubMed]

84. Kondo, S.; Xiao, J.; Satoh, T.; Odamaki, T.; TakaiashiI, S.; Sughara, H.; Yaeshima, T.; Iwatsuki, K.; Kamei, A.; Abe, K. Antiobesity Effects of *Bifidobacterium breve* Strain B-3 Supplementation in a Mouse Model with High-Fat Diet-Induced Obesity. *Biosci. Biotechnol. Biochem.* **2010**, *74*, 1656–1661. [CrossRef] [PubMed]

85. Kondo, S.; Kamei, A.; Xiao, J.Z.; Iwatsuki, K.; Abe, K. *Bifidobacterium breve* B-3 exerts metabolic syndrome-suppressing effects in the liver of diet-induced obese mice: A DNA microarray analysis. *Benef. Microbes* **2013**, *4*, 247–251. [CrossRef] [PubMed]

86. Foster, J.A.; McVey Neufeld, K.-A. Gut-brain axis: How the microbiome influences anxiety and depression. *Trends Neurosci.* **2013**, *36*, 305–312. [CrossRef] [PubMed]

87. Dinan, T.G.; Stanton, C.; Cryan, J.F. Psychobiotics: A Novel Class of Psychotropic. *Biol. Psychiatry* **2013**, *74*, 720–726. [CrossRef] [PubMed]

88. Savignac, H.M.; Kiely, B.; Dinan, T.G.; Cryan, J.F. Bifidobacteria exert strain-specific effects on stress-related behavior and physiology in BALB/c mice. *Neurogastroenterol. Motil.* **2014**, *26*, 1615–1627. [CrossRef] [PubMed]

89. Kobayashi, Y.; Sugahara, H.; Shimada, K.; Mitsuyama, E.; Kuhara, T.; Yasuoka, A.; Kondo, T.; Abe, K.; Xiao, J.Z. Therapeutic potential of *Bifidobacterium breve* strain A1 for preventing cognitive impairment in Alzheimer's disease. *Sci. Rep.* **2017**, *7*, 13510. [CrossRef] [PubMed]

90. Smith, P.M.; Howitt, M.R.; Panikov, N.; Michaud, M.; Gallini, C.A.; Bohlooly-Y, M.; Glickman, J.N.; Garrett, W.S. The Microbial Metabolites, Short-Chain Fatty Acids, Regulate Colonic Treg Cell Homeostasis. *Science* **2013**, *341*, 569–573. [CrossRef] [PubMed]

91. Simopoulos, A.P. The importance of the ratio of omega-6/omega-3 essential fatty acids. *Biomed. Pharmacother.* **2002**, *56*, 365–379. [CrossRef]

92. Salem, N.; Wegher, B.; Mena, P.; Uauy, R. Arachidonic and docosahexaenoic acids are biosynthesized from their 18-carbon precursors in human infants. *Proc. Natl. Acad. Sci. USA* **1996**, *93*, 49–54. [CrossRef] [PubMed]

93. Coakley, M.; Ross, R.P.; Nordgren, M.; Fitzgerald, G.; Devery, R.; Stanton, C. Conjugated linoleic acid biosynthesis by human-derived *Bifidobacterium* species. *J. Appl. Microbiol.* **2002**, *94*, 138–145. [CrossRef]

94. Kritchevsky, D.; Tepper, S.A.; Wright, S.; Tso, P.; Czarnecki, S.K. Influence of Conjugated Linoleic Acid (CLA) on Establishment and Progression of Atherosclerosis in Rabbits. *J. Am. Coll. Nutr.* **2000**, *19*, 472S–477S. [CrossRef] [PubMed]

95. Bassaganya-Riera, J.; Hontecillas, R.; Beitz, D.C. Colonic anti-inflammatory mechanisms of conjugated linoleic acid. *Clin. Nutr.* **2002**, *21*, 451–459. [CrossRef] [PubMed]

96. Wall, R.; Ross, R.P.; Shanahan, F.; Mahony, L.O.; Mahony, C.O.; Coakley, M.; Hart, O.; Lawlor, P.; Quigley, E.M.; Kiely, B.; et al. Metabolic activity of the enteric microbiota in uences the fatty acid composition of murine and porcine liver and adipose tissues. *Am. J. Clin. Nutr.* **2009**, *89*, 1393–1401. [CrossRef] [PubMed]

97. Bolaños, C.A.; Nestler, E.J. Neurotrophic mechanisms in drug addiction. *Neuromol. Med.* **2004**, *5*, 69–83. [CrossRef]

98. Nawa, H.; Takahashi, M.; Patterson, P.H. Cytokine and growth factor involvement in schizophrenia-support for the developmental model. *Mol. Psychiatry* **2000**, *5*, 594–603. [CrossRef] [PubMed]

99. Molteni, R.; Calabrese, F.; Cattaneo, A.; Mancini, M.; Gennarelli, M.; Racagni, G.; Riva, M.A. Acute Stress Responsiveness of the Neurotrophin BDNF in the Rat Hippocampus is Modulated by Chronic Treatment with the Antidepressant Duloxetine. *Neuropsychopharmacology* **2008**, *34*, 1523. [CrossRef] [PubMed]

100. Chapman, C.M.C.; Gibson, G.R.; Rowland, I. Health benefits of probiotics: Are mixtures more effective than single strains? *Eur. J. Nutr.* **2011**, *50*, 1–17. [CrossRef] [PubMed]

101. Timmerman, H.M.; Koning, C.J.M.; Mulder, L.; Rombouts, F.M.; Beynen, A.C. Monostrain, multistrain and multispecies probiotics—A comparison of functionality and efficacy. *Int. J. Food Microbiol.* **2004**, *96*, 219–233. [CrossRef] [PubMed]

102. Stoll, B.J.; Hansen, N.; Fanaroff, A.A.; Wright, L.L.; Carlo, W.A.; Ehrenkranz, R.A.; Lemons, J.A.; Donovan, E.F.; Stark, A.R.; Tyson, J.E.; et al. Late-onset sepsis in very low birth weight neonates: The experience of the NICHD Neonatal Research Network. *Pediatrics* **2002**, *110*, 285–291. [CrossRef] [PubMed]

103. Pessoa-Silva, C.L.; Miyasaki, C.H.; de Almeida, M.F.; Kopelman, B.I.; Raggio, R.L.; Wey, S.B. Neonatal late-onset bloodstream infection: Attributable mortality, excess of length of stay and risk factors. *Eur. J. Epidemiol.* **2001**, *17*, 715–720. [CrossRef] [PubMed]

104. Panigrahi, P.; Gupta, S.; Gewolb, I.H.; Morris, J.G., Jr. Occurrence of Necrotizing Enterocolitis May Be Dependent on Patterns of Bacterial Adherence and Intestinal Colonization: Studies in Caco-2 Tissue Culture and Weanling Rabbit Models. *Pediatr. Res.* **1994**, *36*, 115–121. [CrossRef] [PubMed]
105. Dai, D.; Walker, W.A. Protective nutrients and bacterial colonization in the immature human gut. *Adv. Pediatr.* **1999**, *46*, 353–382. [PubMed]
106. Butel, M.J.; Suau, A.; Campeotto, F.; Magne, F.; Aires, J.; Ferraris, L.; Kalach, N.; Leroux, B.; Dupont, C. Conditions of Bifidobacterial Colonization in Preterm Infants: A Prospective Analysis. *J. Pediatr. Gastroenterol. Nutr.* **2007**, *44*, 577–582. [CrossRef] [PubMed]
107. Jacquot, A.; Neveu, D.; Aujoulat, F.; Mercier, G.; Marchandin, H.; Jumas-Bilak, E.; Picaud, J.-C. Dynamics and Clinical Evolution of Bacterial Gut Microflora in Extremely Premature Patients. *J. Pediatr.* **2011**, *158*, 390–396. [CrossRef] [PubMed]
108. Arboleya, S.; Binetti, A.; Salazar, N.; Fernández, N.; Solís, G.; Hernández-Barranco, A.; Margolles, A.; de los Reyes-Gavilán, C.G.; Gueimonde, M. Establishment and development of intestinal microbiota in preterm neonates. *FEMS Microbiol. Ecol.* **2012**, *79*, 763–772. [CrossRef] [PubMed]
109. Kitajima, H.; Sumida, Y.; Tanaka, R. Early administration of *Bifidobacterium breve* to preterm infants: Randomised controlled trial. *Arch. Dis. Child. Fetal Neonatal Ed.* **1997**, *76*, 101–107. [CrossRef]
110. Li, Y.; Shimizu, T.; Hosaka, A.; Kaneko, N.; Ohtsuka, Y.; Yamashiro, Y. Effects of *Bifidobacterium breve* supplementation on intestinal flora of low birth weight infants. *Pediatr. Int.* **2004**, *46*, 509–515. [CrossRef] [PubMed]
111. Patole, S.; Keil, A.D.; Chang, A.; Nathan, E.; Doherty, D.; Simmer, K.; Esvaran, M.; Conway, P. Effect of *Bifidobacterium breve* M-16V supplementation on fecal bifidobacteria in preterm neonates—A randomised double blind placebo controlled trial. *PLoS ONE* **2014**, *9*, e89511. [CrossRef] [PubMed]
112. Patole, S.K.; Rao, S.C.; Keil, A.D.; Nathan, E.A.; Doherty, D.A.; Simmer, K.N. Benefits of *Bifidobacterium breve* M-16V Supplementation in preterm neonates—A retrospective cohort study. *PLoS ONE* **2016**, *11*, e0150775. [CrossRef] [PubMed]
113. Neu, J.; Walker, W.A. Necrotizing Enterocolitis. *N. Engl. J. Med.* **2011**, *364*, 255–264. [CrossRef] [PubMed]
114. Lin, P.W.; Stoll, B.J. Necrotising enterocolitis. *Lancet* **2006**, *368*, 1271–1283. [CrossRef]
115. Bell, M.J.; Ternberg, J.L.; Feigin, R.D.; Keating, J.P.; Marshall, R.; Barton, L.; Brotherton, T. Neonatal necrotizing enterocolitis. Therapeutic decisions based upon clinical staging. *Ann. Surg.* **1978**, *187*, 1–7. [CrossRef] [PubMed]
116. Jain, L. Necrotizing Enterocolitis Prevention: Art or Science? *Clin. Perinatol.* **2013**, *40*, xiii–xv. [CrossRef] [PubMed]
117. Mai, V.; Young, C.M.; Ukhanova, M.; Wang, X.; Sun, Y.; Casella, G.; Theriaque, D.; Li, N.; Sharma, R.; Hudak, M.; et al. Fecal Microbiota in Premature Infants Prior to Necrotizing Enterocolitis. *PLoS ONE* **2011**, *6*, e20647. [CrossRef] [PubMed]
118. Satoh, Y.; Shinohara, K.; Umezaki, H.; Shoji, H.; Satoh, H.; Ohtsuka, Y.; Shiga, S.; Nagata, S.; Shimizu, T.; Yamashiro, Y. Bifidobacteria prevents necrotizing enterocolitic and infection in preterm infants. *Int. J. Probiot. Prebiot.* **2007**, *2*, 149–154.
119. Lin, J. Too much short chain fatty acids cause neonatal necrotizing enterocolitis. *Med. Hypotheses* **2004**, *62*, 291–293. [CrossRef]
120. Lin, J.; Nafday, S.M.; Chauvin, S.N.; Magid, M.S.; Pabbatireddy, S.; Holzman, I.R.; Babyatsky, M.W. Variable Effects of Short Chain Fatty Acids and Lactic Acid in Inducing Intestinal Mucosal Injury in Newborn Rats. *J. Pediatr. Gastroenterol. Nutr.* **2002**, *35*, 545–550. [CrossRef] [PubMed]
121. Wang, C.; Shoji, H.; Sato, H.; Nagata, S.; Ohtsuka, Y.; Shimizu, T.; Yamashiro, Y. Effects of oral administration of *Bifidobacterium breve* on fecal lactic acid and short-chain fatty acids in low birth weight infants. *J. Pediatr. Gastroenterol. Nutr.* **2007**, *44*, 252–257. [CrossRef] [PubMed]
122. Fujii, T.; Ohtsuka, Y.; Lee, T.; Kudo, T.; Shoji, H.; Sato, H.; Nagata, S.; Shimizu, T.; Yamashiro, Y. *Bifidobacterium breve* enhances transforming growth factor β1 signaling by regulating Smad7 expression in preterm infants. *J. Pediatr. Gastroenterol. Nutr.* **2006**, *43*, 83–88. [CrossRef] [PubMed]
123. Ohtsuka, Y.; Sanderson, I.R. Transforming growth factor-β: An important cytokine in the mucosal immune response. *Curr. Opin. Gastroenterol.* **2000**, *16*, 541–545. [CrossRef] [PubMed]

124. Hikaru, U.; Koichi, S.; Yayoi, S.; Hiromichi, S.; Hiroaki, S.; Yoshikazu, O.; Seigo, S.; Nagata, S.; Toshiaki, S.; Yamashiro, Y. Bifidobacteria prevents preterm infants from developing infection and sepsis. *Int. J. Probiot. Prebiot.* **2010**, *5*, 33–36.
125. Braga, T.D.; Alves, G.; Israel, P.; De Lira, C.; Lima, M.D.C. Efficacy of *Bifidobacterium breve* and *Lactobacillus casei* oral supplementation on necrotizing enterocolitis in very-low-birth-weight preterm infants: A double-blind, randomized, controlled trial 1–3. *J. Clin.* **2011**, *93*, 81–86. [CrossRef] [PubMed]
126. Savino, F.; Pelle, E.; Palumeri, E.; Oggero, R.; Miniero, R. *Lactobacillus reuteri* (American Type Culture Collection Strain 55730) Versus Simethicone in the Treatment of Infantile Colic: A Prospective Randomized Study. *Pediatrics* **2007**, *119*, e124–e130. [CrossRef] [PubMed]
127. Indrio, F.; Di Mauro, A.; Riezzo, G.; Cavallo, L.; Francavilla, R. Infantile colic, regurgitation, and constipation: An early traumatic insult in the development of functional gastrointestinal disorders in children? *Eur. J. Pediatr.* **2015**, *174*, 841–842. [CrossRef] [PubMed]
128. Romanello, S.; Spiri, D.; Marcuzzi, E.; Zanin, A.; Boizeau, P.; Riviere, S.; Vizeneux, A.; Moretti, R.; Carbajal, R.; Mercier, J.C.; et al. Association between Childhood Migraine and History of Infantile Colic. *JAMA* **2013**, *309*, 1607–1612. [CrossRef] [PubMed]
129. Giglione, E.; Prodam, F.; Bellone, S.; Monticone, S.; Beux, S.; Marolda, A.; Pagani, A.; Di Gioia, D.; Del Piano, M.; Mogna, G.; et al. The Association of *Bifidobacterium breve* BR03 and B632 is Effective to Prevent Colics in Bottle-fed Infants. *J. Clin. Gastroenterol.* **2016**, *50*, S164–S167. [CrossRef] [PubMed]
130. Aloisio, I.; Prodam, F.; Giglione, E.; Bozzi Cionci, N.; Solito, A.; Bellone, S.; Baffoni, L.; Mogna, L.; Pane, M.; Bona, G.; et al. Three-Month Feeding Integration with *Bifidobacterium* Strains Prevents Gastrointestinal Symptoms in Healthy Newborns. *Front. Nutr.* **2018**, *5*, 39. [CrossRef] [PubMed]
131. Magne, F.; Puchi Silva, A.; Carvajal, B.; Gotteland, M. The Elevated Rate of Cesarean Section and Its Contribution to Non-Communicable Chronic Diseases in Latin America: The Growing Involvement of the Microbiota. *Front. Pediatr.* **2017**, *5*, 192. [CrossRef] [PubMed]
132. Kuhle, S.; Tong, O.S.; Woolcott, C.G. Association between caesarean section and childhood obesity: A systematic review and meta-analysis. *Obes. Rev.* **2015**, *16*, 295–303. [CrossRef] [PubMed]
133. Van den Berg, M.M.; Benninga, M.A.; Di Lorenzo, C. Epidemiology of Childhood Constipation: A Systematic Review. *Am. J. Gastroenterol.* **2006**, *101*, 2401–2409. [CrossRef] [PubMed]
134. Bongers, M.E.J.; van Wijk, M.P.; Reitsma, J.B.; Benninga, M.A. Long-Term Prognosis for Childhood Constipation: Clinical Outcomes in Adulthood. *Pediatrics* **2010**, *126*, e156–e162. [CrossRef] [PubMed]
135. Tabbers, M.M.; de Milliano, I.; Roseboom, M.G.; Benninga, M.A. Is *Bifidobacterium breve* effective in the treatment of childhood constipation? Results from a pilot study. *Nutr. J.* **2011**, *10*, 19. [CrossRef] [PubMed]
136. Giannetti, E.; Maglione, M.; Alessandrella, A.; Strisciuglio, C.; De Giovanni, D.; Campanozzi, A.; Miele, E.; Staiano, A. A Mixture of 3 Bifidobacteria Decreases Abdominal Pain and Improves the Quality of Life in Children with Irritable Bowel Syndrome. *J. Clin. Gastroenterol.* **2017**, *51*, e5–e10. [CrossRef] [PubMed]
137. Saez-Lara, M.J.; Gomez-Llorente, C.; Plaza-Diaz, J.; Gil, A. The Role of Probiotic Lactic Acid Bacteria and Bifidobacteria in the Prevention and Treatment of Inflammatory Bowel Disease and Other Related Diseasea: A Systematic Review of Randomized Human Clinical Trials. *BioMed Res. Int.* **2015**, *2015*, 505878. [CrossRef] [PubMed]
138. Guandalini, S.; Magazzù, G.; Chiaro, A.; La Balestra, V.; Di Nardo, G.; Gopalan, S.; Sibal, A.; Romano, C.; Canani, R.B.; Lionetti, P.; et al. VSL#3 improves symptoms in children with irritable bowel Syndrome: A multicenter, randomized, placebo-controlled, double-blind, crossover study. *J. Pediatr. Gastroenterol. Nutr.* **2010**, *51*, 24–30. [CrossRef] [PubMed]
139. Miele, E.; Pascarella, F.; Giannetti, E.; Quaglietta, L.; Baldassano, R.N.; Staiano, A. Effect of a probiotic preparation (VSL#3) on induction and maintenance of remission in children with ulcerative colitis. *Am. J. Gastroenterol.* **2009**, *104*, 437–443. [CrossRef] [PubMed]
140. Heyman, M.B.; Kirschner, B.S.; Gold, B.D.; Ferry, G.; Baldassano, R.; Cohen, S.A.; Winter, H.S.; Fain, P.; King, C.; Smith, T.; et al. Children with early-onset inflammatory bowel disease (IBD): Analysis of a pediatric IBD consortium registry. *J. Pediatr.* **2005**, *146*, 35–40. [CrossRef] [PubMed]
141. Turner, D.; Walsh, C.M.; Benchimol, E.I.; Mann, E.H.; Thomas, K.E.; Chow, C.; McLernon, R.A.; Walters, T.D.; Swales, J.; Steinhart, A.H.; et al. Severe paediatric ulcerative colitis: Incidence, outcomes and optimal timing for second-line therapy. *Gut* **2008**, *57*, 331–338. [CrossRef] [PubMed]

142. Dubey, P.A.; Rajeshwari, K.; Chakravarty, A.; Famularo, G. Use of VSL # 3 in the Treatment of Rotavirus Diarrhea in Children: Preliminary results. *J. Clin. Gastroenterol.* **2008**, *42*, 126–129.
143. Sinha, A.; Gupta, S.S.; Chellani, H.; Maliye, C.; Kumari, V.; Arya, S.; Garg, B.S.; Gaur, S.D.; Gaind, R.; Deotale, V.; et al. Role of probiotics VSL#3 in prevention of suspected sepsis in low birthweight infants in India: A randomised controlled trial. *BMJ Open* **2015**, *5*, e006564. [CrossRef] [PubMed]
144. Thibault, H.; Aubert-Jacquin, C.; Goulet, O. Effects of Long-term Consumption of a Fermented Infant Formula (with *Bifidobacterium breve* c50 and *Streptococcus thermophilus* 065) on Acute Diarrhea in Healthy Infants. *J. Pediatr. Gastroenterol. Nutr.* **2004**, *39*, 147–152. [CrossRef] [PubMed]
145. Klemenak, M.; Dolinšek, J.; Langerholc, T.; Di Gioia, D.; Mičetić-Turk, D. Administration of *Bifidobacterium breve* Decreases the Production of TNF-α in Children with Celiac Disease. *Dig. Dis. Sci.* **2015**, *60*, 3386–3392. [CrossRef] [PubMed]
146. Quagliariello, A.; Aloisio, I.; Bozzi Cionci, N.; Luiselli, D.; D'Auria, G.; Martinez-Priego, L.; Pérez-Villarroya, D.; Langerholc, T.; Primec, M.; Mičetić-Turk, D.; et al. Effect of *Bifidobacterium breve* on the Intestinal Microbiota of Coeliac Children on a Gluten Free Diet: A Pilot Study. *Nutrients* **2016**, *8*, 660. [CrossRef] [PubMed]
147. Primec, M.; Klemenak, M.; Di Gioia, D.; Aloisio, I.; Bozzi Cionci, N.; Quagliariello, A.; Gorenjak, M.; Mičetić-Turk, D.; Langerholc, T. Clinical intervention using *Bifidobacterium* strains in celiac disease children reveals novel microbial modulators of TNF-α and short-chain fatty acids. *Clin. Nutr.* **2018**, *4*, 95–101. [CrossRef] [PubMed]
148. Horz, H.-P.; Citron, D.M.; Warren, Y.A.; Goldstein, E.J.C.; Conrads, G. Synergistes Group Organisms of Human Origin. *J. Clin. Microbiol.* **2006**, *44*, 2914–2920. [CrossRef] [PubMed]
149. Rajilić-Stojanović, M.; de Vos, W.M. The first 1000 cultured species of the human gastrointestinal microbiota. *FEMS Microbiol. Rev.* **2014**, *38*, 996–1047. [CrossRef] [PubMed]
150. Schenk, S.; Saberi, M.; Olefsky, J.M. Insulin sensitivity: Modulation by nutrients and inflammation. *J. Clin. Investig.* **2008**, *118*, 2992–3002. [CrossRef] [PubMed]
151. Rocha, V.Z.; Folco, E.J. Inflammatory Concepts of Obesity. *Int. J. Inflam.* **2011**, *2011*, 529061. [CrossRef] [PubMed]
152. Angelakis, E.; Armougom, F.; Million, M.; Raoult, D. The relationship between gut microbiota and weight gain in humans. *Future Microbiol.* **2012**, *7*, 91–109. [CrossRef] [PubMed]
153. Kalliomäki, M.; Carmen Collado, M.; Salminen, S.; Isolauri, E. Early differences in fecal microbiota composition in children may predict overweight. *Am. J. Clin. Nutr.* **2008**, *87*, 534–538. [CrossRef] [PubMed]
154. Yin, Y.N.; Yu, Q.F.; Fu, N.; Liu, X.W.; Lu, F.G. Effects of four Bifidobacteria on obesity in high-fat diet induced rats. *World J. Gastroenterol.* **2010**, *16*, 3394–3401. [CrossRef] [PubMed]
155. Prodam, F.; Archero, F.; Aloisio, I.; Solito, A.; Ricotti, R.; Giglione, E.; Bozzi Cionci, N.; Bellone, S.; Di Gioia, D.; Bona, G. Efficacy of the treatment with Bifidobacterium breve B632 and Bifidobacterium breve BR03 on endocrine response to the oral glucose tolerance test in pediatric obesity: A cross-over double blind randomized controlled trial. In Proceedings of the 39° Congresso Nazionale Società Italiana di Endocrinologia (Endocrinologia 2.0), Rome, Italy, 21–24 June 2017.
156. Watanabe, S.; Narisawa, Y.; Arase, S.; Okamatsu, H.; Ikenaga, T.; Tajiri, Y.; Kumemura, M. Differences in fecal microflora between patients with atopic dermatitis and healthy control subjects. *J. Allergy Clin. Immunol.* **2003**, *111*, 587–591. [CrossRef] [PubMed]
157. Taniuchi, S.; Hattori, K.; Yamamoto, A.; Sasai, M.; Hatano, Y.; Kojima, T.; Kobayashi, Y.; Iwamoto, H.; Yaeshima, T. Administration of *Bifidobacterium* to infants with atopic dermatitis: Changes in fecal microflora and clinical symptoms. *J. Appl. Res.* **2005**, *5*, 387–396.
158. Van Der Aa, L.B.; Heymans, H.S.; Van Aalderen, W.M.; Sillevis Smitt, J.H.; Knol, J.; Ben Amor, K.; Goossens, D.A.; Sprikkelman, A.B. Effect of a new synbiotic mixture on atopic dermatitis in infants: A randomized-controlled trial. *Clin. Exp. Allergy* **2010**, *40*, 795–804. [CrossRef] [PubMed]
159. Knol, J.; Scholtens, P.; Kafka, C.; Steenbakkers, J.; Gro, S.; Helm, K.; Klarczyk, M.; Schöpfer, H.; Böckler, H.-M.; Wells, J. Colon Microflora in Infants Fed Formula with Galacto- and Fructo-Oligosaccharides: More Like Breast-Fed Infants. *J. Pediatr. Gastroenterol. Nutr.* **2005**, *40*, 36–42. [CrossRef] [PubMed]
160. Van Der Aa, L.B.; Van Aalderen, W.M.C.; Heymans, H.S.A.; Henk Sillevis Smitt, J.; Nauta, A.J.; Knippels, L.M.J.; Ben Amor, K.; Sprikkelman, A.B. Synbiotics prevent asthma-like symptoms in infants with atopic dermatitis. *Allergy Eur. J. Allergy Clin. Immunol.* **2011**, *66*, 170–177. [CrossRef] [PubMed]

161. Enomoto, T.; Sowa, M.; Nishimori, K.; Shimazu, S.; Yoshida, A.; Yamada, K.; Furukawa, F.; Nakagawa, T.; Yanagisawa, N.; Iwabuchi, N.; et al. Effects of Bifidobacterial Supplementation to Pregnant Women and Infants in the Prevention of Allergy Development in Infants and on Fecal Microbiota. *Allergol. Int.* **2014**, *63*, 575–585. [CrossRef] [PubMed]
162. Mizuno, T.; Yokoyama, Y.; Nishio, H.; Ebata, T.; Sugawara, G.; Asahara, T.; Nomoto, K.; Nagino, M. Intraoperative Bacterial Translocation Detected by Bacterium-Specific Ribosomal RNA-Targeted Reverse-Transcriptase Polymerase Chain Reaction for the Mesenteric Lymph Node Strongly Predicts Postoperative Infectious Complications After Major Hepatectomy for. *Ann. Surg.* **2010**, *252*, 1013–1019. [CrossRef] [PubMed]
163. Okazaki, T.; Asahara, T.; Yamataka, A.; Ogasawara, Y.; Lane, G.J.; Nomoto, K.; Nagata, S.; Yamashiro, Y. Intestinal microbiota in pediatric surgical cases administered *Bifidobacterium breve*: A randomized controlled trial. *J. Pediatr. Gastroenterol. Nutr.* **2016**, *63*, 46–50. [CrossRef] [PubMed]
164. Umenai, T.; Shime, N.; Asahara, T.; Nomoto, K.; Itoi, T. A pilot study of *Bifidobacterium breve* in neonates undergoing surgery for congenital heart disease. *J. Intensive Care* **2014**, *2*, 36. [CrossRef] [PubMed]
165. Kanamori, Y.; Hashizume, K.; Sugiyama, M.; Morotomi, M.; Yuki, N. Combination therapy with *Bifidobacterium breve, Lactobacillus casei,* and galactooligosaccharides dramatically improved the intestinal function in a girl with short bowel syndrome: A novel synbiotics therapy for intestinal failure. *Dig. Dis. Sci.* **2001**, *46*, 2010–2016. [CrossRef] [PubMed]
166. Sherman, P.; Lichtman, S. Small Bowel Bacterial Overgrowth Syndrome. *Dig. Dis.* **1987**, *5*, 157–171. [CrossRef] [PubMed]
167. Bongaerts, G.P.A.; Tolboom, J.J.M.; Naber, A.H.J.; Sperl, W.J.K.; Severijnen, R.S.V.M.; Bakkeren, J.A.J.M.; Willems, J.L. Role of bacteria in the pathogenesis of short bowel syndrome-associated D-lactic acidemia. *Microb. Pathog.* **1997**, *22*, 285–293. [CrossRef] [PubMed]
168. Kanamori, Y.; Sugiyama, M.; Hashizume, K.; Yuki, N.; Morotomi, M.; Tanaka, R. Experience of long-term synbiotic therapy in seven short bowel patients with refractory enterocolitis. *J. Pediatr. Surg.* **2004**, *39*, 1686–1692. [CrossRef] [PubMed]
169. Kanamori, Y.; Iwanaka, T.; Sugiyama, M.; Komura, M.; Takahashi, T.; Yuki, N.; Morotomi, M.; Tanaka, R. Early use of probiotics is important therapy in infants with severe congenital anomaly. *Pediatr. Int.* **2010**, *52*, 362–367. [CrossRef] [PubMed]
170. Bäckhed, F.; Ding, H.; Wang, T.; Hooper, L.V.; Koh, G.Y.; Nagy, A.; Semenkovich, C.F.; Gordon, J.I. The gut microbiota as an environmental factor that regulates fat storage. *Proc. Natl. Acad. Sci. USA* **2004**, *101*, 15718–15723. [CrossRef] [PubMed]
171. Klastersky, J. A review of chemoprophylaxis and therapy of bacterial infections in neutropenic patients. *Diagn. Microbiol. Infect. Dis.* **1989**, *12*, 201–207. [CrossRef]
172. Resta-Lenert, S.; Barrett, K.E. Live probiotics protect intestinal epithelial cells from the effects of infection with enteroinvasive *Escherichia coli* (EIEC). *Gut* **2003**, *52*, 988–997. [CrossRef] [PubMed]
173. Wada, M.; Nagata, S.; Saito, M.; Shimizu, T.; Yamashiro, Y.; Matsuki, T.; Asahara, T.; Nomoto, K. Effects of the enteral administration of *Bifidobacterium breve* on patients undergoing chemotherapy for pediatric malignancies. *Support. Care Cancer* **2010**, *18*, 751–759. [CrossRef] [PubMed]
174. Minami, J.I.; Kondo, S.; Yanagisawa, N.; Odamaki, T.; Xiao, J.Z.; Abe, F.; Nakajima, S.; Hamamoto, Y.; Saitoh, S.; Shimoda, T. Oral administration of *Bifidobacterium breve* B-3 modifies metabolic functions in adults with obese tendencies in a randomised controlled trial. *J. Nutr. Sci.* **2015**, *4*, e17. [CrossRef] [PubMed]
175. Ishikawa, H.; Matsumoto, S.; Ohashi, Y.; Imaoka, A.; Setoyama, H.; Umesaki, Y.; Tanaka, R.; Otani, T. Beneficial effects of probiotic *Bifidobacterium* and galacto-oligosaccharide in patients with ulcerative colitis: A randomized controlled study. *Digestion* **2011**, *84*, 128–133. [CrossRef] [PubMed]
176. Matts, S.G. The value of rectal biopsy in the diagnosis of ulcerative colitis. *Q. J. Med.* **1961**, *30*, 393–407. [PubMed]
177. Carlson, M.; Raab, Y.; Sevéus, L.; Xu, S.; Hällgren, R.; Venge, P. Human neutrophil lipocalin is a unique marker of neutrophil inflammation in ulcerative colitis and proctitis. *Gut* **2002**, *50*, 501–506. [CrossRef] [PubMed]

178. Kano, M.; Masuoka, N.; Kaga, C.; Sugimoto, S.; Iizuka, R.; Manabe, K.; Sone, T.; Oeda, K.; Nonaka, C.; Miazaki, K.; et al. Consecutive Intake of Fermented Milk Containing *Bifidobacterium breve* Strain Yakult and Galacto-oligosaccharides Benefits Skin Condition in Healthy Adult Women. *Biosci. Microbiota Food Health* **2013**, *21*, 33–39. [CrossRef] [PubMed]
179. Cheng, T.; Hitomi, K.; van Vlijmen-Willems, I.M.J.J.; de Jongh, G.J.; Yamamoto, K.; Nishi, K.; Watts, C.; Reinheckel, T.; Schalkwijk, J.; Zeeuwen, P.L.J.M. Cystatin M/E Is a High Affinity Inhibitor of Cathepsin V and Cathepsin L by a Reactive Site That Is Distinct from the Legumain-binding Site: A novel clue for the role of cystatin M/E in epidermal cornification. *J. Biol. Chem.* **2006**, *281*, 15893–15899. [CrossRef] [PubMed]
180. Brigidi, P.; Vitali, B.; Swennen, E.; Bazzocchi, G.; Matteuzzi, D. Effects of probiotic administration upon the composition and enzymatic activity of human fecal microbiota in patients with irritable bowel syndrome or functional diarrhea. *Res. Microbiol.* **2001**, *152*, 735–741. [CrossRef]
181. Mobley, H.L.; Hausinger, R.P. Microbial ureases: Significance, regulation, and molecular characterization. *Microbiol. Rev.* **1989**, *53*, 85–108. [PubMed]
182. Pronio, A.; Montesani, C.; Butteroni, C.; Vecchione, S.; Mumolo, G.; Vestri, A.; Vitolo, D.; Boirivant, M. Probiotic administration in patients with ileal pouch-anal anastomosis for ulcerative colitis is associated with expansion of mucosal regulatory cells. *Inflamm. Bowel Dis.* **2008**, *14*, 662–668. [CrossRef] [PubMed]
183. Kühbacher, T.; Ott, S.J.; Helwig, U.; Mimura, T.; Rizzello, F.; Kleessen, B.; Gionchetti, P.; Blaut, M.; Campieri, M.; Fölsch, U.R.; et al. Bacterial and fungal microbiota in relation to probiotic therapy (VSL#3) in pouchitis. *Gut* **2006**, *55*, 833–841. [CrossRef] [PubMed]
184. Bibiloni, R.; Fedorak, R.N.; Tannock, G.W.; Madsen, K.L.; Gionchetti, P.; Campieri, M.; De Simone, C.; Sartor, R.B. VSL#3 probiotic-mixture induces remission in patients with active ulcerative colitis. *Am. J. Gastroenterol.* **2005**, *100*, 1539–1546. [CrossRef] [PubMed]
185. Venturi, A.; Gionchetti, P.; Rizzello, F.; Johansson, R.; Zucconi, E.; Brigidi, P.; Matteuzzi, D.; Campieri, M. Impact on the composition of the faecal flora by a new probiotic preparation: Preliminary data on maintenance treatment of patients with ulcerative colitis. *Aliment. Pharmacol. Ther.* **1999**, *13*, 1103–1108. [CrossRef] [PubMed]
186. Tursi, A.; Brandimarte, G.; Giorgetti, G.M.; Forti, G.; Modeo, M.E.; Gigliobianco, A. Low-dose balsalazide plus a high-potency probiotic preparation is more effective than balsalazide alone or mesalazine in the treatment of acute mild-to-moderate ulcerative colitis. *Med. Sci. Monit.* **2004**, *10*, PI126–PI131. [PubMed]
187. Tursi, A.; Brandimarte, G.; Papa, A.; Giglio, A.; Elisei, W.; Giorgetti, G.M.; Forti, G.; Morini, S.; Hassan, C.; Pistoia, M.A.; et al. Treatment of relapsing mild-to-moderate ulcerative colitis with the probiotic VSL3 as adjunctive to a standard pharmaceutical treatment: A double-blind, randomized, placebo-controlled study. *Am. J. Gastroenterol.* **2010**, *105*, 2218–2227. [CrossRef] [PubMed]
188. Wong, R.K.; Yang, C.; Song, G.H.; Wong, J.; Ho, K.Y. Melatonin Regulation as a Possible Mechanism for Probiotic (VSL#3) in Irritable Bowel Syndrome: A Randomized Double-Blinded Placebo Study. *Dig. Dis. Sci.* **2014**, *60*, 186–194. [CrossRef] [PubMed]
189. Kim, H.J.; Camilleri, M.; Mckinzie, S. A Randomized Controlled Trial of a Probiotic, VSL#3, on Gut Transit and Symptoms in Diarrhoea-Predominant Irritable Bowel Syndrome. *Aliment. Pharmacol. Ther.* **2003**, *17*, 895–904. [CrossRef] [PubMed]
190. Michail, S.; Kenche, H. Gut Microbiota is Not Modified by Randomized, Double-Blind, Placebo-Controlled Trial of VSL#3 in Diarrhea-Predominant Irritable Bowel Syndrome. *Probiot. Antimicrob. Proteins* **2011**, *3*, 1–7. [CrossRef] [PubMed]

© 2018 by the authors. Licensee MDPI, Basel, Switzerland. This article is an open access article distributed under the terms and conditions of the Creative Commons Attribution (CC BY) license (http://creativecommons.org/licenses/by/4.0/).

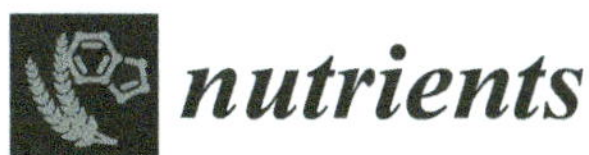

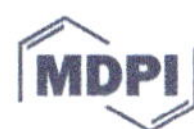

Article

A Randomized, Placebo-Controlled, Pilot Clinical Trial to Evaluate the Effect of Supplementation with Prebiotic Synergy 1 on Iron Homeostasis in Children and Adolescents with Celiac Disease Treated with a Gluten-Free Diet

Klaudia Feruś [1], Natalia Drabińska [2], Urszula Krupa-Kozak [2] and Elżbieta Jarocka-Cyrta [1,*]

1 Department of Pediatrics, Gastroenterology and Nutrition, Collegium Medicum Faculty of Medicine, University of Warmia & Mazury, Oczapowskiego 2 Str., 10-719 Olsztyn, Poland; klaudiaferus@o2.pl

2 Department of Chemistry and Biodynamics of Food, Institute of Animal Reproduction and Food Research of Polish Academy of Sciences, Tuwima 10 Str., 10-748 Olsztyn, Poland; n.drabinska@pan.olsztyn.pl (N.D.); u.krupa-kozak@pan.olsztyn.pl (U.K.-K.)

* Correspondence: ejarocka@op.pl; Tel.: +48-89-539-33-69

Received: 16 October 2018; Accepted: 16 November 2018; Published: 21 November 2018

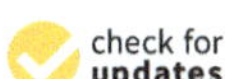

Abstract: Iron deficiency anemia (IDA) occurs in 15–46% of patients with celiac disease (CD), and in some cases, it may be its only manifestation. Studies in animal models have shown that prebiotics, including inulin, may help to increase intestinal absorption of iron. The aim of this study was to evaluate the effect of a prebiotic, oligofructose-enriched inulin (Synergy 1), on iron homeostasis in non-anemic children and adolescents with celiac disease (CD) in association with a gluten-free diet (GFD). Thirty-four CD patients (4–18 years old) were randomized into two groups receiving Synergy 1 (10 g/day) or a placebo (maltodextrin) for three months. Before and after intervention, blood samples were collected from all patients for assessment of blood morphology, biochemical parameters and serum hepcidin concentration. We found that serum hepcidin concentration after the intervention was significantly decreased by 60.9% ($p = 0.046$) in the Synergy 1 group, whereas no significant difference was observed in the placebo group. No differences in morphological and biochemical blood parameters (including ferritin, hemoglobin and C-reactive protein (CRP)) were observed after intervention in either group. Given that hepcidin decrease may improve intestinal iron absorption, these results warrant further investigation in a larger cohort and especially in patients with IDA.

Keywords: celiac disease; iron deficiency anemia; gluten-free diet; inulin; prebiotics; iron absorption; hepcidin

---

1. Introduction

Celiac disease (CD) is a small intestine enteropathy that is triggered by the ingestion of storage proteins (gluten) from wheat, barley or rye. It occurs in genetically predisposed individuals at any age, at a frequency of 1:100 [1–4]. Characteristic features of CD include a massive lymphocytic infiltration of the lamina propria and atrophy of intestinal villi. Consequently, there is a significant reduction of the intestinal absorption surface, leading to malabsorption of macro- and micronutrients [2,4,5].

Iron deficiency anemia (IDA) is a common finding in children and adults with CD, with an estimated prevalence at diagnosis between 15% and 46% [6]. Anemia may accompany the intestinal presentation of CD, but it can also be the only manifestation of the disease. As such, the possibility of CD should be considered in patients with refractory anemia after other possible causes have been excluded [7]. Iron absorption and distribution is tightly controlled. Hepcidin, a 25-amino-acid peptide hormone produced in the liver, is a central regulator of systemic iron homeostasis. Iron deficiency and hypoxia can decrease hepcidin production, while the pro-inflammatory cytokine IL-6 increases hepcidin expression. Increased serum levels of hepcidin contribute to anemia in chronic diseases [8,9].

Previous studies have shown that the main cause of IDA in CD patients is the limited iron absorption, as a consequence of chronic damage of the intestinal mucosa [6]. Other authors have highlighted the role of chronic mucosal inflammation [10], and the presence of mutations in genes encoding proteins involved in iron absorption [11,12].

The only known therapy for celiac disease is a lifelong gluten-free diet (GFD). Adherence to a GFD leads to recovery of the intestinal mucosa, thereby normalizing nutrient absorption. In most patients, a 6-month period is adequate for nutritional absorption to improve [13]. Normalization of iron and hemoglobin levels depends on the severity of the disease at presentation, compliance to GFD, and bioavailability of dietary iron. In the majority of patients, anemia resolves after approximately one year of a GFD, but persistent IDA is observed in about 8% of patients despite a GFD and even up to 20.5% according to some reports [14,15]. Evaluation of serum CD-associated antibodies, such as anti-tissue transglutaminase antibodies, and the assessment of clinical symptoms, are the most commonly used methods to assess CD patients during follow-up. However, these antibodies often decrease and/or disappear regardless of histological healing and GFD adherence [16]. In one study, complete histological recovery after one year of well-followed GFD in adults was only obtained in 66% of patients [17]. Moreover, GFD itself may result in further deficiencies, including fibre, B vitamins, iron, and trace minerals [18,19]. Decreased iron intake while following a GFD has been reported [20]. All abovementioned clinical circumstances can influence the availability and absorption rate of iron and result in prolonged iron deficiency. Thus, additional safe and easily accepted therapeutic options to improve the iron status in CD patients are needed.

Prebiotics, typically oligosaccharides, such as fructo- and galactooligosaccharides (FOS and GOS) or inulin, have been shown to improve bioavailability of minerals, and to enhance iron absorption in animal studies [21,22].

The aim of this study was to evaluate the effect of oligofructose-enriched inulin (Synergy 1) on iron homeostasis in CD children following a GFD. We posited that Synergy 1 supplementation would result in an improvement of blood morphology and other parameters relative to iron homeostasis.

2. Materials and Methods

2.1. Study Design

We performed a single-center, randomized, placebo-controlled, double-blind study in patients diagnosed with CD and treated with a GFD. The intervention consisted of introducing oligofructose-enriched inulin (Synergy 1) into the diet for 12 weeks. We assessed the impact of the intervention on nutritional status, morphological and biochemical blood parameters and gut microbiota. Details of the study protocol have been previously described by Krupa-Kozak et al. [23]. Results regarding nutritional status, gut microbiota composition, and short-chain fatty acids concentration in the stool have been previously reported elsewhere [24].

2.2. Participants Selection

Participants were enrolled among consecutive patients with celiac disease, aged 4–18 years, treated with a gluten-free diet for at least 6 months prior to enrolment, treated and followed-up at the Department of Paediatrics, Gastroenterology and Nutrition Medical Faculty of University of Warmia and Masuria in Children's Hospital, Olsztyn, Poland. CD was diagnosed according to criteria created by the European Society for Paediatric Gastroenterology, Hepatology and Nutrition (ESPGHAN 2012 criteria) [25]. All patients had positive ($\geq$8 AU/mL) anti-transglutaminase 2 antibodies at the time of diagnosis. To confirm the diagnosis, endoscopy with small bowel biopsies was performed in all patients and the specimens were interpreted according to the Marsh criteria [25]. Among the 96 patients who met the inclusion criteria (Table 1), a consent to participate in the study was obtained for 34 patients.

Table 1. Participant selection criteria.

Inclusion Criteria	Exclusion Criteria
Diagnosed Celiac Disease Gluten-free diet for at least 6 months Age: 4–18 years old Normalization of Tissue Transglutaminase Antibody (TTGA) level Written consent from parents/caregivers	Iron deficiency anemia [1] Iron deficiency [2] Immunoglobulin A (IgA) deficiency Treatment with oral formulas in the 2 months prior to the study Therapy by antibiotics or probiotics/prebiotics in the 2 months prior to the study Chronic inflammatory disorders

[1] Iron deficiency anemia was defined as a hemoglobin level below WHO range for sex and age. [2] iron deficiency was defined as a ferritin level <12 ng/mL [26].

2.3. Ethics

Parents and caregivers were informed about potential benefits and risks and signed a written consent form during the enrollment visit. Experimental design and all procedures were approved by the Bioethics Committee of the Faculty of Medical Sciences of the University of Warmia and Mazury in Olsztyn (permission No. 23/2015 of 16 June 2015). The study was registered in the ClinicalTrials database (NCT03064997) [27].

2.4. Intervention

Patients (n = 34) were randomly assigned to the placebo group (n = 16) or the Synergy 1 group (n = 18) [23]. The intervention lasted 3 months. Participants in the control group received maltodextrin (7 g orally/day; Maltodextrin DE 20, Hotrimex, Konin, Poland), while participants in the examination group received oligofructose-enriched inulin (10 g orally/day; Orafti® Synergy 1, Beneo, Tienen, Belgium). Patients, parents/caregivers, and all investigators except N.D. (who was in charge of the treatment distribution) were blinded to the allocated experimental group. Maltodextrin was the placebo of choice, as it is digested in the small intestine and thus does not exert local effects in the colon, contrarily to prebiotics. During the study, patients were required to record adherence to supplementation, side effects, if any, and the intake of other substances, i.e., antibiotic, probiotic, or prebiotic. The nutritional value of the diet during study and adherence to GFD were monitored using a validated food frequency questionnaire (FFQ-6) [28].

2.5. Sample Collection

Blood samples were collected from all participants at two time points: before and after the intervention. Complete blood count and biochemical parameters (C-reactive protein (CRP) and ferritin) were analyzed according to standard procedures of the hospital laboratory, as previously described [23]. Serum hepcidin levels were measured using a commercial ELISA kit (FRG Instruments GmbH, Nuremberg, Germany).

2.6. Statistical Analysis

All below analyses were performed in duplicate and the data were analyzed using the Statistica 12 software (StatSoft, Tulsa, OK, USA). A difference with a p-value < 0.05 was considered statistically significant. Normality of quantitative variables was tested by the Shapiro–Wilk W test. Quantitative variables with a normal distribution were expressed as mean ± SD, while quantitative variables which showed a non-normal distribution were expressed as a median (P25-P75). Differences in characteristics between groups were tested with the parametric Student's t-test or the non-parametric Mann–Whitney U test, as appropriate. Differences within groups before and after intervention were determined with the Student's t-test for paired samples or the Wilcoxon signed-rank test, as appropriate.

3. Results

3.1. Study Population

Thirty-four children and adolescents (mean age 10 years; 62% females; all anthropometric details summarized in Table 2), were included in the study. The duration of the GFD prior to enrolment ranged between seven months to nine years but showed no significant difference between Synergy 1 and the placebo group ($p = 0.608$). Thirty patients completed the study (88.2%), while four children were excluded from the analysis due to non-compliance in the test protocol.

Table 2. Participant anthropometric data.

	Total Sample		Intervention Group (Synergy 1)		Placebo Group (Maltodextrin)	
N	30		17 (56.6%)		13 (63.4%)	
Gender (G–girls, B–boys)	G = 18 (60%) B = 12 (40%)		G = 10 (58.8%) B = 7 (41.2%)		G = 8 (61.5%) B = 5 (38.5%)	
Age (years)	4–18 Average = 10		4–18 Average = 10		4–16 Average = 10	
	T0 [a]	**T1 [b]**	**T0**	**T1**	**T0**	**T1**
Weight (kg)	15.0–78.0 Av = 35.8	15.7–77.5 Av = 37.6	15.0–78.0 Av = 35.8	15.7–77.5 Av = 37.6	16.3–66.8 Av = 33.7	17.0–71.5 Av = 36.2
Height (cm)	103.0–183.0 Av = 139.6	104.5–184.5 Av = 141.4	104.5–183.0 Av = 141.5	108.0–184.5 Av = 142.4	103.0–172.0 Av = 137.1	104.5–172.6 Av = 139.7
BMI (kg/m^2)	12.5–28.4 Av = 17.1	12.7–29.0 Av = 17.3	12.5–23.5 Av = 17.1	12.7–23.6 Av = 17.3	13.7–28.4 Av = 17.0	13.4–29.0 Av = 17.3

[a] T0—baseline; [b] T1—after three-month intervention.

The safety profile and side effects of Synergy 1 in this trial have been previously described [24]. Briefly, no severe side effects were noted during the three-month intervention with Synergy 1 and there was no significant difference in the frequency of reported symptoms between the two experimental groups. The levels of anti-tissue transglutaminase antibodies (tTGA) were measured before and after intervention. In all patients, tTGA titers before and after intervention were within the recommended level (<8.0 AU/mL). All patients had adequate adherence to GFD according to the FFQ-6 questionnaire.

3.2. Morphological and Biochemical Parameters of Blood

Morphological and biochemical blood parameters at baseline were comparable between the Synergy 1 and the placebo group. No statistically significant difference in those parameters was observed before and after intervention in either of the two experimental groups (Table 3).

3.3. Hepcidin

Serum hepcidin concentrations at baseline (T0) were comparable between the two groups ($p = 0.547$). Hepcidin levels in the Synergy 1 group were significantly lower after 3-months intervention than at baseline (median: 1.73 (1.31–3.14) versus 4.42 (1.89–8.64), respectively; $p = 0.046$), accounting for a 60.9% decrease. Conversely, no significant difference in hepcidin concentration was observed between T1 and T0 in the placebo group (median: 2.43 (0.91–3.87) versus 2.99 (1.23–5.09), respectively) (Figure 1). There was no significant difference between the Synergy 1 and placebo group after the intervention ($p = 0.645$).

Table 3. Morphological and biochemical parameters before (T0) and after (T1) the intervention, expressed as mean ± SD.

Morphology Parameters	Synergy 1 Group		Placebo Group		Synergy 1: T0 vs. T1 [1] (*p* Value)	Placebo: T0 vs. T1 [1] (*p* Value)	T1: Synergy 1 vs. Placebo (*p* Value)
	T0	T1	T0	T1			
Red Blood Cell ($10^6/mm^3$)	4.63 ± 0.37	4.69 ± 0.34	4.58 ± 0.37	4.57 ± 0.34	0.274	0.851	0.359
Hemoglobin (g/dL)	13.22 ± 0.99	13.13 ± 1.09	13.12 ± 0.99	12.89 ± 1.09	0.912	0.297	0.565
Hematocrit (%)	39.11 ± 2.95	39.65 ± 3.22	38.94 ± 2.95	38.93 ± 3.22	0.314	0.838	0.559
Mean Cell Volume (μm^3)	84.50 ± 4.18	84.63 ± 4.33	85.19 ± 4.18	84.92 ± 4.33	1.000	0.779	0.283
Mean Cell Hemoglobin (pg)	28.48 ± 1.53	27.65 ± 1.17	28.65 ± 1.53	28.13 ± 1.17	0.139	0.052	0.102
Red Blood Cell Distribution Width (%)	12.64 ± 0.71	12.91 ± 0.92	12.99 ± 0.71	13.22 ± 0.92	0.247	0.308	0.695
Platelets ($10^3/mm^3$)	290.28 ± 64.15	314.63 ± 55.51	301.38 ± 64.15	315.77 ± 55.51	0.299	0.197	0.957
White Blood Cell ($10^3/mm^3$)	6.29 ± 1.64	6.57 ± 1.78	6.59 ± 1.64	6.65 ± 1.78	0.721	0.844	0.283
Biochemical parameters							
C-reactive protein (CRP) (mg/dL)	0.14 ± 0.08	0.11 ± 0.07	0.10 ± 0.08	0.12 ± 0.07	0.582	0.100	0.660
Ferritin (ng/mL)	25.78 ± 14.48	22.94 ± 13.94	27.62 ± 14.48	23.08 ± 13.94	0.507	0.107	0.742

[1] Comparison within groups using Student's *t*-test or the Wilcoxon test, as appropriate.

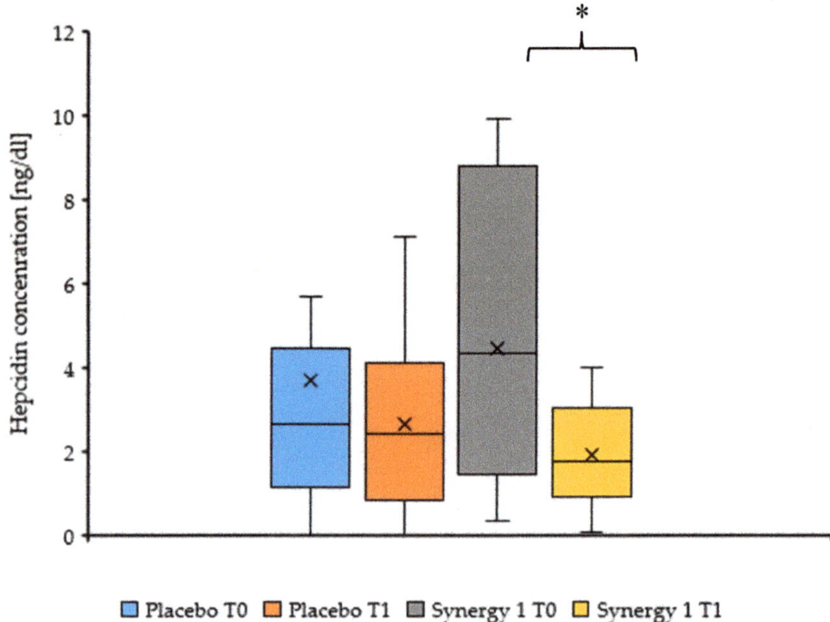

Figure 1. Serum hepcidin concentration before (T0) and after (T1) intervention, expressed as a median (cross) (P25-P75) (box). * $p = 0.046$.

4. Discussion

To our knowledge, this is the first prospective, randomized, placebo-controlled, double-blind study of the effects of oligofructose-enriched inulin (Synergy 1) on iron homeostasis in CD patients treated with a GFD. Our key finding was a significant decrease in plasma hepcidin concentration after 3 months of treatment with Synergy 1 (10 g daily), whereas no such effect was observed in the placebo group. Hepcidin downregulates duodenal iron absorption and decreases iron storage release by modulating cellular export via ferroportin [11]. Hepcidin production disorders result in impaired iron homeostasis: Hepcidin deficiency may cause iron overload, while excess is associated with IDA [8,9]. Thus, the observed decrease in hepcidin levels upon the Synergy 1 treatment could potentially help improve iron absorption in CD children and adolescents.

To confirm this hypothesis, a positive effect of Synergy 1 on ferritin levels would need to be demonstrated. Plasma ferritin concentration is the most sensitive indicator of iron storage capacity in IDA. In our study, the Synergy 1 treatment did not alter ferritin or haemoglobin levels. However, in patients with normal iron stores, ferritin levels are finely regulated to avoid excessive iron absorption and accumulation in the organism [7]. Given that the present study was conducted on non-anemic children and adolescents, the potential effect of Synergy 1 on ferritin and on haemoglobin levels cannot be properly evaluated. Further prospective studies are warranted, focusing on CD children with IDA and especially on those with refractory IDA, to verify whether Synergy 1 can indeed increase iron absorption and whether it could have a clinical benefit in this setting. As a secondary finding, our results show that Synergy 1 does not cause excessive iron accumulation or iron deficiency in non-anemic CD patients, thus supporting a safe profile of this prebiotic in regards to iron homeostasis in non-anemic individuals.

One possible explanation of the observed decrease in hepcidin is the potential anti-inflammatory effect of prebiotics, which has been previously reported in animal models. In a study by Marciano et al. [22], supplementation of anemic growing rats with oligofructose, but not with inulin, led to decreased TNF-α, IL-6 and IL-10 expression in the cecum and to a decrease in urinary hepcidin. In another study, inulin and oligofructose supplementation led to a downregulation of pro-inflammatory genes in colonic tissue of young anemic pigs [29]. Although the Synergy 1 treatment did not influence CRP levels in our study, pro-inflammatory cytokines were not measured.

The beneficial role of prebiotics on iron absorption could have important clinical implications, but so far, results from different model systems have been discrepant. Many animal studies suggest a positive effect [22,29,30]. For example, in rats, a beneficial effect of FOS supplementation on iron absorption was observed in both iron-deficient animals [22,31] and in growing rats with a normal iron status [32]. In vitro experiments on the human cell line Caco-2, a widely-used model for studying absorptive proprieties of the intestinal mucosa, have yielded inconsistent results: in two studies, prebiotics did not improve iron bioavailability from milk- or soy-based yogurts [33,34], while in two other studies, iron bioavailability from iron-fortified cereal biscuits [35] and from the commercial Young Child Formula® [36] were significantly improved by prebiotic supplementation. In humans, no positive results are available to date. In healthy men aged 20–30 years, iron absorption measured using a stable isotope technique was 20% higher in individuals supplemented daily with FOS (15 g/day for 21 days) than in the control group, but the results did not reach statistical significance [37]. In women with anemia, supplementation with 20 g of inulin per day for four weeks did not cause an increase of iron absorption, although changes in gut microbiota composition and a decrease of fecal pH were observed [38].

Although our work reveals a potential link between prebiotic supplementation and hepcidin levels, prebiotics may also enhance iron absorption in other ways, including a direct effect on iron transporter expression [22] and their potential to decrease systemic inflammation [22,29]. Moreover, fermentation of indigestible oligosaccharides increases the production of fatty acids by *Bifidobacteria* spp. and lowers the fecal pH, which in turn can improve iron solubility and enhance its absorption [21,38]. The potential effect of prebiotics on iron status could also be a more complex process, affecting not only absorption but also the stage of transfer, storage, and recycling [22,29,30].

Healing of the intestinal mucosa is a critical step towards recovering normal absorption of macro- and micro-nutrients. However, CD patients with anemia usually show a more severe enteropathy than non-anemic patients and their intestinal mucosa may take longer to heal [38].

Our study has some limitations, including a small cohort size, inclusion of patients within a wide age range, and a relatively short intervention duration. Thus, these findings need to be validated on a larger cohort, including patients with IDA, and measuring additional parameters, such as pro-inflammatory cytokines, with the potential to elucidate the mechanisms of hepcidin changes in this setting. Intestinal histological healing in children after GFD has also been shown to occur earlier and to a greater extent than in adults [39]. Thus, further research is needed to establish the potential role of Synergy-1 in iron hemostasis in adult CD patients.

5. Conclusions

We have previously shown that oligofructose-enriched inulin (Synergy 1) was a safe and well-tolerated prebiotic in children and adolescents with CD in association with a GFD. Here, we found that a three-month intervention with Synergy 1 (10 g orally/day) led to a significant decrease of serum hepcidin concentrations by 60.9% ($p = 0.046$) in those patients, whereas no significant difference was observed in the placebo group. Given that hepcidin decrease may improve iron absorption, these promising results warrant further investigation in a larger cohort, including patients with iron deficiency anemia, who represent the potential target group for this type of treatment.

Author Contributions: U.K.-K. conceived the study. U.K.-K., N.D., K.F. and E.J.-C. were involved in designing of the study; N.D. and E.J.-C. carried out the study and collected samples; N.D. performed the main part of the experiments; N.D. and K.F. analyzed the data; K.F. drafted the manuscript; E.J.-C. and N.D. contributed to the further writing of the manuscript. All authors read and approved the final version of the manuscript.

Funding: This research received no external funding.

Acknowledgments: We wish to sincerely thank all the patients who participated in this study. The research was supported by statutory funds of the Department of Chemistry and Biodynamics of Food at the Institute of Animal Reproduction and Food Research, Polish Academy of Science, Poland (GW20).

Conflicts of Interest: The authors declare no conflict of interest.

References

1. Guandalini, S.; Assiri, A. Celiac disease: A review. *JAMA Pediatr.* **2014**, *168*, 272–278. [CrossRef] [PubMed]
2. Dickson, B.C.; Streutker, C.J.; Chetty, R. Coeliac disease: An update for pathologists. *J. Clin. Pathol.* **2006**, *59*, 1008–1016. [CrossRef] [PubMed]
3. Crocker, H.; Jenkinson, C.; Churchman, D.; Peters, M. The Coeliac Disease Assessment Questionnaire (CDAQ): Development of a patient-reported outcome measure. *Value Health* **2016**, *9*, A595. [CrossRef]
4. Schumann, M.; Siegmund, B.; Schulzke, J.D.; Fromm, M. Celiac Disease: Role of the Epithelial Barrier. *Cell. Mol. Gastroenterol. Hepatol.* **2017**, *3*, 150–162. [CrossRef] [PubMed]
5. Roma, E.; Roubani, A.; Kolia, E.; Panayiotou, J.; Zellos, A.; Syriopoulou, V.P. Dietary compliance and life style of children with coeliac disease. *J. Hum. Nutr. Diet.* **2010**, *23*, 176–182. [CrossRef] [PubMed]
6. Efthymakis, K.; Milano, A.; Laterza, F.; Serio, M.; Neri, M. Iron deficiency anemia despite effective gluten-free diet in celiac disease: Diagnostic role of small bowel capsule endoscopy. *Dig. Liver Dis.* **2017**, *49*, 412–416. [CrossRef] [PubMed]
7. Freeman, H.J. Iron deficiency anemia in celiac disease. *World J. Gastroenterol.* **2015**, *21*, 9233–9238. [CrossRef] [PubMed]
8. Nemeth, E.; Ganz, T. The role of hepcidin in iron metabolism. *Acta Haematol.* **2009**, *122*, 78–86. [CrossRef] [PubMed]
9. Choi, H.S.; Song, S.H.; Lee, J.H.; Kim, H.-J.; Yang, H.R. Serum hepcidin levels and iron parameters in children with iron deficiency. *Korean J. Hematol.* **2012**, *47*, 286–292. [CrossRef] [PubMed]
10. Harper, J.W.; Holleran, S.F.; Ramakrishnan, R.; Bhagat, G.; Green, P.H.R. Anemia in celiac disease is multifactorial in etiology. *Am. J. Hematol.* **2007**, *82*, 996–1000. [CrossRef] [PubMed]
11. Gulec, S.; Anderson, G.J.; Collins, J.F. Mechanistic and regulatory aspects of intestinal iron absorption. *AJP Gastrointest. Liver Physiol.* **2014**, *307*, G397–G409. [CrossRef] [PubMed]
12. Elli, L.; Poggiali, E.; Tomba, C.; Andreozzi, F.; Nava, I.; Bardella, M.T.; Campostrini, N.; Girelli, D.; Conte, D.; Cappellini, M.D. Does TMPRSS6 RS855791 polymorphism contribute to iron deficiency in treated celiac disease. *Am. J. Gastroenterol.* **2015**, *110*, 200–202. [CrossRef] [PubMed]
13. Garcia-Manzanares, A.; Lucendo, A.J. Nutritional and dietary aspects of celiac disease. *Nutr. Clin. Pract.* **2011**, *26*, 163–173. [CrossRef] [PubMed]
14. Rubio-Tapia, A.; Hill, I.D.; Kelly, C.P.; Calderwood, A.H.; Murray, J.A. ACG clinical guidelines: Diagnosis and management of celiac disease. *Am. J. Gastroenterol.* **2013**, *108*, 656–676. [CrossRef] [PubMed]
15. Deora, V.; Aylward, N.; Sokoro, A.; El-Matry, W. Serum vitamins and minerals at diagnosis an follow-up in children with celiac disease. *J. Pediatr. Gastroenterol. Nutr.* **2017**, *65*, 185–189. [CrossRef] [PubMed]
16. Galli, G.; Esposito, G.; Lahner, E.; Pilozzi, E.; Corleto, V.D.; Di Giulio, E.; Aloe Spiriti, M.A.; Annibale, B. Histological recovery and gluten-free diet adherence: A prospective 1-year follow-up study of adult patients with coeliac disease. *Aliment. Pharmacol. Ther.* **2014**, *40*, 639–647. [CrossRef] [PubMed]
17. Bardella, M.T.; Velio, P.; Cesana, B.M. Coeliac disease: A histological follow-up study. *Histopathology* **2007**, *50*, 465–471. [CrossRef] [PubMed]
18. Vici, G.; Belli, L.; Biondi, M.; Polzonetti, V. Gluten free diet and Nutrient deficiencies: A revive. *Clin. Nutr.* **2016**, *35*, 1236–1241. [CrossRef] [PubMed]
19. Theethira, T.G.; Dennis, M.; Leffler, D.A. Nutritional consequences of celiac disease and gluten-free diet. *Expert Rev. Gastroenterol. Hepatol.* **2014**, *8*, 123–129. [CrossRef] [PubMed]
20. Thomson, T.; Dennis, M.; Higgins, L.A.; Lee, A.R.; Sharrett, M.K. Gluten-free diet survey: Are Americans with celiac disease consuming recommended amounts of fiber, iron, calcium and grain foods? *J. Hum. Nutr. Diet.* **2005**, *18*, 163–169. [CrossRef] [PubMed]

21. Yeung, C.K.; Glahn, R.E.; Welch, R.M.; Miller, D.D. Prebiotics and Iron Bioavailability-Is There a Connection? *J. Food Sci.* **2005**, *70*, R88–R92. [CrossRef]
22. Marciano, R.; Santamarina, A.B.; De Santana, A.A.; Silva, M.D.L.C.; Amancio, O.M.S.; Do Nascimento, C.M.D.P.O.; Oyama, L.M.; De Morais, M.B. Effects of prebiotic supplementation on the expression of proteins regulating iron absorption in anaemic growing rats. *Br. J. Nutr.* **2015**, *113*, 901–908. [CrossRef] [PubMed]
23. Krupa-Kozak, U.; Drabińska, N.; Jarocka-Cyrta, E. The effect of oligofructose-enriched inulin supplementation on gut microbiota, nutritional status and gastrointestinal symptoms in paediatric coeliac disease patients on a gluten-free diet: Study protocol for a pilot randomized controlled trial. *Nutr. J.* **2017**, *16*, 47. [CrossRef] [PubMed]
24. Drabińska, N.; Jarocka-Cyrta, E.; Markiewicz, L.H.; Krupa-Kozak, U. The Effect of Oligofructose-Enriched Inulin on Faecal Bacterial Counts and Microbiota-Associated Characteristics in Celiac Disease Children Following a Gluten-Free Diet: Results of a Randomized, Placebo-Controlled Trial. *Nutrients* **2018**, *10*, 201. [CrossRef] [PubMed]
25. Husby, S.; Koletzko, I.R.; Korponay-Szabo, M.L.; Mearin, A.P.; Shamir, R.; Troncone, R.; Giersiepen, K.; Branksi, D.; Catasssi, C.; Lelgeman, M.; et al. European Society for Pediatric Gastroenterology, Hepatology, and Nutrition Guidelines for the Diagnosis of Coeliac Disease. *J. Pediatr. Gastroenterol. Nutr.* **2012**, *54*, 136–160. [CrossRef] [PubMed]
26. WHO. *Iron Deficiency Anaemia: Assessment, Prevention, and Control. A Guide for Programme Managers*; World Health Organization: Geneva, Switzerland, 2001.
27. U.S. National Institutes of Health. Available online: https://clinicaltrials.gov/ (accessed on 27 February 2017).
28. Yasuda, K.; Dawson, H.D.; Wasmuth, E.V.; Roneker, C.A.; Chen, C.; Urban, J.F.; Welch, R.M.; Miller, D.D.; Lei, X.G. Supplemental Dietary Inulin Influences Expression of Iron and Inflammation Related Genes in Young Pigs. *J. Nutr.* **2009**, *139*, 2018–2023. [CrossRef] [PubMed]
29. Patterson, J.K.; Yasuda, K.; Welch, R.M.; Miller, D.D.; Lei, X.G. Supplemental Dietary Inulin of Variable Chain Lengths Alters Intestinal Bacterial Populations in Young Pigs. *J. Nutr.* **2010**, *140*, 2158–2161. [CrossRef] [PubMed]
30. Ohta, A.; Ohtsuki, M.; Baba, S.; Takizawa, T.; Adachi, T.; Kimura, S. Effects of fructooligosaccharides on the absorption of iron, calcium and magnesium in iron-deficient anemic rats. *J. Nutr. Sci. Vitaminol.* **1995**, *41*, 281–291. [CrossRef] [PubMed]
31. Delzenne, N.; Aertssens, J.; Verplaetse, H.; Roccaro, M.; Roberfroid, M. Effect of fermentable fructo-oligosaccharides on mineral, nitrogen and energy digestive balance in the rat. *Life Sci.* **1995**, *57*, 1579–1587. [CrossRef]
32. Laparra, J.M.; Tako, E.; Glahn, R.P.; Miller, D.D. Supplemental inulin does not enhance iron bioavailability to Caco-2 cells from milk- or soy-based, probiotic-containing, yogurts but incubation at 37 °C does. *Food Chem.* **2008**, *109*, 122–128. [CrossRef] [PubMed]
33. Laparra, J.M.; Glahn, R.P.; Miller, D.D. Assessing potential effects of inulin and probiotic bacteria on Fe availability from common beans (*Phaseolus vulgaris* L.) to Caco-2 cells. *J. Food Sci.* **2009**, *74*, 40–46. [CrossRef] [PubMed]
34. Vitali, D.; Radić, M.; Cetina-Čižmek, B.; Vedrina Dragojević, I. Caco-2 cell uptake of Ca, Mg and Fe from biscuits as affected by enrichment with pseudocereal/inulin mixtures. *Acta Aliment.* **2011**, *40*, 480–489. [CrossRef]
35. Christides, T.; Ganis, J.C.; Sharp, P.A. In vitro assessment of iron availability from commercial Young Child Formulae supplemented with prebiotics. *Eur. J. Nutr.* **2018**, *57*, 669–678. [CrossRef] [PubMed]
36. Van den Heuvel, E.G.H.M.; Schaafsma, G.; Muys, T.; Van Dokkum, W. Nondigestible oligosaccharides do not interfere with calcium and nonheme-iron absorption in young, healthy men. *Am. J. Clin. Nutr.* **1998**, *67*, 445–451. [CrossRef] [PubMed]
37. Petry, N.; Egli, I.; Chassard, C.; Lacroix, C.; Hurrell, R. Inulin modifies the bifidobacteria population, fecal lactate concentration, and fecal pH but does not influence iron absorption in women with low iron status. *Am. J. Clin. Nutr.* **2012**, *96*, 325–331. [CrossRef] [PubMed]

38. Abu Daya, H.; Lebwohl, B.; Lewis, S.K.; Green, P.H. Celiac disease patients presenting with anemia have more severe disease than those presenting with diarrhea. *Clin. Gastroenterol. Hepatol.* **2013**, *11*, 1472–1477. [CrossRef] [PubMed]
39. Rubio-Tapia, A.; Rahim, M.W.; See, J.A.; Lahr, B.D.; Wu, T.T.; Murray, J.A. Mucosal recovery and mortality in adults with celiac disease after treatment with a gluten-free diet. *Am. J. Gastroenterol.* **2010**, *105*, 1412–1420. [CrossRef] [PubMed]

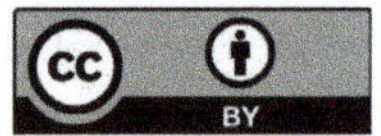

© 2018 by the authors. Licensee MDPI, Basel, Switzerland. This article is an open access article distributed under the terms and conditions of the Creative Commons Attribution (CC BY) license (http://creativecommons.org/licenses/by/4.0/).

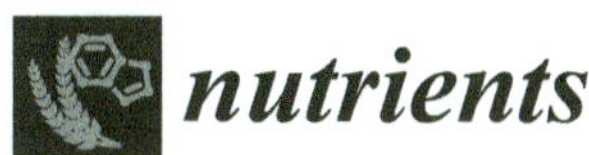

Review

Probiotics in Celiac Disease

Fernanda Cristofori [1], Flavia Indrio [2], Vito Leonardo Miniello [2], Maria De Angelis [3] and Ruggiero Francavilla [2,4,*]

1 Paediatric Department, "SS Annunziata" Hospital, 74100 Taranto, Italy; fernandacristofori@gmail.com
2 Department of Paediatrics, Paediatric Hospital Giovanni XXIII, Via Amendola 207, 70126 Bari, Italy; flaviaindrio1@gmail.com (F.I.); vito.miniello@libero.it (V.L.M.)
3 Department of Soil, Plant and Food Sciences, University of Bari Aldo Moro, 70126 Bari, Italy; maria.deangelis@uniba.it
4 Pediatric Section, Department of Interdisciplinary Medicine, University of Bari Aldo Moro, 70124 Bari, Italy
* Correspondence: rfrancavilla@gmail.com or ruggiero.francavilla@uniba.it; Tel.: +39-080-5592063

Received: 30 September 2018; Accepted: 15 November 2018; Published: 23 November 2018 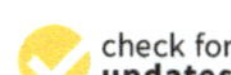

Abstract: Recently, the interest in the human microbiome and its interplay with the host has exploded and provided new insights on its role in conferring host protection and regulating host physiology, including the correct development of immunity. However, in the presence of microbial imbalance and particular genetic settings, the microbiome may contribute to the dysfunction of host metabolism and physiology, leading to pathogenesis and/or the progression of several diseases. Celiac disease (CD) is a chronic autoimmune enteropathy triggered by dietary gluten exposure in genetically predisposed individuals. Despite ascertaining that gluten is the trigger in CD, evidence has indicated that intestinal microbiota is somehow involved in the pathogenesis, progression, and clinical presentation of CD. Indeed, several studies have reported imbalances in the intestinal microbiota of patients with CD that are mainly characterized by an increased abundance of *Bacteroides* spp. and a decrease in *Bifidobacterium* spp. The evidence that some of these microbial imbalances still persist in spite of a strict gluten-free diet and that celiac patients suffering from persistent gastrointestinal symptoms have a desert gut microbiota composition further support its close link with CD. All of this evidence gives rise to the hypothesis that probiotics might play a role in this condition. In this review, we describe the recent scientific evidences linking the gut microbiota in CD, starting from the possible role of microbes in CD pathogenesis, the attempt to define a microbial signature of disease, the effect of a gluten-free diet and host genetic assets regarding microbial composition to end in the exploration of the proof of concept of probiotic use in animal models to the most recent clinical application of selected probiotic strains.

Keywords: probiotics; microbiota; celiac disease; gluten free diet

---

1. Introduction

Celiac disease (CD) is a lifelong immune mediated enteropathy initiated by exposure to dietary gluten in individuals carrying human leucocyte antigen (HLA)-DQ2 or DQ8 [1]. Loss of gluten tolerance may occur at the time of its introduction into the diet or at any time in life, and the underlying mechanism is still under research. The role for an environmental component in CD pathogenesis is supported by: (a) HLA and non-HLA genes explain only 55% of disease susceptibility, (b) the concordance of celiac disease in monozygotic twins is around 80%, and (c) the incidence on this condition is rapidly increasing [2–4].

Intestinal microbiota could be somehow involved in the pathogenesis of CD and/or in its progression and/or in the development of clinical manifestation [5–9]. Briefly, gut microbiota can impact on the pathogenesis of CD in different ways: (a) modulating the digestion of gluten peptides both generating toxic and/or tolerogenic peptides that might impact on the acquisition of dietary tolerance to antigen, (b) influencing the intestinal permeability through zonulin release and tight junction expression, (c) promoting the maturation of the mucosal epithelium, and (d) regulating the activity of the immune system via expression of cytokines and pro-inflammatory or anti-inflammatory peptides [10].

In the last decade, several studies have reported imbalances in the intestinal microbiota of patients with CD, even though the literature shows that there is not a univocal microbial signature of CD [11]. It is also matter of debate whether dysbiosis plays a role in the pathogenesis of the disease, or whether it is just a consequence of CD inflammation; however, the intestinal dysbiosis often persists irrespective of the adherence to a gluten-free diet (GFD), and in part is also related to this particular diet. Finally, the identification of intestinal dysbiosis in CD, with the evidence supporting a role for gut microbiota in regulating key aspects of innate and adaptive immunity and the persistence of dysbiosis despite a prolonged GFD, have led to a hypothesis suggesting the clinical use of probiotics.

The aim of this review is to describe the recent scientific evidence on the role of gut microbiota in CD, and the proof of concept for the use of probiotics in CD patients.

2. Gut Microbiota and Risk of Developing Celiac Disease

Microbiota has a crucial role in the maturation of the immune system, being pivotal for the development of protective/tolerogenic immune responses [12]. Current evidence shows that environmental agents and/or endogenous signals may cause dysbiosis, which is responsible for a breakdown of immune homeostasis and an increase in the risk of immune conditions such as CD, among others [13].

There are several early life events that may prime a dysregulated gut microbiota, starting from the mode of delivery. After vaginal delivery, the colonization of the newborn is characterized mainly by *Lactobacilli*, *Prevotella*, and *Bifidobacteria* [14,15], while after cesarean section (C-section), the infant flora is mainly influenced by environmental and maternal skin bacteria [16]. This might explain an increased risk of CD in C-section newborns, as reported by previous studies [17,18].

Breastfeeding is a second factor that might impact gut microbiota composition; indeed, the presence of human maternal oligosaccharides supports the survival and growth of a healthy microbiota. Retrospective studies have shown that the duration of breastfeeding and particularly gluten introduction during breastfeeding reduce or delays CD onset [19]. However, both these evidence have been recently questioned and not confirmed, so the issue is still debated [20–22], and the issue may be more complicated than initially thought. De Palma et al. studied 164 newborns (born in a family with a first-degree relative with CD) divided according to HLA genotype and modality of feeding (breast versus formula), and found a different gut colonization according to with the type of feeding. Overall, they showed that carrying the HLA predisposition was associated with increased numbers of *Bacteroides fragilis* and *Staphylococcus*, and decreased *Bifidobacterium*, and that these differences were increased by formula as compared to breastfeeding. These results support the idea that gut microbiota composition is a multiplayer game where both feeding type and HLA genotype are key regulators [23]. Another variable can complicate this issue: evidence that breast milk samples from mothers with CD as compared to those without CD have lower titers of interleukin12p70, transforming growth factor-β1, and secretory immunoglobulin A (IgA), and a decrease in the *Bifidobacterium* and *Bacteroides fragilis* groups. This study supports the hypothesis that the reduction of immune-protective compounds and *Bifidobacterium* species can reduce the protection conferred by breastfeeding, thus increasing the child's risk of CD [24].

That a particular genetic asset could play a role in shaping gut microbiota in early life is further supported by a recent study. De Palma et al. studied the faecal microbiota of 22 breastfed infants (born in a family with a first-degree relative with CD), and found that carrying a high (HLA-DQ2) as compared to a low genetic risk (non-HLA-DQ2/8) was followed by the presence of higher proportions of Firmicutes and Proteobacteria (*Corynebacterium*, *Gemella*, unclassified *Clostridiaceae*, unclassified *Enterobacteriaceae,* and *Raoultella*) and lower proportions of *Actinobacteria* (*Bifidobacterium* and unclassified Bifidobacteriaceae). These results highlight that a specific host genotype might modulate the gut microbiota composition of infants and contribute to an increasing disease risk [25]. The possibility that a particular genotype can shape the gut microbial composition is supported by genome-wide association studies that have identified 39 non-HLA CD risk loci. Interestingly, some of these genes related to immune functions and bacterial colonization and disease-associated single nucleotide polymorphism (SNPs) involved in the regulation of microbiota handling may explain the role of genes in gut microbiota composition [26].

In order to investigate the role of gut microbiota (and their products—metabolome) as contributory factors leading to the onset of CD, a large international study: "Celiac Disease Genomic, Environmental, Microbiome, and Metabolomic Study (CDGEMM) is ongoing in the United States (USA), Italy and Spain. CDGEMM is a prospective, longitudinal observational cohort study of infants with a first-degree family member with CD that aims to investigate if the time of gluten introduction, microbiota composition, and genetic asset are involved in the loss of gluten tolerance, and identify and validate specific microbiota and metabolic profiles that are mechanistically linked to gut functions (including permeability, immune function, and stem cell niche biology) and can anticipate a loss of gluten tolerance in genetically predisposed individuals. This study will be the proof of concept to plan preventive interventions to induce gluten immune tolerance and possibly prevent CD [27].

3. Microbiota in Celiac Patient

As shown in Table 1, in the last 10 years, several studies [28–51] have been performed evaluating fecal, salivary, and duodenal microbiota in CD patients. Interestingly, Collado et al. have shown a correlation between bacterial species found in both biopsies and feces of CD patients indicating that the fecal microbiota is comparable to the small intestine microbiota, and may have a diagnostic value [31].

Table 1. Scientific findings of the last 10 years on salivary, duodenal, and fecal microbiota in celiac patients.

Author	Population	Age	Saliva Samples	Duodenal Biopsies	Fecal Samples	Methods	Results in CD Patients
Collado et al. [28]	26 CD vs. 23 HC	Children	No	No	Yes	Colture and FISH	↑ *Bacteroides–Prevotella, Clostriudium hystoliticum, Eubacterium rectale–C. coccoides, Atopobium and Staphylococcus*
Sanz et al. [29]	10 CD vs. 10 HC	Children	No	No	Yes	Culture DGGE	*L. curvatus, Leuconostoc mesenteroides* only in CD
Nadal et al. [30]	20 CD vs. 10 CD-GFD vs. 8 HC	Children	No	Yes	No	FISH Flow citometry	↓ Ratio of *Lactobacillus–Bifidobacterium to Bacteroides–E. coli* ↑ Gram-negative
Collado et al. [31]	8 CD vs. 8 CD vs. 8 HC	Children	No	Yes	Yes	real-time PCR	↑ *Bacteroides, C. leptum, E. coli, Staphylococcus* ↓ *Bifidobacteria*
Di Cagno et al. [32]	7 CD vs. 7 CD-GFD vs. 7 HC	Children	No	No	Yes	real time PCR DGGE	↓ Ratio of cultivable lactic acid bacteria and *Bifidobacterium* to *Bacteroides* and *enterobacteria* ↓ *Lactobacillus*
Ou et al [33]	45 CD vs. 18 HC	Children	No	Yes	No	16S rDNA sequencing	↑ *Haemophilus, Streptococcus, Neisseria*
Schippa et al. [34]	20 CD before and after GFD vs. 10 HC	Children	No	Yes	No	16S rDNA sequencing TTGE	↑ *Bacteroides vulgatus* and *Escherichia coli*
De Palma et al. [35]	24 CD vs. 18 CD-GFD vs. 20 HC	Children	No	No	Yes	FISH flow cytometry	↓ Gram-positive to Gram-negative bacteria ratio ↓ *Bifidobacterium, Clostridium histolyticum, C. lituseburense* and *Faecalibacterium prausnitzii* ↑ *Bacteroides–Prevotella*

Table 1. *Cont.*

Author	Population	Age	Saliva Samples	Duodenal Biopsies	Fecal Samples	Methods	Results in CD Patients
Sanchez et al. [36]	20 CD vs. 12 CD-GFD vs. 8 HC	Children	No	Yes	No	DGGE	↑ *Bacteroides dorei* ↓ *Bacteroides distasonis, Bacteroides fragilis/Bacteroides thetaiotaomicron, Bacteroides uniformis*, and *Bacteroides ovatus* ↑ *Bifidobacterium adolescentis Bifidobacterium animalis* subsp *lactis*
Di Cagno et al. [37]	19 CD vs. 15 HC	Children	No	Yes	Yes	DGGE	↓ *Lactobacillus, Enterococcus*, and *Bifidobacteria*
Nistal et al. [38]	10 CD vs. 11 CD-GFD vs. 11 HC	Adults	No	No	Yes	DGGE	↑ *B. bifidum and catenulatum*
Nistal et al. [39]	13 CD vs. 5 CD-GFD vs. 10 HC	Children Adults	No	Yes	No	16SrRNA gene sequencing	↓ *Streptococcus* and *Prevotella*
Sanchez et al. [40]	20 CD vs. 20 CD-GFD vs. 20 HC	Children	No	No	Yes	PCR DNA sequencing	↑ *Staphylococcus epidermidis Staphylococcus haemolyticus* ↓ *S. aureus*
Acar et al. [41]	35 CD vs. 35 HC	Children	Yes	No	No	CRT Bacteria	↓ Salivary mutans streptococci and lactobacilli colonization
De Meij et al. [42]	21 CD vs. 21 HC	Children	No	Yes	No	IS-pro, profiling method	No differences
Sanchez et al. [43]	32 CD vs. 17 CD-GFD vs. 8 HC	Children	No	Yes	No	Colture 16S rRNA gene sequencing	↑ Proteobacteria, Enterobacteriaceae, and Staphylococcaceae ↓ Streptococcaceae, Firmicutes
Wacklin et al. [44]	33 CD (either symptomatic or asymptomatic) vs. 18 HC	Adults	No	Yes	No	16S rRNA gene sequencing	↑ Proteobacteria, such as *Acinetobacter* and *Neisseria*, in patient with GI symptoms. ↓ microbial diversity in GI symptoms or anemia
Cheng et al [45]	10 CD vs. 9 HC	Children	No	Yes	No	qRT-PCR	No differences *Haemophilus* ssp. and *Serratia* ssp. had relatively higher abundance in CD
Francavilla et al. [46]	13 CD-GFD vs. 13 HC	Children	Yes	No	No	16S rRNA gene sequencing	↑ Lachnospiraceae, Gemellaceae, and *Streptococcus sanguinis* Bacteroidetes ↓ *Streptococcus thermophilus*
Wacklin et al. [47]	18 CD-GFD symptomatic vs. 18 CD-GFD asymptomatic	Adults	No	Yes	No	16S rRNA gene sequencing	↑ Proteobacteria ↓ *Bacteroides* and Firmicutes
Giron-Fernandez Crehuet et al. [48]	11 A-CD vs. 11 HC	Children	No	Yes	No	DGGE	*Lactobacillus* genus
D'Argenio et al. [49]	20 A-CD vs. 6 CD-GFD vs. 15 HC	Adults	No	Yes	No	16S rRNA gene sequencing metagenomics	↑ Proteobacteria ↓ Firmicutes and Actinobacteria ↑ *Neisseria* genus (*Neisseria flavescens*)
Quagliariello et al. [50]	40 A-CD vs. 16 HC	Children	No	No	Yes	16S rRNA gene sequencing Quantitative PCR (qPCR)	↓ Firmicutes/Bacteroidetes ratio, ↓ Actinobacteria and Euryarchaeota
Tian et al. [51]	21 CD-GFD vs. 8 RCD vs. 20 HC	Adults	Yes	No	No	16S rRNA gene sequencing	Bacteroidetes (CD > RCD), Actinobacteria (CD < RCD), Fusobacteria (CD > RCD)

A-CD: active celiac disease, CD-GFD: celiac disease on gluten-free diet, GI: gastrointestinal, RCD: refractory celiac disease, HC: healthy controls, FISH: fluorescent in situ hybridization, TTGE: temporal temperature gradient gel electrophoresis, DGGE: denaturing gradient gel electrophoresis; qPCR: quantitative PCR; qRT-PCR: quantitative reverse-transcriptase-PCR; ↓ Decrease; ↑ Increase.

Among the various studies, results may vary, which is due to huge differences in terms of microbiological methods, sample sizes, and patients' characteristics. Nevertheless, there is substantial agreement on the presence of an imbalance between pro-inflammatory and anti-inflammatory species, with a prevalence of the former.

We investigated the fecal microbiota of children with active CD (A-CD) and after (T-CD) GFD and of healthy children (HC) showing a reduction of *Lactobacill*us in A-CD, but not in T-CD, that was similar to that of HC. Using gas chromatography mass spectrometry solid-phase microextraction analysis, we found a profound variation of the mean concentrations of volatile organic compounds with short chain fatty acids being more represented in HC [32]. In a subsequent study, we analyzed the duodenal microbiota of 19 T-CD and 15 HC, and found a higher diversity of *Eubacteria* and lower counts of *Bifidobacteria* in T-CD as compared to HC children. According to the most recent scientific evidences, the CD patients' microbiota seems to be characterized by an increased abundance of *Bacteroides* spp., *E. Coli*, *Proteobacteria*, and *Staphylococcus* and a decrease in *Bifidobacterium* spp. and *Lactobacillus* [52]. This result supports the knowledge that a long-lasting GFD did not completely restore the microbiota of CD children [37].

A study by Wacklin et al. suggested that the microbiota might have a role in the clinical manifestation of the disease. Indeed, the authors demonstrated that CD patients with gastrointestinal symptoms compared to those without and controls have different microbiota compositions (more abundant in *Proteobacteria* phylum versus more abundant in *Firmicutes* phylum, respectively) [44]. Moreover, alterations of microbiota may have pathogenic implication, leading to persistent gastrointestinal symptoms, despite a strict GFD. Indeed, the same group found that CD patients on a GFD who are still symptomatic have a reduced microbial richness and a different duodenal microbiota colonization in comparison with asymptomatic patients (higher relative abundance of *Proteobacteria* and a lower abundance of *Bacteroidetes* and *Firmicutes*), showing that intestinal dysbiosis might be responsible for the persistence of symptoms, even while adhering to a strict GFD [47].

4. Gluten-Free Diet and Gut Microbiota

At present, a strict GFD is the only available treatment [53] and, although evidence exists on the comparison between the gut microbiota of CD patients on a GFD or a gluten-containing diet (GCD) and/or controls, very few data are available in prospectively followed CD patients before and after GFD.

GFD is only partially effective in restoring the gut microbiota: indeed, while higher numbers of *Enterobacteria* or *Staphylococci* are restored, other alterations such as decreased *Bifidobacteria* and *Lactobacilli* and increased *Bacteroides*, *Enterobacteriaceae* and virulent *E. coli* still are persistent [54].

On the other hand, a GFD can itself influence gut microbiota composition. De Palma et al. studied the effects of a month of GFD on the composition of the gut microbiota in 10 healthy subjects, and found a significant decrease of *Bifidobacterium*, *Clostridium lituseburense*, and *Faecalibacterium prausnitzii*, and an increase of Enterobacteriaceae and *Escherichia coli* counts [54]. The analysis of the daily energy and nutrient intake before and after the GFD found no significant differences in dietary intake, except for a significant reduction in polysaccharide intake, leading the authors to conclude that a natural reduction in polysaccharide intake (fructans), which have prebiotic action and constitute one of the main energy sources for commensal components of the gut microbiota [55], might explain the reductions in beneficial gut bacteria populations. Therefore, a GFD itself rather than CD may be responsible for gut microbiota unbalance.

5. Probiotics Supplementation

Most of the evidence on the effect of probiotics in CD comes from animal models. Experiments using transgenic non-obese diabetic-DQ8 mice are the proof of concept that the microbiota shape the gluten-related immune-mediated mucosal damage. In germ-free conditions, mice develop a more aggressive gluten-induced pathology as compared with mice colonized with altered Schaedler flora (benign microbiota) that is deprived of opportunistic pathogens. However, in the presence of a microbiota with opportunistic pathogens or in the case of perturbations secondary to antibiotic use, mice develop gluten-induced severe pathology. These results reinforce the pivotal effect of gut microbiota in the inflammatory response that is associated with gluten ingestion [56].

Mouse models have demonstrated that probiotics can modulate innate and adaptive immunity, and reduce gliadin-induced inflammation [57–59].

Lindfors K et al. studied whether *Lactobacillus fermentum* or *Bifidobacterium lactis* are able to reduce the toxic effects of gluten-derived peptides in intestinal cell culture (Caco-2) conditions. They showed that *Bifidobacterium lactis* was able to inhibit the gliadin-induced derangement of epithelial permeability, and speculated that this probiotic could counteract the harmful effects of toxic gliadin epitopes [60].

Papista C et al. investigated the influence of probiotics in a model of gluten sensitivity (BALB/c mice); the authors were able to show that the *Saccharomyces boulardii KK1* strain hydrolyzed the gliadin toxic peptides, and its consumption was followed by improved enteropathy and a decrease of histological damage and pro-inflammatory cytokine production [59].

Laparra J.M. et al. studied the use of *Bifidobacterium longum CECT 7347* in an animal model of gliadin-induced enteropathy. The authors showed that the administration of this particular strain reduces the production of pro-inflammatory cytokines and the mediated immune response [61].

The idea that the effect played by probiotics is strain-specific is supported by the work of D'Arienzo et al., who studied the effect of *Lactobacillus* and *Bifidobacterium lactis* strains in transgenic mice expressing human DQ8, and found an increased antigen-specific tumor necrosis factor (TNF) secretion showing that probiotics may have pro-inflammatory rather than suppressive effects [62].

Despite the encouraging data deriving from in vitro studies, few in vivo data are available on probiotics supplementation in patients with CD (Table 2).

Table 2. Main evidence on the use of probiotics in patients with celiac disease.

Author	RCT	Population	Used Strain	Time of Administration	Findings in Probiotics Group
Smecuol et al. [63]	Yes	22 A-CD (12 *probiotic* vs. 10 placebo)	*Bifidobacterium infantis* Natren life start	3 weeks	Improvement in GI symptoms (indigestion, constipation, and gastroesophageal reflux) ↓ Final/baseline IgA tTG and IgA DGP antibody concentration ratios ↑ Serum macrophage inflammatory protein-1β No differences in intestinal permeability No significant changes in cytokines and chemokines production
Pinto-Sánchez et al. [64]	No	24 A-CD no treatment vs. 12 A-CD probiotic treatment vs. 5 CD-GFD	*Bifidobacterium infantis* Natren life start	3 weeks	↓ Paneth cell counts ↓ α-defensin-5
Olivares et al. [65]	Yes	36 A-CD (18 *B. longum* + GFD vs. 18 placebo + GFD)	*Bifidobacterium longum* CECT 7347	3 months	↑ Height percentile ↓ Peripheral $CD3^+$ T lymphocytes concentration ↓ TNF-α levels ↓ *Bacteroides fragilis* and Enterobacteriaceae ↑ Harmless to potentially harmful bacteria ratio No differences in GI symptoms
Quagliarello et al. [50]	Yes	40 A-CD children (20 probiotic and 20 placebo) vs. 16 HC	*Bifidobacterium breve strains* (B632 and BR03)	3 months	↑ Actinobacteria Re-establishment Firmicutes/Bacteroidetes ratio.
Harnett et al. [66]	Yes	45 CD-GFD with symptoms (23 probiotic and 22 placebo)	multispecies probiotic VSL#3 (450 billion viable lyophilized bacteria *Streptococcus thermophilus, Bifidobacterium breve, Bifidobacterium longum, Bifidobacterium infantis, Lactobacillus acidophilus, Lactobacillus plantarum, Lactobacillus paracasei*, and *Lactobacillus delbrueckii subsp. Bulgaricus)*	12 weeks	No differences in the fecal microbiota counts No differences in symptoms severity

Table 2. *Cont.*

Author	RCT	Population	Used Strain	Time of Administration	Findings in Probiotics Group
Klemenak et al. [67]	Yes	49 CD-GFD (24 probiotic and 25 placebo) 18 HC	*Bifidobacterium breve strains* (BR03 and B632)	3 months	↓ TNF-alpha levels (not persistent)
Primec et al. [68]	Yes	40 CD (20 probiotic and 20 placebo) 16 HC	*Bifidobacterium breve strains* (BR03 and B632)	3 months	Negative relationship between Firmicutes and pro-inflammatory TNF-α.
Francavilla et al. [69]	Yes	109 CD-GFD with IBS symptoms (54 probiotic vs. 55 placebo)	mixture of 5 *Lactobacillus casei* LMG 101/37 P-17504 *Lactobacillus plantarum* CECT 4528, *Bifidobacterium animalis subsp. lactis* Bi1 LMG P-17502, *Bifidobacterium breve* Bbr8 LMG P-17501 *Bifidobacterium breve* Bl10 LMG P-17500	6 weeks	Improvement in GI symptoms ↑ *Bifidobacteria* (persistent)

A-CD: active celiac disease; CD-GFD: celiac disease on gluten-free diet; HC: healthy controls; GI: gastrointestinal, IgA: immunoglobulin A; tTG: antitransglutaminase; DGP: deamidated gliadin peptide; TNF: tumor necrosis factor; ↓ Decrease; ↑ Increase.

Smecuol et al. investigated the effects of *Bifidobacterium infantis* Natren life start strain (NLS-SS), randomizing 22 patients with A-CD to receive the probiotic or placebo while on a GCD, showing that this probiotic led to a significant improvement in GI symptoms. However, they found no effect on cytokines and growth factors, neither on celiac serology nor gut permeability [63].

The same group speculated that the favorable effect that was observed could be due to its influence on innate immunity. Thus, they tested the effect of *Bifidobacterium infantis* NLS-SS by assessing Paneth cells and macrophage counts and human α-defensin 5 (HD5) expression in duodenal biopsies of CD patients on a GFD. The results of this second study demonstrated that patients that assumed *Bifidobacterium infantis* NLS-SS experience a decrease in the expression of the antimicrobial peptide HD5, which is paralleled by a decrease in Paneth cells counts [64].

In a recent randomized control trial, Olivares at al. demonstrated in children with a new diagnosis of CD that the administration of *Bifidobacterium longum* CECT 7347 for three months, when associated with a GFD, was able to determine a height percentile increase compared with a placebo, as well as lower peripheral $CD3^{+}$ T lymphocytes concentration and slightly reduced TNF-α levels; moreover, the treatment with *Bifidobacterium longum* CECT 7347 was associated with a significant decrease in the *Bacteroides fragilis* group and *Enterobacteriaceae* and a higher ratio of harmless to potentially harmful bacteria. However, the authors did not find any improvement of gastrointestinal symptoms [65].

Quagliarello et al. performed a RCT in 49 CD children to evaluate the efficacy of three months of administration of two *Bifidobacterium breve* strains (B632 and BR03) on the re-establishment of eubiosis in CD children on a GFD, demonstrating that supplementation induces an increase of Actinobacteria as well as a restoration of the Firmicutes/Bacteroidetes ratio [50].

On the contrary, Harnett et al. randomized 45 CD patients on a GFD, with persistent symptoms, to receive VSL#3 (5 g) or placebo, and found no differences in the fecal microbiota counts, and symptoms severity after two weeks of supplementation [66].

Klemenak et al. investigated the effect of two *Bifidobacterium breve* strains (BR03 and B632) on serum interleukin-10 and TNF-α levels in 49 children with CD on GFD, demonstrating lower levels of TNF-α after three months of daily use; no difference was found for interleukin (IL)-10 levels [67].

In 2018, Primec M. et al. performed a double-blind placebo-controlled study enrolling 40 CD and 16 healthy children. CD children were randomized to receive placebo or a mixture of two *Bifidobacterium breve* strains (DSM 16604 and DSM 24706) for three months. The authors showed that this probiotic mixture was able to modulate the production of acetic acid and total short-chain fatty acids (SCFAs), promoting a potential role in microbiome restoration [68].

Finally, our group recently performed a large prospective, randomized study in 109 CD patients strictly adherent to a GFD with irritable bowel syndrome (IBS) symptoms. Enrolled patients were randomized to probiotics (mixture of five strains of lactic acid bacteria and *bifidobacteria*:

Lactobacillus casei LMG 101/37 P-17504 (5 Å~ 109 CFU/sachet), *Lactobacillus plantarum* CECT 4528 (5 Å~ 109 CFU/sachet), *Bifidobacterium animalis* subsp. *lactis* Bi1 LMG P-17502 (3.4 Å~ 109 CFU/sachet), *Bifidobacterium breve* Bbr8 LMG P-17501 (3.4 Å~ 109 CFU/sachet), *Bifidobacterium breve* Bl10 LMG P-17500 (3.4 Å~ 109 CFU/sachet)), or placebo for six weeks, and then followed up for six more weeks. Our results showed that the probiotic mix under study is effective in ameliorating the severity of IBS symptoms measured by IBS severity score (IBS-SS). After six weeks of treatment, we found a significantly higher proportion of treatment success (a decrease of at least 50% of IBS-SS), at both intention-to-treat (14.8% versus 3.6%; $p < 0.04$) and per protocol analysis (15.3% versus 3.8%; $p < 0.04$) [69]. A recent meta-analysis has shown that CD patients with GI symptoms have a higher prevalence of small intestinal bacterial overgrowth (SIBO) as compared to controls (28% versus 10%), although the difference does not reach statistical significance, and the analysis is affected by the large heterogeneity of the studies [70]. At present, no studies have been conducted to investigate whether probiotic administration might have an impact on SIBO in CD patients, nor have we explored this in our trial. However, we were able to show a positive modulation of gut microbiota with an increase of *bifidobacteria* still detectable six weeks after the discontinuation of probiotics [69].

6. Conclusions

Gut microbiota is an essential mediator of health, and its imbalance might be followed by an alteration of microbiota functions with a negative impact on health. Research in the last 10 years has shed new light on the role of the gut microbiota in CD and the complex relation between its composition, genetic background, GFD, and the persistence of clinical symptoms. Although many critical issues remain to be defined, some aspects are now clear. (a) Gut microbiota participate and mediate the gluten related inflammation. (b) As of yet, there is not a definite microbial signature of disease, although some microbial alterations are consistently reported, both in biopsies and fecal samples (abundance of *Bacteroides* spp., a decrease in *Bifidobacterium* spp.). (c) Some alterations of gut microbial composition revert to normal, while others are sustained by a GFD, and might be in part responsible for the persistence of symptoms in this population. (d) Selected probiotics with clinical proven efficacy might be of help in controlling gluten-mediated inflammation and ameliorating clinical symptoms (Figure 1).

With the increasing prevalence of people that adopt the gluten-free regimen, it is mandatory to define the intimate link between gut microbiota and gluten-related disorders in order to explore new possible avenues to offer a valid dietetic counseling to this expanding population and possibly in the future to identify new strategies for prevention and treatment.

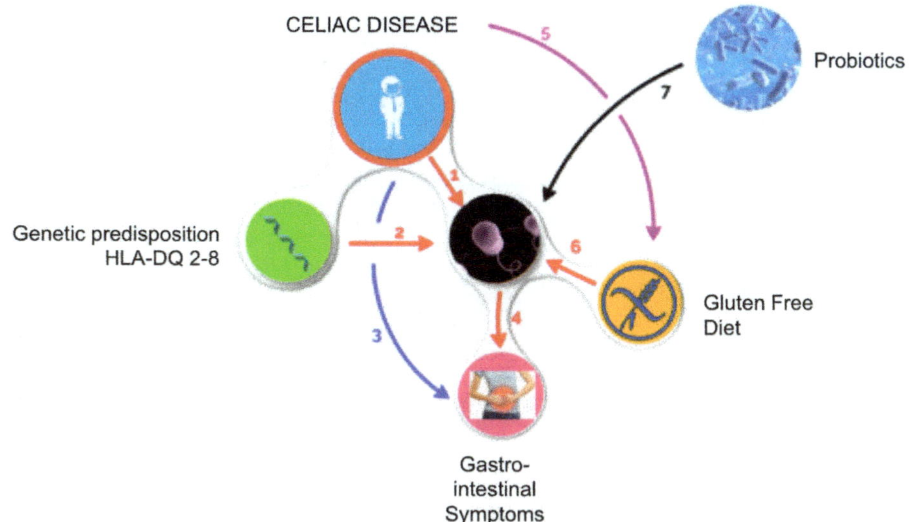

Figure 1. Mechanism of action of probiotics in controlling GI symptoms in celiac patients. Recent data have shown that patients with celiac disease (CD) have an altered gut microbiota (GM), (1) and that carrying the genetic predisposition (HLA-DQ-2 or DQ-8) may predispose individuals to a state of dysbiosis. (2) Patients with CD usually have GI symptoms (3) that can persist to a strict gluten-free diet (GFD); moreover, the alteration of GM can be one of the main causes of the persistence of GI symptoms. (4) CD requires that a patient follow a rigorous GFD (5) and a natural reduction in polysaccharide intake (fructans), which have prebiotic action, and constitute one of the main energy sources for commensals of the GM that might further worsen gut dysbiosis. (6) In turn, this reinforces the persistence of GI symptoms. (7). If we consider that most of the variables of this complex equation are fixed (genetic predisposition, CD, need for a GFD, the presence of GI symptoms), the only variable on which we can operate is the GM: therefore, the adoption of a probiotic supplementation that restores the imbalance in the GM of a celiac patient might be a reasonable therapeutic option.

Author Contributions: All of the authors reviewed the available literature, wrote the paper, has approved the submitted version and agrees to be personally accountable for the author's own contributions and for ensuring that questions related to the accuracy or integrity of any part of the work.

Funding: This research received no external funding.

Conflicts of Interest: R.F., F.I., M.D.A. are the inventors of the probiotic mixture used in the study [69] patent N 0001425900, released on 17 November 2016 (Italy). The remaining authors declare that they have nothing to disclose.

References

1. Green, P.H.; Cellier, C. Celiac disease. *N. Engl. J. Med.* **2007**, *357*, 1731–1743. [CrossRef] [PubMed]
2. Ludvigsson, J.F.; Rubio-Tapia, A.; van Dyke, C.T.; Melton, L.J., 3rd; Zinsmeister, A.R.; Lahr, B.D.; Murray, J.A. Increasing incidence of celiac disease in a North American population. *Am. J. Gastroenterol.* **2013**, *108*, 818–824. [CrossRef] [PubMed]
3. Murray, J.A.; Van Dyke, C.; Plevak, M.F.; Dierkhising, R.A.; Zinsmeister, A.R.; Melton, L.J., 3rd. Trends in the identification and clinical features of celiac disease in a North American community, 1950–2001. *Clin. Gastroenterol. Hepatol.* **2003**, *1*, 19–27. [CrossRef] [PubMed]
4. White, L.E.; Merrick, V.M.; Bannerman, E.; Russell, R.K.; Basude, D.; Henderson, P.; Wilson, D.C.; Gillett, P.M. The rising incidence of celiac disease in Scotland. *Pediatrics* **2013**, *132*, e924–e931. [CrossRef] [PubMed]

5. Galipeau, H.J.; McCarville, J.L.; Huebener, S.; Litwin, O.; Meisel, M.; Jabri, B.; Sanz, Y.; Murray, J.A.; Jordana, M.; Alaedini, A.; et al. Intestinal microbiota modulates gluten-induced immunopathology in humanized mice. *Am. J. Pathol.* **2015**, *185*, 2969–2982. [CrossRef] [PubMed]
6. Sellitto, M.; Bai, G.; Serena, G.; Fricke, W.F.; Sturgeon, C.; Gajer, P.; White, J.R.; Koenig, S.S.; Sakamoto, J.; Boothe, D.; et al. Proof of concept of microbiome-metabolome analysis and delayed gluten exposure on celiac disease autoimmunity in genetically at-risk infants. *PLoS ONE* **2012**, *7*, 33387. [CrossRef] [PubMed]
7. Conte, M.P.; Schippa, S.; Zamboni, I.; Penta, M.; Chiarini, F.; Seganti, L.; Osborn, J.; Falconieri, P.; Borrelli, O.; Cucchiara, S. Gut-associated bacterial microbiota in paediatric patients with inflammatory bowel disease. *Gut* **2006**, *55*, 1760–1767. [CrossRef] [PubMed]
8. Maynard, C.L.; Elson, C.O.; Hatton, R.D.; Weaver, C.T. Reciprocal interactions of the intestinal microbiota and immune system. *Nature* **2012**, *489*, 231–241. [CrossRef] [PubMed]
9. Becker, S.; Oelschlaeger, T.A.; Wullaert, A.; Vlantis, K.; Pasparakis, M.; Wehkamp, J.; Stange, E.F.; Gersemann, M. Bacteria regulate intestinal epithelial cell differentiation factors both in vitro and in vivo. *PLoS ONE* **2013**, *8*, e55620. [CrossRef]
10. Cénit, M.C.; Olivares, M.; Codoner-Franch, P.; Sanz, Y. Intestinal microbiota and celiac disease: Cause, consequence or coevolution? *Nutrients* **2015**, *7*, 6900–6923. [CrossRef] [PubMed]
11. Verdu, E.F.; Galipeau, H.J.; Jabri, B. Novel players in coeliac disease pathogenesis: Role of the gut microbiota. *Nat. Rev. Gastroenterol. Hepatol.* **2015**, *12*, 497–506. [CrossRef] [PubMed]
12. Sommer, F.; BaÅNckhed, F. The gut microbiota—Masters of host development and physiology. *Nat. Rev. Microbiol.* **2013**, *11*, 227–238. [CrossRef] [PubMed]
13. Belkaid, Y.; Hand, T.W. Role of the microbiota in immunity and inflammation. *Cell* **2014**, *157*, 121–141. [CrossRef] [PubMed]
14. Neu, J.; Rushing, J. Cesarean versus vaginal delivery: Long-term infant outcomes and the hygiene hypothesis. *Clin. Perinatol.* **2011**, *38*, 321–331. [CrossRef] [PubMed]
15. Dominguez-Bello, M.G.; Costello, E.K.; Contreras, M.; Magris, M.; Hidalgo, G.; Fierer, N.; Knight, R. Delivery mode shapes the acquisition and structure of the initial microbiota across multiple body habitats in newborns. *Proc. Natl. Acad. Sci. USA* **2010**, *107*, 11971–11975. [CrossRef] [PubMed]
16. Francavilla, R.; Cristofori, F.; Tripaldi, M.E.; Indrio, F. Intervention for Dysbiosis in Children Born by C-Section. *Ann. Nutr. Metab.* **2018**, *73* (Suppl. 3), 33–39. [CrossRef] [PubMed]
17. Decker, E.; Hornef, M.; Stockinger, S. Cesarean delivery is associated with celiac disease but not inflammatory bowel disease in children. *Gut Microbes* **2011**, *2*, 91–98. [CrossRef] [PubMed]
18. Adlercreutz, E.H.; Wingren, C.J.; Vincente, R.P.; Merlo, J.; Agardh, D. Perinatal risk factors increase the risk of being affected by both type 1 diabetes and coeliac disease. *Acta Paediatr.* **2015**, *104*, 178–184. [CrossRef] [PubMed]
19. Akobeng, A.K.; Ramanan, A.V.; Buchan, I.; Heller, R.F. Effect of breast feeding on risk of coeliac disease: A systematic review and meta-analysis of observational studies. *Arch. Dis. Child.* **2006**, *91*, 39–43. [CrossRef] [PubMed]
20. Dydensborg Sander, S.; Hansen, A.V.; Størdal, K.; Andersen, A.N.; Murray, J.A.; Husby, S. Mode of delivery is not associated with celiac disease. *Clin. Epidemiol.* **2018**, *10*, 323–332. [CrossRef] [PubMed]
21. Aronsson, C.A.; Lee, H.-S.; Liu, E.; Uusitalo, U.; Hummel, S.; Yang, J.; Hummel, M.; Rewers, M.; She, J.-X.; Simell, O.; et al. Age at gluten introduction and risk of celiac disease. *Pediatrics* **2015**, *135*, 239–245. [CrossRef] [PubMed]
22. Størdal, K.; White, R.A.; Eggesbø, M. Early feeding and risk of celiac disease in a prospective birth cohort. *Pediatrics* **2013**, *132*, e1202–e1209. [CrossRef] [PubMed]
23. Palma, G.D.; Capilla, A.; Nova, E.; Castillejo, G.; Varea, V.; Pozo, T.; Garrote, J.A.; Polanco, I.; López, A.; Ribes-Koninckx, C.; et al. Influence of milk-feeding type and genetic risk of developing coeliac disease on intestinalbmicrobiota of infants: The PROFICEL study. *PLoS ONE* **2012**, *7*, e30791. [CrossRef] [PubMed]
24. Olivares, M.; Albrecht, S.; De Palma, G.; Ferrer, MD.; Castillejo, G.; Schols, HA.; Sanz, Y. Human milk composition differs in healthy mothers and mothers with celiac disease. *Eur. J. Nutr.* **2015**, *54*, 119–128. [CrossRef] [PubMed]
25. Olivares, M.; Neef, A.; Castillejo, G.; Palma, G.D.; Varea, V.; Capilla, A.; Palau, F.; Nova, E.; Marcos, A.; Polanco, I.; et al. The HLA-DQ2 genotype selects for early intestinal microbiota composition in infants at high risk of developing coeliac disease. *Gut* **2015**, *64*, 406–417. [CrossRef] [PubMed]

26. Dieli-Crimi, R.; Cénit, M.C.; Núñez, C. The genetics of celiac disease: A comprehensive review of clinical implications. *J. Autoimmun.* **2015**, *64*, 26–41. [CrossRef] [PubMed]
27. Leonard, M.M.; Camhi, S.; Huedo-Medina, T.B.; Fasano, A. Celiac Disease Genomic, Environmental, Microbiome, and Metabolomic (CDGEMM) Study Design: Approach to the Future of Personalized Prevention of Celiac Disease. *Nutrients* **2015**, *7*, 9325–9336. [CrossRef] [PubMed]
28. Collado, M.C.; Calabuig, M.; Sanz, Y. Differences between the fecal microbiota of coeliac infants and healthy controls. *Curr. Issues Intest. Microbiol.* **2007**, *8*, 9–14. [PubMed]
29. Sanz, Y.; Sanchez, E.; Marzotto, M.; Calabuig, M.; Torriani, S.; Dellaglio, F. Differences in faecal bacterial communities in coeliac and healthy children as detected by PCR and denaturing gradient gel electrophoresis. *FEMS Immunol. Med. Microbiol.* **2007**, *51*, 562–568. [CrossRef] [PubMed]
30. Nadal, I.; Donat, E.; Ribes-Koninckx, C.; Calabuig, M.; Sanz, Y. Imbalance in the composition of the duodenal microbiota of children with coeliac disease. *J. Med. Microbiol.* **2007**, *56*, 1669–1674. [CrossRef] [PubMed]
31. Collado, MC.; Donat, E.; Ribes-Koninckx, C.; Calabuig, M.; Sanz, Y. Specific duodenal and faecal bacterial groups associated with paediatric coeliac disease. *J. Clin. Pathol.* **2009**, *62*, 264–269. [CrossRef] [PubMed]
32. Di Cagno, R.; Rizzello, C.G.; Gagliardi, F.; Ricciuti, P.; Ndagijimana, M.; Francavilla, R.; Guerzoni, M.E.; Crecchio, C.; Gobbetti, M.; De Angelis, M. Different fecal microbiotas and volatile organic compounds in treated and untreated children with celiac disease. *Appl. Environ. Microbiol.* **2009**, *75*, 3963–3971. [CrossRef] [PubMed]
33. Ou, G.; Hedberg, M.; Horstedt, P.; Baranov, V.; Forsberg, G.; Drobni, M.; Sandström, O.; Wai, S.N.; Johansson, I.; Hammarström, M.L.; et al. Proximal small intestinal microbiota and identification of rod-shaped bacteria associated with childhood celiac disease. *Am. J. Gastroenterol.* **2009**, *104*, 3058–3067. [CrossRef] [PubMed]
34. Schippa, S.; Iebba, V.; Barbato, M.; Di Nardo, G.; Totino, V.; Checchi, M.P.; Longhi, C.; Maiella, G.; Cucchiara, S.; Conte, M.P. A distinctive "microbial signature" in celiac pediatric patients. *BMC Microbiol.* **2010**, *10*, 175. [CrossRef] [PubMed]
35. De Palma, G.; Nadal, I.; Medina, M.; Donat, E.; Ribes-Koninckx, C.; Calabuig, M.; Sanz, Y. Intestinal dysbiosis and reduced immunoglobulin-coated bacteria associated with coeliac disease in children. *BMC Microbiol.* **2010**, *10*, 63. [CrossRef] [PubMed]
36. Sanchez, E.; Donat, E.; Ribes-Koninckx, C.; Calabuig, M.; Sanz, Y. Intestinal Bacteroides species associated with coeliac disease. *J. Clin. Pathol.* **2010**, *63*, 1105–1111. [CrossRef] [PubMed]
37. Di Cagno, R.; De Angelis, M.; De Pasquale, I.; Ndagijimana, M.; Vernocchi, P.; Ricciuti, P.; Gagliardi, F.; Laghi, L.; Crecchio, C.; Guerzoni, M.E.; et al. Duodenal and faecal microbiota of celiac children: Molecular, phenotype and metabolome characterization. *BMC Microbiol.* **2011**, *11*, 219. [CrossRef] [PubMed]
38. Nistal, E.; Caminero, A.; Vivas, S.; Ruiz de Morales, J.M.; Sáenz de Miera, L.E.; Rodríguez-Aparicio, L.B.; Casqueiro, J. Differences in faecal bacteria populations and faecal bacteria metabolism in healthy adults and celiac disease patients. *Biochimie* **2012**, *94*, 1724–1729. [CrossRef] [PubMed]
39. Nistal, E.; Caminero, A.; Herran, A.R.; Arias, L.; Vivas, S.; de Morales, J.M.; Calleja, S.; de Miera, L.E.; Arroyo, P.; Casqueiro, J. Differences of small intestinal bacteria populations in adults and children with/without celiac disease: Effect of age, gluten diet, and disease. *Inflamm. Bowel Dis.* **2012**, *18*, 649–656. [CrossRef] [PubMed]
40. Sanchez, E.; Ribes-Koninckx, C.; Calabuig, M.; Sanz, Y. Intestinal *Staphylococcus* spp. and virulent features associated with coeliac disease. *J. Clin. Pathol.* **2012**, *65*, 830–834. [CrossRef] [PubMed]
41. Acar, S.; Yetkiner, A.A.; Ersin, N.; Oncag, O.; Aydogdu, S.; Arikan, C. Oral findings and salivary parameters in children with celiac disease: A preliminary study. *Med. Princ. Pract.* **2012**, *21*, 129–133. [CrossRef] [PubMed]
42. De Meij, T.G.J.; Budding, A.E.; Grasman, M.E.; Kneepkens, C.M.F.; Savelkoul, P.H.M.; Mearin, M.L. Composition and diversity of the duodenal mucosa-associated microbiome in children with untreated coeliac disease. *Scand. J. Gastroenterol.* **2013**, *48*, 530–536. [CrossRef] [PubMed]
43. Sanchez, E.; Donat, E.; Ribes-Koninckx, C.; Fernandez-Murga, M.L.; Sanz, Y. Duodenal-mucosal bacteria associated with celiac disease in children. *Appl. Environ. Microbiol.* **2013**, *79*, 5472–5479. [CrossRef] [PubMed]
44. Wacklin, P.; Kaukinen, K.; Tuovinen, E.; Collin, P.; Lindfors, K.; Partanen, J.; Mäki, M.; Mättö, J. The duodenal microbiota composition of adult celiac disease patients is associated with the clinical manifestation of the disease. *Inflamm. Bowel Dis.* **2013**, *19*, 934–941. [CrossRef] [PubMed]

45. Cheng, J.; Kalliomaki, M.; Heilig, H.G.H.J.; Palva, A.; Lähteenoja, H.; de Vos, W.M.; Salojärvi, J.; Satokari, R. Duodenal microbiota composition and mucosal homeostasis in pediatric celiac disease. *BMC Gastroenterol.* **2013**, *13*, 113. [CrossRef] [PubMed]
46. Francavilla, R.; Ercolini, D.; Piccolo, M.; Vannini, L.; Siragusa, S.; De Filippis, F.; De Pasquale, I.; Di Cagno, R.; Di Toma, M.; Gozzi, G.; et al. Salivary microbiota and metabolome associated with celiac disease. *Appl. Environ. Microbiol.* **2014**, *80*, 3416–3425. [CrossRef] [PubMed]
47. Wacklin, P.; Laurikka, P.; Lindfors, K.; Collin, P.; Salmi, T.; Lähdeaho, M.L.; Saavalainen, P.; Mäki, M.; Mättö, J.; Kurppa, K.; et al. Altered duodenal microbiota composition in celiac disease patients suffering from persistent symptoms on a long-term gluten-free diet. *Am. J. Gastroenterol.* **2014**, *109*, 1933–1941. [CrossRef] [PubMed]
48. Giron Fernandez-Crehuet, F.; Tapia-Paniagua, S.; Morinigo Gutierrez, M.A.; Navas-López, V.M.; Juliana Serrano, M.; Blasco-Alonso, J.; Sierra Salinas, C. The duodenal microbiota composition in children with active coeliac disease is influenced by the degree of enteropathy. *An. Pediatr. (Barc.)* **2016**, *84*, 224–230. [CrossRef] [PubMed]
49. D'Argenio, V.; Casaburi, G.; Precone, V.; Pagliuca, C.; Colicchio, R.; Sarnataro, D.; Discepolo, V.; Kim, S.M.; Russo, I.; Del Vecchio Blanco, G.; et al. Metagenomics Reveals Dysbiosis and a Potentially Pathogenic, N. flavescens Strain in Duodenum of Adult Celiac Patients. *Am. J. Gastroenterol.* **2016**, *111*, 879–890. [CrossRef] [PubMed]
50. Quagliariello, A.; Aloisio, I.; Bozzi Cionci, N.; Luiselli, D.; D'Auria, G.; Martinez-Priego, L.; Pérez-Villarroya, D.; Langerholc, T.; Primec, M.; Mičetić-Turk, D.; et al. Effect of Bifidobacterium breve on the Intestinal Microbiota of Coeliac Children on a Gluten Free Diet: A Pilot Study. *Nutrients* **2016**, *8*, 660. [CrossRef] [PubMed]
51. Tian, N.; Faller, L.; Leffler, D.A.; Kelly, C.P.; Hansen, J.; Bosch, J.A.; Wei, G.; Paster, B.J.; Schuppan, D.; Helmerhorst, E.J. Salivary Gluten Degradation and Oral Microbial Profiles in Healthy Individuals and Celiac Disease Patients. *Appl. Environ. Microbiol.* **2017**, 83. [CrossRef] [PubMed]
52. Sanz, Y. Microbiome and gluten. *Ann. Nutr. Metab.* **2015**, *2*, 28–41. [CrossRef] [PubMed]
53. Guandalini, S.; Assiri, A. Celiac disease: A review. *JAMA Pediatr.* **2014**, *168*, 272–278. [CrossRef] [PubMed]
54. De Palma, G.; Nadal, I.; Collado, M.C.; Sanz, Y. Effects of a gluten-free diet on gut microbiota and immune function in healthy adult human subjects. *Br. J. Nutr.* **2009**, *102*, 1154–1160. [CrossRef] [PubMed]
55. Jackson, F.W. Effects of a gluten-free diet on gut microbiota and immune function in healthy adult human subjects-comment by Jackson. *Br. J. Nutr.* **2010**, *104*, 773. [CrossRef] [PubMed]
56. Galipeau, H.; McCarville, J.L.; Moeller, S.; Murray, J.; Alaedini, A.; Jabri, B.; Verdu, E. Gluten-induced responses in NOD/DQ8 mice are influenced by bacterial colonization. *Gastroenterology* **2014**, *146* (Suppl. 1). [CrossRef]
57. D'Arienzo, R.; Maurano, F.; Luongo, D.; Mazzarella, G.; Stefanile, R.; Troncone, R.; Auricchio, S.; Ricca, E.; David, C.; Rossi, M. Adjuvant effect of Lactobacillus casei in a mouse model of gluten sensitivity. *Immunol. Lett.* **2008**, *119*, 78–83. [CrossRef] [PubMed]
58. D'Arienzo, R.; Stefanile, R.; Maurano, F.; Mazzarella, G.; Ricca, E.; Troncone, R.; Auricchio, S.; Rossi, M. Immunomodulatory effects of Lactobacillus casei administration in a mouse model of gliadin-sensitive enteropathy. *Scand. J. Immunol.* **2011**, *74*, 335–341. [CrossRef] [PubMed]
59. Papista, C.; Gerakopoulos, V.; Kourelis, A.; Sounidaki, M.; Kontana, A.; Berthelot, L.; Moura, I.C.; Monteiro, R.C.; Yiangou, M. Gluten induces coeliac-like disease in sensitised mice involving IgA, CD71 and transglutaminase 2 interactions that are prevented by probiotics. *Lab. Investig.* **2012**, *92*, 625–635. [CrossRef] [PubMed]
60. Lindfors, K.; Blomqvist, T.; Juuti-Uusitalo, K.; Stenman, S.; Venäläinen, J.; Mäki, M.; Kaukinen, K. Live probiotic Bifidobacterium lactis bacteria inhibit the toxic effects induced by wheat gliadin in epithelial cell culture. *Clin. Exp. Immunol.* **2008**, *152*, 552–558. [CrossRef] [PubMed]
61. Laparra, J.M.; Olivares, M.; Gallina, O.; Sanz, Y. Bifidobacterium longum CECT 7347 modulates immune responses in a gliadin-induced enteropathy animal model. *PLoS ONE* **2012**, *7*, e30744. [CrossRef] [PubMed]
62. D'Arienzo, R.; Maurano, F.; Lavermicocca, P.; Ricca, E.; Rossi, M. Modulation of the immune response by probiotic strains in a mouse model of gluten sensitivity. *Cytokine* **2009**, *48*, 254–259. [CrossRef] [PubMed]

63. Smecuol, E.; Hwang, H.J.; Sugai, E.; Corso, L.; Cherñavsky, A.C.; Bellavite, F.P.; González, A.; Vodánovich, F.; Moreno, M.L.; Vázquez, H.; et al. Exploratory, randomized, double-blind, placebo-controlled study on the effects of Bifidobacterium infantis Natren life start strain super strain in active celiac disease. *J. Clin. Gastroenterol.* **2013**, *47*, 139–147. [CrossRef] [PubMed]
64. Pinto-Sánchez, M.I.; Smecuol, E.C.; Temprano, M.P.; Sugai, E.; González, A.; Moreno, M.L.; Huang, X.; Bercik, P.; Cabanne, A.; Vázquez, H.; et al. Bifidobacterium infantis NLS Super Strain Reduces the Expression of α-Defensin-5, a Marker of Innate Immunity, in the Mucosa of Active Celiac Disease Patients. *J. Clin. Gastroenterol.* **2017**, *51*, 814–817. [CrossRef] [PubMed]
65. Olivares, M.; Castillejo, G.; Varea, V.; Sanz, Y. Double-blind, randomised, placebo-controlled intervention trial to evaluate the effects of Bifidobacterium longum CECT 7347 in children with newly diagnosed coeliac disease. *Br. J. Nutr.* **2014**, *112*, 30–40. [CrossRef] [PubMed]
66. Harnett, J.; Myers, S.P.; Rolfe, M. Probiotics and the microbiome in celiac disease: A randomised controlled trial. *Evid. Based. Complement. Altern. Med.* **2016**, *2016*, 9048574. [CrossRef] [PubMed]
67. Klemenak, M.; Dolinšek, J.; Langerholc, T.; Di Gioia, D. Administration of Bifidobacterium breve Decreases the Production of TNF-α in Children with Celiac Disease. *Dig. Dis. Sci.* **2015**, *60*, 3386–3392. [CrossRef] [PubMed]
68. Primec, M.; Klemenak, M.; Di Gioia, D.; Aloisio, I.; Bozzi Cionci, N.; Quagliariello, A.; Gorenjak, M.; Mičetić-Turk, D.; Langerholc, T. Clinical intervention using Bifidobacterium strains in celiac disease children reveals novel microbial modulators of TNF-α and short-chain fatty acids. *Clin. Nutr.* **2018**. [CrossRef] [PubMed]
69. Francavilla, R.; Piccolo, M.; Francavilla, A.; Polimeno, L.; Semeraro, F.; Cristofori, F.; Castellaneta, S.; Barone, M.; Indrio, F.; Gobbetti, M.; et al. Clinical and Microbiological Effect of a Multispecies Probiotic Supplementation in Celiac Patients with Persistent IBS-type Symptoms: A Randomized, Double-Blind, Placebo-controlled, Multicenter Trial. *J. Clin. Gastroenterol.* **2018**. [CrossRef] [PubMed]
70. Losurdo, G.; Marra, A.; Shahini, E.; Girardi, B.; Giorgio, F.; Amoruso, A.; Pisani, A.; Piscitelli, D.; Barone, M.; Principi, M.; et al. Small intestinal bacterial overgrowth and celiac disease: A systematic review with pooled-data analysis. *Neurogastroenterol. Motil.* **2017**, *29*. [CrossRef] [PubMed]

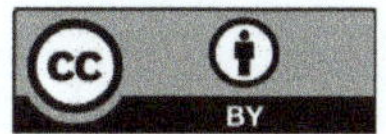

© 2018 by the authors. Licensee MDPI, Basel, Switzerland. This article is an open access article distributed under the terms and conditions of the Creative Commons Attribution (CC BY) license (http://creativecommons.org/licenses/by/4.0/).

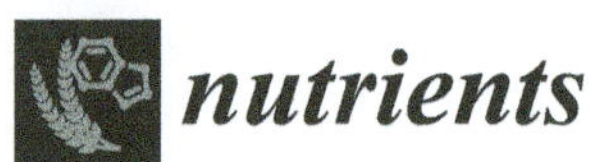

Review

Probiotics on Pediatric Functional Gastrointestinal Disorders

Anna Pärtty [1,2,*], Samuli Rautava [1,2] and Marko Kalliomäki [1,2]

1 Department of Pediatrics, University of Turku, 20521 Turku, Finland; samrau@utu.fi (S.R.); markal@utu.fi (M.K.)
2 Department of Pediatrics and Adolescent Medicine, Turku University Hospital, 20521 Turku, Finland
* Correspondence: aklein@utu.fi; Tel.: +358-407-237-781

Received: 26 October 2018; Accepted: 27 November 2018; Published: 29 November 2018

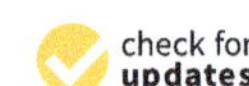

Abstract: The potential association between gut microbiota perturbations and childhood functional gastrointestinal disturbances opens interesting therapeutic and preventive possibilities with probiotics. The aim of this review was to evaluate current evidence on the efficacy of probiotics for the management of pediatric functional abdominal pain disorders, functional constipation and infantile colic. Thus far, no single strain, combination of strains or synbiotics can be recommended for the management of irritable bowel syndrome, functional abdominal pain or functional constipation in children. However, *Lactobacillus reuteri* DSM 17938 may be considered for the management of breastfed colic infants, while data on other probiotic strains, probiotic mixtures or synbiotics are limited in infantile colic.

Keywords: probiotics; functional gastrointestinal disorders; functional abdominal pain disorders; functional constipation; infantile colic

---

1. Introduction

The role of the intestinal microbiota in health and disease has been the focus of intensive research during the past decades. This interest has largely resulted from studies indicating differences in gut microbiota between healthy individuals and patients afflicted with non-communicable disease. Particularly, various chronic gastrointestinal disorders such as functional gastrointestinal disorders (FGID), colic crying, inflammatory bowel disease, and celiac disease have been associated with perturbations in gut microbiota composition. While these associations offer no proof of causality or direction, they serve as starting points for research aiming to establish whether gut microbiota disturbances might predispose one to or be involved in the causal complex leading to disease. The association between dysbiosis and functional gastrointestinal disorders in children and infants has raised great interest in modulating the gut microbiota composition and activity as a promising therapeutic and preventive option. The aim of this review was to evaluate current evidence on the efficacy of probiotic interventions for the management and prevention of functional gastrointestinal disorders, especially focusing on pediatric functional abdominal pain disorders, functional constipation and infantile colic.

2. Intestinal Microbial Colonization in Early Life

Neonatal gut colonization is a stepwise process which is affected by genetic and maternal influences and, perhaps more profoundly, by environmental and dietary exposures. Recent reports from clinical and experimental studies suggest that intestinal colonization may begin already during fetal life by microbes present in the intrauterine environment [1,2]. These findings, while extremely interesting, need further confirmation in large clinical studies with methodological rigor to exclude the possibility of contamination during sample acquisition and all steps during sample preparation, processing and analysis.

Human neonates receive an important inoculum of colonizing microbes during vaginal delivery. While maternal vaginal microbes, primarily lactobacilli, transiently colonize the neonatal gut [3], it is evident that the maternal gut is the most important source of early colonizing bacteria to the neonate [4]. The significance of vaginal delivery to healthy gut colonization is underscored by data suggesting aberrant gut colonization patterns in infants born by caesarean section delivery as compared to those born vaginally [5]. After birth, gut colonization progresses in a stepwise manner and bifidobacteria soon dominate the gut microbiota of breastfed infants [6,7]. This is thought to primarily result from breast milk components, including glycoproteins and particularly human milk oligosaccharides (HMOs), which selectively enhance the growth of bifidobacteria [8]. This notion is supported by the fact that *Bifidobacterium longum* subspecies *infantis*, a microbe capable of utilizing a variety of HMOs, is practically universally encountered in breastfed infant microbiota throughout the world [9–11]. Moreover, the gut microbiota of infants fed with cow's milk-based formula devoid of HMOs exhibits more diversity and a lower abundance of bifidobacteria [12]. While breastfeeding is associated with reduced risk of chronic non-communicable diseases including type II diabetes mellitus and obesity [13], the contribution of gut microbiota modulation to these health impacts is currently not known.

The infant and child gut microbiota gradually shifts to resemble that of adults and a stable, adult-like gut microbiota is thought to be established by the age of 2–3 years. The introduction of solid foods and particularly the cessation of breastfeeding are major driving forces of gut microbiota maturation [4]. It is noteworthy, however, that the mature gut microbiota exhibits considerable differences depending on geographical area [14]. The contribution of dietary practices most likely outweighs the effect of genetic differences in explaining this phenomenon. Throughout the maturation process, detrimental exposures and particularly antibiotic use may cause profound disturbances in gut microecology. The potential clinical significance of these temporary perturbations is illustrated by epidemiological studies suggesting an association between early-life antibiotic exposure and chronic disorders including overweight and obesity, asthma and inflammatory bowel disease [15].

3. Functional Gastrointestinal Disorders and Gut Microbiota

Since the early 1990s, the Rome foundation, a group of experts in functional gastrointestinal disorders (FGIDs), has collected the summary of knowledge among the FGIDs into the Rome criteria [16]. The most recent version, the Rome IV criteria, categorizes FGIDs among children and adolescents into three main classes based on the prime symptoms, i.e., functional nausea and vomiting disorders, functional abdominal pain disorders and functional defecation disorders. Functional nausea and vomiting disorders include cyclic vomiting syndrome, functional nausea and vomiting, rumination syndrome, and aerophagia. Functional abdominal pain disorders are classified into four groups: functional dyspepsia, irritable bowel syndrome (IBS), abdominal migraine, and functional abdominal pain (FAP)—not otherwise specified, whereas functional constipation and non-retentive fecal incontinence belong to the functional defecation syndromes [17].

According to the Rome IV criteria, infant colic is recurrent and presents with prolonged periods of crying, fussing or irritability in otherwise healthy infants under the age of 5 months. Colic crying resolves by the first five months of life and occurs without obvious cause and cannot be prevented or resolved [18]. However, the most widely accepted definition was penned by Wessel in 1954 as "paroxysms of irritability, fussing or crying lasting for a total of more than three hours a day and occurring on more than three days in any one week" in an otherwise healthy and thriving infant (19).

Since the Rome criteria are based on a systemic review of the literature and are widely adopted, we decided to concentrate here on only randomized clinical probiotic studies where the criteria have been used. However, in most of the colic studies, the "Wessel rule of three" has been used as the diagnostic criteria of infantile colic [19], and thus we included studies using those criteria as well. Moreover, the focus is on functional abdominal pain disorders, functional constipation and infantile colic since clinical trials in the field have been done almost exclusively with children with those disorders, as recently systemically reviewed [20,21]. In addition, in this review, we focused on the studies where these disorders were the primary outcome.

Given the association between early gut microbiota composition and chronic disease later in childhood, it is intriguing to hypothesize that disturbances in gut colonization might also play a role in the etiology and pathogenesis of childhood functional gastrointestinal disorders. The data regarding gut microbiota perturbations related to irritable bowel syndrome (IBS) and other functional gastrointestinal disorders in adults are not easy to interpret due to discrepant findings, despite attempts to adhere to generally accepted diagnostic criteria. The extrapolation of results obtained from an adult population to apply to children should always be done with caution. Only a few studies have systematically investigated gut microbiota composition or activity in children with functional gastrointestinal disorders.

In a case-control study of 22 school-aged children with IBS as defined by the Rome III criteria and 22 healthy controls, a fecal microbiota analysis by sequencing the 16S ribosomal RNA gene revealed that IBS was associated with a greater relative abundance of Proteobacteria, and particularly Gammaproteobacteria [22]. Rigsbee and colleagues [23] reported significant differences in gut microbiota composition between 22 school-aged children newly diagnosed with diarrhea-prominent IBS (IBS-D) fulfilling the Rome II criteria and 22 healthy children. Using several molecular methods (microarrays, 16S rRNA gene sequencing, quantitative PCR and fluorescent in situ-hybridization) they showed differing abundances of several bacterial genera between children with and without IBS-D. In contrast, no significant differences in fecal microbiota profiles or relative abundances of specific taxa were detected between 76 children aged between 4 and 17 years with functional constipation as defined by the Rome III criteria as compared to 61 healthy children of similar age [24]. Nonetheless, the children with functional constipation could be distinguished from the healthy matched controls by the ridge regression analysis of the fecal microbiota.

Whilst some studies suggest gut microbiota differences between pediatric patients with IBS and healthy children, it is not at all certain whether the gut microbiota plays a causal role in the pathogenesis of IBS. We are not aware of any reports with fecal samples obtained before the onset of IBS. However, a recent register-based study of more than 2 million individuals, of whom more than 14,000 had been diagnosed with IBS [25], suggests that caesarean section delivery is associated with a slightly increased risk of developing IBS (adjusted odds ratio (OR) 1.09, 95% confidence interval (CI) 1.03–1.16). This increase in risk, albeit small on an individual level, may at least in part be attributable to the aberrant gut colonization associated with caesarean section delivery. More circumstantial evidence for the connection between early gut microbiota perturbations and later functional gastrointestinal disorders may be drawn from a birth cohort study of more than 2700 children from Sweden [26], in which antibiotic use in the first or second year of life was associated with increased risk of recurrent abdominal pain in later childhood in girls. However, the association was not detected in boys.

The most comprehensive data on the association between gut microbiota alterations and functional gastrointestinal disorders are currently those regarding infantile colic. As early as 1994, Lehtonen and colleagues have reported based on culture methods that infants with colic were more often colonized by clostridia than healthy age-matched control infants, and that the difference was no longer detectable later at the age of three months [27]. Through the use of a modern microarray method in a case-control study of 12 infants with colic and 12 healthy age-matched controls with serial fecal samples, de Weerth and co-workers demonstrated that gut microbiota alterations are detectable already in the first weeks of life in infants who later develop colic [28]. Colic was specifically associated with the enrichment of Proteobacteria including *Escherichia*, *Klebsiella* and *Pseudomonas*, whereas the phyla Firmicutes and Actinobacteria were more prevalent in infants who did not develop colic. A decreased abundance of Actinobacteria and especially Bifidobacteria in the feces of infants with colic was recently confirmed by the 16S rRNA gene sequencing of fecal samples obtained from 37 infants with colic and 28 healthy controls [29]. Taken together, these data suggest not only that infantile colic is associated with altered gut microbiota composition but also that aberrant gut colonization precedes and may be causally related to the development of colic. This notion is corroborated by a recent report suggesting that maternal intrapartum antibiotic treatment, which is known to affect neonatal gut colonization, is more prevalent in infants who later develop colic [30].

4. Probiotics

The potential association between gut microbiota perturbations and functional gastrointestinal disturbances in children opens interesting therapeutic and preventive possibilities. The modification of the gut microbiota composition and activity by dietary interventions is currently an active area of research. Probiotics are one of the most commonly used treatment modalities.

Probiotics have been defined as live micro-organisms that, when administered in adequate amounts, confer a health benefit to the host [31]. It is important to note that, in order to be named a probiotic, the microbe in question must have evidence-based health effects. It is equally important to realize that probiotic effects are strain and species-specific. Clinical or mechanistic probiotic effects cannot be extrapolated to apply to other, even closely related microbes. This should also be borne in mind when devising or interpreting systematic reviews and meta-analyses of clinical probiotic studies.

The mechanisms of action of probiotics appear to be complex. It is often assumed that probiotics function by modulating the gut microbiota, but the evidence for this conjecture is sparse and the definition of probiotics cited above makes no reference to the gut microbiota. Specific probiotics have been shown to effective in reducing the risk and treatment of gastrointestinal disorders such as childhood infectious diarrhea [32,33], but it is not evident that these beneficial effects entail an impact on gut microecology. Moreover, there are clinical trials indicating that probiotic intervention on the pregnant and breastfeeding mother significantly reduces the occurrence of atopic dermatitis in high-risk infants with no effect on the infant gut microbiota composition [34,35]. Intriguingly, clinical and experimental studies have demonstrated that specific probiotics have direct effects on host physiological processes involving digestion and gut barrier function, immune responses, metabolism, nociception and behavior. It is therefore not surprising that probiotics have in some clinical trials shown clinical benefit in reducing the risk of diseases such as respiratory tract infections or otitis media [36], which have little to do with the gut microbiota. Based on all of this, it is paramount that determining the efficacy of probiotic interventions should be based on clinical criteria and not surrogate outcomes such as effects on gut microbiota.

4.1. Probiotics in the Management Pediatric Functional Abdominal Pain Disorders

Several clinical observations suggest that dysbiosis is a hallmark of IBS. First, symptoms in a substantial proportion of IBS patients are preceded by gastroenteritis or a round of antibiotics [37,38]. Moreover, rifaximin, the nonabsorbable antibiotic, has been shown to be effective in the treatment of adult patients with diarrhea-predominant irritable bowel syndrome (IBS-D) [39], although it was ineffective in children with chronic abdominal pain [40]. Indeed, gut microbiota alterations have found both in adults (reviewed in [41]) and children (reviewed above), thus offering a rationale for the therapeutic manipulation of gut microbiota in this group of patients.

Lactobacillus reuteri DSM 17938 has been the most widely studied probiotic in the field. Its effect has been investigated in 5 randomized clinical studies in children with FAP or IBS. In the first study, Romana et al. [42] compared the *Lactobacillus reuteri* with a placebo in 60 children. A significant reduction in pain intensity was found only in the probiotic group whereas a comparable significant reduction in pain frequency was shown in both groups. However, all these data were only graphically shown, without numeric presentation, limiting the interpretation of the findings [43]. Eftekhari et al. [43] did not find any significant differences between probiotic and placebo groups in severity of pain in 80 children with FAP despite a similar significant decrease within the groups as compared to the baseline. These studies both consisted of four weeks of intervention and follow-up.

Weizman et al. [44] evaluated the effect of *Lactobacillus reuteri* DSM 17938 with placebo in 101 children with FAP. At the end of the 4-week intervention, both the frequency and severity of pain were significantly lower in the probiotic group than in the placebo arm. After the 4-week follow-up, only the latter difference remained significant between the groups [44]. Jadresin et al. [45] studied *Lactobacillus reuteri* DSM 17938 in comparison to placebo in 55 children with FAP or IBS during a 16-week trial. Children in the probiotic group had more days without pain as compared to the placebo group during the study period. The intensity of pain was also less severe in the second and fourth month among the former group. However, absence from school or activities did not differ between the groups [45]. In the most recent study, Maragkoudaki et al. [46] compared *Lactobacillus reuteri* DSM 17938 to placebo in 54 children with FAP. Both the probiotic and placebo significantly reduced pain intensity and frequency from the baseline, but there was no significant difference between the groups. In addition, absence from school and use of analgesics were comparable between the groups [46].

The use of *Lactobacillus rhamnosus* GG in the management of pediatric FGIDs has been evaluated in three randomized clinical studies [17]. Bauserman et al. [47] found no difference in the change of abdominal pain severity between probiotic and placebo groups in 64 children with IBS. The number of responders was also similar between the groups. Abdominal distension was the only remaining symptom which was significantly less often present in the probiotic than the placebo group at the end of the 6-week study [47]. Gawronska et al. [48] investigated the effect of *Lactobacillus* GG versus placebo in 20 children with functional dyspepsia, 37 children with IBS and 47 children with FAP. Comparable amounts of patients (25% in probiotic and 9% in placebo group) reported no pain at the end of the 4-week study period. However, IBS patients receiving the probiotic were significantly more often without pain than patients on placebo (33% versus 5%) [48]. In the largest trial so far, Francavilla et al. [49] compared *Lactobacillus* GG versus placebo in 83 patients with IBS and 58 patients with FAP. They found that after a 4-week run-in and 8-week intervention, both pain intensity and frequency were significantly smaller in children with probiotic than those with placebo. These differences remained stable during the 8-week follow-up. Moreover, treatment was more often successful (i.e., at least 50% decrease both in pain intensity and frequency from the baseline) in the probiotic than the placebo group (72% vs. 53%) [49].

In addition to the above-mentioned studies, three trials have been conducted where other probiotic strains or combination of strains have been tested against placebo in children with functional abdominal disorders. Guandalini et al. [50] evaluated VSL#3 (a mixture of 8 strains) versus placebo in a crossover study of 67 children with IBS. Abdominal pain had decreased in both groups by the end of the 6-week intervention, but significantly more in the VSL#3 group. At week 6, the last week of the intervention, disruption of family life was assessed to be decreased more in the probiotic than placebo group [50]. Basturk et al. [51] investigated the effect of *Bifidobacterium lactis* B94 versus prebiotic inulin versus a synbiotic (inulin and *Bifidobacterium lactis* B94) in 71 children with IBS. The resolution of all symptoms during a 4-week trial was found in comparable amounts in the probiotic (39%) and synbiotic (29%) groups, but less often in those on inulin (12%). Giannetti et al. [52] studied a mixture of *Bifidobacterium infantis* M63, *Bifidobacterium breve* M16-V and *Bifidobacterium longum* BB36 in a crossover study of 50 children with IBS and 28 children with functional dyspepsia. They reported that abdominal pain disappeared significantly more often in the probiotic than placebo group in patients with IBS but not in those with functional dyspepsia. Again, quality of life improved significantly more often only in IBS patients on probiotics as compared to the same patients on placebo [52].

4.2. Probiotics in the Management of Pediatric Functional Constipation

Banaszkiewicz and Szajewska [53] investigated the effect of *Lactobacillus rhamnosus* GG versus placebo as an adjunct to lactulose in 84 children with constipation. Treatment success (at least 3 spontaneous bowel movements per week) was comparable between the groups both at the end of the 12-week intervention and 12 weeks later. Bu et al. [54] compared *Lactobacillus casei rhamnosus* Lcr35, magnesium oxide and placebo in 45 children with constipation in a 4-week trial. Lactulose and glycerin enema were allowed if stool passage was not noted for 3 and 5 days, respectively. The patients on probiotic and magnesium oxide had a higher defecation frequency, higher treatment success and fewer hard stools and less need for glycerin enema as compared to the placebo group [54].

Coccorullo et al. [55] studied the effect of an oil suspension with *Lactobacillus reuteri* DSM 17,938 or placebo in 44 infants with constipation in an 8-week intervention. Significantly more patients passed at least 5 stools a week in the probiotic than the placebo group at weeks 2, 4 and 8. Stool consistency did not differ between the groups [55]. Guerra et al. [56] evaluated a goat yogurt containing *Bifidobacterium longum* versus the yogurt alone in 59 children with constipation in a 10-week crossover intervention. When all the crossover data were analyzed, significant differences were observed between the groups in defecation frequency, defecation pain and abdominal pain. However, the authors did not state whether the difference was in favor of the probiotic goat yogurt or goat yogurt alone. In addition, all the results were presented graphically only [56]. Tabbers et al. [57] compared the effect of a fermented milk containing *Bifidobacterium lactis* DN-173 010 with a non-fermented milk-based dairy product in 159 constipated children. The rate of responders was similar in both groups. Moreover, stool frequency, pain during defecation, abdominal pain and bisacodyl use were comparable between the groups. However, flatulence was reported significantly less often during the 3-week study among those on the probiotic product [57].

Sadeghzadeh et al. [58] investigated the effect of lactulose plus a mixture of 7 probiotic strains versus lactulose plus placebo in 56 children with functional constipation during a 4-week intervention. Stool frequency and stool consistency improved in both groups, but significantly more so in those on lactulose plus probiotic. Russo et al. [59] studied polyethylene glycol 4000 plus a combination of three *Bifidobacteria* versus polyethylene glycol 4000 alone in 55 constipated children during an 8-week intervention. They reported that stool frequency and stool consistency improved in both groups as compared to baseline. However, no significant differences were detected between the groups [59]. Wojtyniak et al. [60] compared *Lactobacillus casei rhamnosus* LCR35 to a placebo in 94 children with constipation. Treatment success (at least 3 spontaneous stools per week without fecal soiling) was comparable between the groups although stool frequency was significantly lower in the probiotic group [60]. In the latest trial, the effect of *Lactobacillus reuteri* DSM 17938 and macrogol versus macrogol and matching placebo were studied in 129 constipated children for 8 weeks [61]. Stool frequency increased in almost all the patients and in comparable amount in both groups. Moreover, there were no significant differences between the groups in the number of patients with hard stools, painful defecation, large stools, fecal soling or abdominal pain [61].

In their comprehensive systemic reviews, Wegh et al. [20] and Wojtyniak and Szajewska [21] assessed the methodological quality and potential risks of bias of most of the studies reviewed above [42–60]. All in all, a relatively high risk of bias was found [20,21]. In addition, interventions and follow-up were short-term, the study populations were fairly small and heterogeneous as to their study design, probiotic strain and dose, duration of intervention and follow-up, and outcome measures. Therefore, no single strain or combination of strains can be recommended in the management of IBS, FAP or functional constipation in children. This is in accordance with a recent systematic review where potential dietary, pharmacological and psychological interventions of functional abdominal pain disorders in children were evaluated [62]. Probiotics were found to be effective if all the studies with different strains or combinations of them were pooled together: the odds ratio for improvement in pain was 1.61 (95% CI 1.15–2.27) for probiotics compared to placebo. When different strains were analyzed separately, the effect was not as clear, making a recommendation for clinical practice unjustified [62].

4.3. Probiotics in the Management of Infantile Colic

As altered gut microbiota, dysbiosis has been proposed to play a part in the pathophysiology of colic, probiotic bacteria have been suggested as a promising treatment for colic crying. Most intervention studies have examined the role of one specific probiotic, *Lactobacillus reuteri* DSM 17938. However, there are a handful of studies examining the role of other *Lactobacillus* spp. or mixture of different probiotics or synbiotics.

A recent systematic review and meta-analysis included altogether seven randomized controlled trials (471 participants) with a low risk of bias [63]. Five included randomized controlled trials (RCTs) involving 349 infants evaluated the effect of *L. reuteri* DSM 17938 at daily dose of 10^8 colony-forming unit (CFU) given for 21 or 28 days [64–68]. *L. reuteri* was associated with treatment success (relative risk (RR) 1.67, 95% CI 1.10–2.81, number needed to treat (NNT) 5, 95% CI 4–8) and reduced crying times at the end of intervention (mean difference (MD)-49 min, 95% CI−66–33), nevertheless the effect was mainly seen in exclusively breastfed infants.

In accordance, an individual participant data meta-analysis (IPDMA), pooling raw data from four individual trials involving 345 infants [64–67] to create sufficient power for sub-group analysis, suggests that *L. reuteri* DSM 17,938 is effective in treating breastfed infants with colic, but not formula-fed infants [69]. The probiotic group was almost twice as likely than the placebo group to experience treatment success and averaged less crying and/or fussing time than the placebo group. Moreover, the intervention effects were dramatic in breastfed infants (NNT 2.6, 95% CI 2.0–3.6), but were insignificant in formula-fed infants. All the infants included in the meta-analysis were exclusively or predominantly breastfed, except the infants participating in the largest Australian trial, which included both breast and formula-fed infants. The gut microbiota composition of breastfed and formula-fed infants is distinct, and this might therefore explain the better effectiveness of probiotic intervention in breastfed infants. On the other hand, the superior effectiveness of *L. reuteri* in breastfed infants might also be explained by the direct effects of microbes or oligosaccharides in breast milk.

After publishing these two meta-analyses, two more RCTs with *L. reuteri* DSM 17938 in treating infantile colic in breastfed infants have been published [70,71]. A study with 60 colic infants showed *L. reuteri* significantly decreasing daily crying time during a 30-day intervention period [70], while a small trial with only 20 colic infants found no significant difference in daily crying time between the probiotic and placebo group [71].

Only one small RCT has examined the role of *Lactobacillus rhamnosus* GG (LGG) in treating infant colic during a 28-day intervention [72]. A study with 30 breast and formula-fed colic infants found no difference in daily crying time between infants receiving probiotic or placebo. However, it is interesting to note that the study suggested LGG to be effective by parental report, but not by the validated prospectively recorded Baby Day Diary. This finding emphasizes the importance of using uniform validated methods in measuring infant crying.

A recent RCT with a mixture of 8 different probiotic bacterial strains in 53 exclusively breastfed colic infants showed that the probiotic-mixture group had less crying per day than the placebo group at the end of 3-week treatment period [73]. In addition, a higher rate of infants from the probiotic-mixture group responded to treatment at end of the study. Interestingly, the probiotic intervention did not modify the gut microbiota composition compared to placebo in this study. However, the observation from a metabolomics perspective showed that the fecal molecular profile differed in connection with the treatment. Dupont et al. investigated the effect of a probiotic-supplemented (*L. rhamnosus* and *B. infantis*) and alpha-enriched formula versus standard formula on daily crying in 66 colic infants during a 1-month intervention period [74]. The study found no differences for crying duration between the probiotic and placebo groups.

There are two RCT investigating the role of synbiotics—the combination of probiotics and prebiotics—in treating infant colic. A trial with 50 breastfed colic infants receiving a synbiotic (containing *L. casei, L. rhamnosus, S. thermophiles, B. breve, L. acidophilus, B. infants, L. bulgariucs* and fructo-oligosaccharides) or placebo for 30 days demonstrated that treatment success was significantly higher in the synbiotic group compared with placebo at day 7 and 30 [75]. Another trial with 60 colic infants investigated the effect of intervention formula (containing *B. lactis* BB12, galacto-oligosaccaharides combined with reduced lactose and partial whey hydrolysate) on daily crying amount compared to standard formula [76]. During the 1-month intervention period, daily crying duration decreased significantly more in infants receiving synbiotics than standard formula.

Taken together, the role of mixtures of probiotics and synbiotics in the treatment of colic crying is promising, but still indefinite, due to the variation in the used probiotic strains, and more data is therefore needed before any conclusions can be drawn.

Thus far, two studies have examined the role of pro- and prebiotics in preventing infant colic as the primary outcome. A large RCT with 589 term infants studied the effect of *L. reuteri* 17938 or placebo during the first 90 days of life in preventing the onset of colic, gastroesophageal reflux and constipation [77]. The study concluded that daily administration of *L. reuteri* significantly reduces daily crying duration at an age of 1 monthcompared to the placebo, and the effect was sustained at 3 months. In addition, the number of regurgitations per day was significantly lower and the number of evacuations per day higher in infants receiving *L. reuteri* compared to placebo. Another randomized controlled trial of 94 preterm infants (gestational age 32–36 weeks) investigated the effects of *L. rhamnosus* GG versus galacto-ologosaccharides versus placebo in preventing infant colic during the first 2 months of life [78]. A total of 27 out of 94 infants were classified as excessive criers at the age of 2 months, while this was significantly less in the probiotic and prebiotic group than in the placebo group (19% vs. 19% vs. 47%).

5. Conclusions

Infantile colic seems to be both associated with and preceded by altered gut microbiota composition, suggesting that dysbiosis may be causally related to the development of the condition. As regards older children's FGIDs, gut microbiota alterations have only been described in children with IBS, although their exact role in the pathogenesis remain unclear. So far, in addition to *Lactobacillus reuteri* DSM 17938 in the treatment of breastfed infant's colic, no other probiotic or combination of them for the management of pediatric FGIDs can be recommended (Table 1). Further clinical studies among children with these disorders should preferably focus both on relevant clinical outcomes and gut microbiota composition and function together in order to get a more comprehensive view of the role of the gut microbiota in these common maladies.

Table 1. Probiotics in children with functional gastrointestinal disorders. Summary of the RCT trials included in the review, quality of evidence and recommendation for clinical practice.

Disorder	Number of RCTs (No. of Children Altogether)					Quality of Evidence	Recommendation for Clinical Practice
	Probiotic Strain						
	L. reuteri *DSM17938*	*L. rhamnosus* GG	Other Single Strains	Mixtures of Probiotics	Synbiotics		
Treatment of functional abdominal pain disorders	5 RCT [42–46] (n = 350)	3 RCT [47–49] (n = 309)	1 RCT * [51] (n = 71)	2 RCT [50,52] (n = 145)	1 RCT * [51] (n = 71)	Low Not enough data High risk of bias in many of the studies [20,21]	No single strain or combination of strains can be recommended for the management of functional abdominal pain disorders [20,21]
Treatment of functional constipation	2 RCT [55,61] (n = 173)	1 RCT [53] (n = 84)	3 RCT [54,56,57,60] (n = 35)	2 RCT [58,59] (n = 111)		Low Not enough data High risk of bias in many of the studies [20,21]	No single strain or combination of strains can be recommended for the management of functional constipation [20,21]
Treatment of Infantile colic	7 RCT [64–68,70,71] (n = 429)	1 RCT [72] (n = 30)		2 RCT [73,74] (n = 119)	2 RCT [75,76] (n = 110)	Good Low risk of bias in most of the studies with *L. reuteri.* [63]	*L. reuteri* DSM 17938 at daily dose of 10^8 CFU may be considered for the management of breastfed colic infants. Data on other probiotics or formula-fed infants are limited [63,69]
Prevention of Infantile colic	1 RCT [77] (n = 589)	1 RCT [78] (n = 94)				Moderate Low risk of bias Data mostly from one study	No single strain can be recommended for the prevention of infantile colic, although there are promising data on *L. reuteri* DSM 17938 [77,78]

RCT=randomized controlled trial, *L. Lactobacillus*, * Same RCT.

Author Contributions: Each author (A.P., S.R. and M.K.) have made substantial contributions to the conception and design of the work, have drafted the work and substantively revised it; and has approved the submitted version and agrees to be personally accountable for the author's own contributions and for ensuring that questions related to the accuracy or integrity of any part of the work, even ones in which the author was not personally involved, are appropriately investigated, resolved, and documented in the literature.

Funding: This research received no external funding.

Conflicts of Interest: None of the authors have any conflict of interest.

References

1. Collado, M.C.; Rautava, S.; Aakko, J.; Isolauri, E.; Salminen, S. Human gut colonisation may be initiated in utero by distinct microbial communities in the placenta and amniotic fluid. *Sci. Rep.* **2016**, *6*, 23129. [CrossRef] [PubMed]
2. Martinez, K.A., 2nd; Romano-Keeler, J.; Zackular, J.P.; Moore, D.J.; Brucker, R.M.; Hooper, C.; Meng, S.; Brown, M.; Mallal, S.; Reese, J.; et al. Bacterial DNA is present in the fetal intestine and overlaps with that in the placenta in mice. *PLoS ONE* **2018**, *13*, e0197439. [CrossRef] [PubMed]
3. Matsumiya, Y.; Kato, N.; Watanabe, K.; Kato, H. Molecular epidemiological study of vertical transmission of vaginal Lactobacillus species from mothers to newborn infants in Japanese, by arbitrarily primed polymerase chain reaction. *J. Infect. Chemother.* **2002**, *8*, 43–49. [CrossRef] [PubMed]
4. Bäckhed, F.; Roswall, J.; Peng, Y.; Feng, Q.; Jia, H.; Kovatcheva-Datchary, P.; Li, Y.; Xia, Y.; Xie, H.; Zhong, H.; et al. Dynamics and stabilization of the human gut microbiome during the first year of life. *Cell. Host Microbe* **2015**, *17*, 690–703. [CrossRef] [PubMed]
5. Jakobsson, H.E.; Abrahamsson, T.R.; Jenmalm, M.C.; Harris, K.; Quince, C.; Jernberg, C.; Björkstén, B.; Engstrand, L.; Andersson, A.F. Decreased gut microbiota diversity, delayed Bacteroidetes colonisation and reduced Th1 responses in infants delivered by caesarean section. *Gut* **2014**, *63*, 559–566. [CrossRef] [PubMed]
6. Harmsen, H.J.; Wildeboer-Veloo, A.C.; Raangs, G.C.; Wagendorp, A.A.; Klijn, N.; Bindels, J.G.; Welling, G.W. Analysis of intestinal flora development in breast-fed and formula-fed infants by using molecular identification and detection methods. *J. Pediatr. Gastroenterol. Nutr.* **2000**, *30*, 61–67. [CrossRef] [PubMed]
7. Roger, L.C.; Costabile, A.; Holland, D.T.; Hoyles, L.; McCartney, A.L. Examination of faecal Bifidobacterium populations in breast- and formula-fed infants during the first 18 months of life. *Microbiology* **2010**, *156*, 3329–3341. [CrossRef] [PubMed]
8. Bode, L. Human milk oligosaccharides: Every baby needs a sugar mama. *Glycobiology* **2012**, *22*, 1147–1162. [CrossRef] [PubMed]
9. Underwood, M.A.; German, J.B.; Lebrilla, C.B.; Mills, D.A. Bifidobacterium longum subspecies infantis: Champion colonizer of the infant gut. *Pediatr. Res.* **2015**, *77*, 229–235. [CrossRef] [PubMed]
10. Grześkowiak, Ł.; Collado, M.C.; Mangani, C.; Maleta, K.; Laitinen, K.; Ashorn, P.; Isolauri, E.; Salminen, S. Distinct gut microbiota in southeastern African and northern European infants. *J. Pediatr. Gastroenterol. Nutr.* **2012**, *54*, 812–816. [CrossRef] [PubMed]
11. Grześkowiak, Ł.; Sales Teixeira, T.F.; Bigonha, S.M.; Lobo, G.; Salminen, S.; Ferreira, C.L. Gut Bifidobacterium microbiota in one-month-old Brazilian newborns. *Anaerobe* **2015**, *35*, 54–58. [CrossRef] [PubMed]
12. Azad, M.B.; Konya, T.; Persaud, R.R.; Guttman, D.S.; Chari, R.S.; Field, C.J.; Sears, M.R.; Mandhane, P.J.; Turvey, S.E.; Subbarao, P.; et al. Impact of maternal intrapartum antibiotics, method of birth and breastfeeding on gut microbiota during the first year of life: A prospective cohort study. *BJOG* **2016**, *123*, 983–993. [CrossRef] [PubMed]
13. Victora, C.G.; Bahl, R.; Barros, A.J.; França, G.V.; Horton, S.; Krasevec, J.; Murch, S.; Sankar, M.J.; Walker, N.; Rollins, N.C. Lancet Breastfeeding Series Group. Breastfeeding in the 21st century: Epidemiology, mechanisms, and lifelong effect. *Lancet* **2016**, *387*, 475–490. [CrossRef]
14. De Filippo, C.; Cavalieri, D.; Di Paola, M.; Ramazzotti, M.; Poullet, J.B.; Massart, S.; Collini, S.; Pieraccini, G.; Lionetti, P. Impact of diet in shaping gut microbiota revealed by a comparative study in children from Europe and rural Africa. *Proc. Natl. Acad. Sci. USA* **2010**, *107*, 14691–14696. [CrossRef] [PubMed]
15. Turta, O.; Rautava, S. Antibiotics, obesity and the link to microbes—What are we doing to our children? *BMC Med.* **2016**, *14*, 57. [CrossRef] [PubMed]

16. Drossman, D.A. Functional gastrointestinal disorders: History, pathophysiology, clinical features, and Rome IV. *Gastroenterology* **2016**, *150*, 1262–1279. [CrossRef] [PubMed]
17. Rasquin, A.; Di Lorenzo, C.; Forbes, D.; Guiraldes, E.; Hyams, J.S.; Staiano, A.; Walker, L.S. Childhood functional gastrointestinal disorders: Child/adolescent. *Gastroenterology* **2016**, *150*, 1456–1468. [CrossRef] [PubMed]
18. Benninga, M.A.; Faure, C.; Hyman, P.E.; St James Roberts, I.; Schechter, N.L.; Nurko, S. Childhood Functional Gastrointestinal Disorders: Neonate/Toddler. *Gastroenterology* **2016**, *150*, 443–1455. [CrossRef] [PubMed]
19. Wessel, M.A.; Cobb, J.C.; Jackson, E.B.; Harris, G.S.; Detwiler, A.C. Paroxysmal fussing in infancy, sometimes called colic. *Pediatrics* **1954**, *14*, 421–435.
20. Wegh, C.A.M.; Benninga, M.A.; Tabbers, M.M. Effectiveness of probiotics in children with functional abdominal pain disorders and functional constipation. A systematic review. *J. Clin. Gastroenterol.* **2018**. [Epub ahead of print]. [CrossRef] [PubMed]
21. Wojtyniak, K.; Szajewska, H. Systematic review: Probiotics for functional constipation. *Eur. J. Pediatr.* **2017**, *176*, 1155–1162. [CrossRef] [PubMed]
22. Saulnier, D.M.; Riehle, K.; Mistretta, T.A.; Diaz, M.A.; Mandal, D.; Raza, S.; Weidler, E.M.; Qin, X.; Coarfa, C.; Milosavljevic, A.; et al. Gastrointestinal microbiome signatures of pediatric patients with irritable bowel syndrome. *Gastroenterology* **2011**, *141*, 1782–1791. [CrossRef] [PubMed]
23. Rigsbee, L.; Agans, R.; Shankar, V.; Kenche, H.; Khamis, H.J.; Michail, S.; Paliy, O. Quantitative profiling of gut microbiota of children with diarrhea-predominant irritable bowel syndrome. *Am. J. Gastroenterol.* **2012**, *107*, 1740–1751. [CrossRef] [PubMed]
24. De Meij, T.G.; de Groot, E.F.; Eck, A.; Budding, A.E.; Kneepkens, C.M.; Benninga, M.A.; van Bodegraven, A.A.; Savelkoul, P.H. Characterization of Microbiota in Children with Chronic Functional Constipation. *PLoS ONE* **2016**, *11*, e0164731. [CrossRef] [PubMed]
25. Olén, O.; Stephansson, O.; Backman, A.S.; Törnblom, H.; Simrén, M.; Altman, M. Pre- and perinatal stress and irritable bowel syndrome in young adults—A nationwide register-based cohort study. *Neurogastroenterol. Motil.* **2018**, *30*, e13436. [CrossRef] [PubMed]
26. Uusijärvi, A.; Bergström, A.; Simrén, M.; Ludvigsson, J.F.; Kull, I.; Wickman, M.; Alm, J.; Olén, O. Use of antibiotics in infancy and childhood and risk of recurrent abdominal pain–a Swedish birth cohort study. *Neurogastroenterol. Motil.* **2014**, *26*, 841–850. [CrossRef] [PubMed]
27. Lehtonen, L.; Korvenranta, H.; Eerola, E. Intestinal microflora in colicky and noncolicky infants: Bacterial cultures and gas-liquid chromatography. *J. Pediatr. Gastroenterol. Nutr.* **1994**, *19*, 310–314. [CrossRef] [PubMed]
28. De Weerth, C.; Fuentes, S.; Puylaert, P.; de Vos, W.M. Intestinal microbiota of infants with colic: Development and specific signatures. *Pediatrics* **2013**, *131*, 550–558. [CrossRef] [PubMed]
29. Rhoads, J.M.; Collins, J.; Fatheree, N.Y.; Hashmi, S.S.; Taylor, C.M.; Luo, M.; Hoang, T.K.; Gleason, W.A.; Van Arsdall, M.R.; Navarro, F.; et al. Infant colic represents gut inflammation and dysbiosis. *J. Pediatr.* **2018**. [CrossRef] [PubMed]
30. Leppälehto, E.; Pärtty, A.; Kalliomäki, M.; Löyttyniemi, E.; Isolauri, E.; Rautava, S. Maternal Intrapartum Antibiotic Administration and Infantile Colic: Is there a Connection? *Neonatology* **2018**, *114*, 226–229. [CrossRef] [PubMed]
31. Hill, C.; Guarner, F.; Reid, G.; Gibson, G.R.; Merenstein, D.J.; Pot, B.; Morelli, L.; Canani, R.B.; Flint, H.J.; Salminen, S.; et al. Expert consensus document. The International Scientific Association for Probiotics and Prebiotics consensus statement on the scope and appropriate use of the term probiotic. *Nat. Rev. Gastroenterol. Hepatol.* **2014**, *11*, 506–514. [CrossRef] [PubMed]
32. Goldenberg, J.Z.; Lytvyn, L.; Steurich, J.; Parkin, P.; Mahant, S.; Johnston, B.C. Probiotics for the prevention of pediatric antibiotic-associated diarrhea. *Cochrane Database Syst. Rev.* **2015**, *12*, CD004827. [CrossRef] [PubMed]
33. Szajewska, H.; Skórka, A.; Ruszczyński, M.; Gieruszczak-Białek, D. Meta-analysis: Lactobacillus GG for treating acute gastroenteritis in children—Updated analysis of randomised controlled trials. *Aliment. Pharmacol. Ther.* **2013**, *38*, 467–476. [CrossRef] [PubMed]
34. Dotterud, C.K.; Storrø, O.; Johnsen, R.; Oien, T. Probiotics in pregnant women to prevent allergic disease: A randomized, double-blind trial. *Br. J. Dermatol.* **2010**, *163*, 616–623. [CrossRef] [PubMed]

35. Dotterud, C.K.; Avershina, E.; Sekelja, M.; Simpson, M.R.; Rudi, K.; Storrø, O.; Johnsen, R.; Øien, T. Does Maternal Perinatal Probiotic Supplementation Alter the Intestinal Microbiota of Mother and Child? *J. Pediatr. Gastroenterol. Nutr.* **2015**, *61*, 200–207. [CrossRef] [PubMed]
36. Rautava, S.; Salminen, S.; Isolauri, E. Specific probiotics in reducing the risk of acute infections in infancy—A randomised, double-blind, placebo-controlled study. *Br. J. Nutr.* **2009**, *101*, 1722–1726. [CrossRef] [PubMed]
37. Klem, F.; Wadhwa, A.; Prokop, L.J.; Sundt, W.J.; Farrugia, G.; Camilleri, M.; Singh, S.; Grover, M. Prevalence, risk factors, and outcome of irritable bowel syndrome after infectious enteritis: A systematic review and meta-analysis. *Gastroenterology* **2017**, *152*, 1042–1052. [CrossRef] [PubMed]
38. Maxwell, P.R.; Rink, E.; Kumar, D.; Mendall, M.A. Antibiotics increase functional abdominal symptoms. *Am. J. Gastroenterol.* **2002**, *97*, 104–108. [CrossRef] [PubMed]
39. Lembo, A.; Pimentel, M.; Rao, S.S.; Schoenfeld, P.; Cash Weinstock, L.B.; Paterson, C.; Bortey, E.; Forbes, W.P. Repeat treatment with rifaximin is safe and effective in patients with diarrhea-predominant irritable bowel syndrome. *Gastoenterology* **2016**, *151*, 1113–1121. [CrossRef] [PubMed]
40. Collins, B.S.; Lin, H.C. Double-blind, placebo-controlled antibiotic treatment study of small intestinal bacterial overgrowth in children with chronic abdominal pain. *J. Pediatr. Gastroenterol. Nutr.* **2011**, *52*, 382–386. [CrossRef] [PubMed]
41. Rajilic-Stojanovic, M.; Jonkers, D.M.; Salonen, A.; Inte Hanevik, K.; Raes, J.; Jalanka, J.; de Vos, W.M.; Manichanh, C.; Golic, N.; Enck, P.; et al. Intestinal microbiota and diet in IBS: Causes, consequences, or epiphenomena? *Am. J. Gastroenterol.* **2015**, *110*, 278–287. [CrossRef] [PubMed]
42. Romano, C.; Ferrau, V.; Cavataio, F.; Iacono, G.; Spina, M.; Lionetti, E.; Comisi, F.; Famiani, A.; Comito, D. *Lactobacillus reuteri* in children with functional abdominal pain (FAP). *J. Paediatr. Child Health* **2014**, *50*, 68–70. [CrossRef] [PubMed]
43. Eftekhari, K.; Vahedi, Z.; Kamali Aghdam, M.; Noemi Diaz, D. A randomized double-blind placebo-controlled trial of *Lactobacillus reuteri* for chronic functional abdominal pain in children. *Iran. J. Pediatr.* **2015**, *25*, e2616. [CrossRef] [PubMed]
44. Weizman, Z.; Abu-Abed, J.; Binsztok, M. *Lactobacillus reuteri* 17938 for the management of functional abdominal pain in childhood: A randomized, double-blind placebo-controlled trial. *J. Pediatr.* **2016**, *174*, 160–164. [CrossRef] [PubMed]
45. Jadresin, O.; Hojsak, I.; Misak, Z.; Kekez, A.J.; Trbojević, T.; Ivković, L.; Kolaček, S. *Lactobacillus reuteri* 17938 in the treatment of functional abdominal pain in children: RCT study. *J. Pediatr. Gastroenterol. Nutr.* **2017**, *64*, 925–929. [CrossRef] [PubMed]
46. Maragkoudaki, M.; Chouliaras, G.; Orel, R.; Horvath, A.; Szajewska, H.; Papadopoulou, A. *Lactobacillus reuteri* DSM 17938 and a placebo both significantly reduced symptoms in children with functional abdominal pain. *Acta Paediatr.* **2017**, *106*, 1857–1862. [CrossRef] [PubMed]
47. Bauserman, M.; Michail, S. The use of *Lactobacillus* GG in irritable bowel syndrome in children: A double-blind randomized control trial. *J. Pediatr.* **2005**, *147*, 197–201. [CrossRef] [PubMed]
48. Gawronska, A.; Dziechciarz, P.; Horvath, A.; Szajewska, H. Randomized double-blind placebo-controlled trial of *Lactobacillus* GG for abdominal pain disorders in children. *Aliment. Pharmacol. Ther.* **2007**, *25*, 177–184. [CrossRef] [PubMed]
49. Francavilla, R.; Miniello, V.; Magista, A.M.; De Canio, A.; Bucci, N.; Gagliardi, F.; Lionetti, E.; Castellaneta, S.; Polimeno, L.; Peccarisi, L.; et al. A randomized controlled trial of *Lactobacillus* GG in children with functional abdominal pain. *Pediatrics* **2010**, *126*, 1445–1452. [CrossRef] [PubMed]
50. Guandalini, S.; Magazzu, G.; Chiaro, A.; La Balestra, V.; Di Nardo, G.; Gopalan, S.; Sibal, A.; Romano, C.; Canani, R.B.; Lionetti, P.; et al. VSL#3 improves symptoms in children with irritable bowel syndrome: A multicenter, randomized, double-blind, placebo-controlled, crossover study. *J. Pediatr. Gastroenterol. Nutr.* **2010**, *51*, 24–30. [CrossRef] [PubMed]
51. Basturk, A.; Artan, R.; Yilmaz, A. Efficacy of synbiotic, probiotic, and prebiotic treatments for irritable bowel syndrome in children: A randomized controlled trial. *Turk. J. Gastroenterol.* **2016**, *27*, 439–443. [CrossRef] [PubMed]
52. Giannetti, E.; Maglione, M.; Alessandrella, A.; Strisciuglio, C.; De Giovanni, D.; Campanozzi, A.; Miele, E.; Staiano, A. A mixture of 3 Bifidobacteria decreases abdominal pain and improves the quality of life in

children irritable bowel syndrome: Multi-center, randomized, double-blind, placebo-controlled, crossover trial. *J. Clin. Gastroenterol.* **2017**, *51*, 10–15. [CrossRef] [PubMed]

53. Banaszkiewicz, A.; Szajewska, H. Ineffectiveness of Lactobacillus GG as an adjunct to lactulose for the treatment of constiopation in children: A double-blind placebo-controlled randomized trial. *J. Pediatr.* **2005**, *146*, 364–396. [CrossRef] [PubMed]
54. Bu, L.N.; Chang, M.H.; Ni, Y.H.; Chen, H.L.; Cheng, C.C. Lactobacillus casei rhamnosus Lcr 35 in children with chronic constipation. *Pediatr. Int.* **2007**, *49*, 485–490. [CrossRef] [PubMed]
55. Coccorullo, P.; Strisciuglio, C.; Martinelli, M.; Miele, E.; Greco, L.; Staiano, A. *Lactobacillus reuteri* (17938) in infants with functional chronic constipation: A double-blind, randomized, placebo-controlled study. *J. Pediatr.* **2010**, *157*, 598–602. [CrossRef] [PubMed]
56. Guerra, P.V.P.; Lima, L.N.; Souza, T.C.; Mazochi, V.; Penna, F.J.; Silva, A.M.; Nicoli, J.R.; Guimarães, E.V. Periatric functional constipation treatment with *Bifidobacterium*-containing yogurt: A crossover, double-blind, controlled trial. *World J. Gastroenterol.* **2011**, *17*, 3916–3921. [CrossRef] [PubMed]
57. Tabbers, M.M.; Chmielewska, A.; Roseboom, M.G.; Crastes, N.; Perrin, C.; Reitsma, J.B.; Norbruis, O.; Szajewska, H.; Benninga, M.A. Fermented milk containing Bifidobacterium lactis DN-173 010 in childhood constipation: A randomized, double-blind, controlled trial. *Pediatrics* **2011**, *127*, 1392–1399. [CrossRef] [PubMed]
58. Sadeghzadeh, M.; Rabieefar, A.; Khoshnevisasl, P.; Mousavinasab, N.; Eftekhari, K. The effect of probiotics on childhood constipation: A randomized controlled double blind clinical trial. *Int. J. Pediatr.* **2014**, *2014*, 937212. [CrossRef] [PubMed]
59. Russo, M.; Giugliano, F.P.; Quitadamo, P.; Mancusi, V.; Miele, E.; Staiano, A. Efficacy of a mixture of probiotic agents as complimentary therapy for chronic functional constipation in childhood. *Ital. J. Pediatr.* **2017**, *43*, 24. [CrossRef] [PubMed]
60. Wojtyniak, K.; Horvath, A.; Dziechciarz, P.; Szajewska, H. *Lactobacillus casei rhamnosus* Lcr35 in the management of functional constipation in children: A randomized trial. *J. Pediatr.* **2017**, *184*, 101–105. [CrossRef] [PubMed]
61. Wegner, A.; Banaszkiewicz, A.; Kierkus, J.; Landowski, P.; Korlatowicz-Bilar, A.; Wiecek, S.; Kwiecien, J.; Gawronska, A.; Dembinski, L.; Czaja-Bulsa, G.; et al. The effectiveness of Lactobacillus reuteri DSM 17938 as an adjunct to macrogol in the treatment of functional constipation in children. A randomized, double-blind, placebo-controlled, multicentre trial. *Clin. Res. Hepatol. Gastroenterol.* **2018**, *42*, 494–500. [CrossRef] [PubMed]
62. Abbott, R.A.; Martin, A.E.; Tamsin, V.; Bethel, A.; Whear, R.S.; Thompson Coon, J.; Logan, S. Recurrent abdominal pain in children: Summary evidence from 3 systematic reviews of treatment effectiveness. *J. Pediatr. Gastroenterol. Nutr.* **2018**, *67*, 23–33. [CrossRef] [PubMed]
63. Dryl, R.; Szajewska, H. Probiotics for management of infantile colic: A systematic review of randomized controlled trials. *Arch. Med. Sci.* **2018**, *14*, 1137–1143. [CrossRef] [PubMed]
64. Savino, F.; Cordisco, L.; Tarasco, V.; Palumeri, E.; Calabrese, R.; Oggero, R.; Roos, S.; Matteuzzi, D. Lactobacillus reuteri DSM 17938 in infantile colic: A randomized, double-blind, placebo-controlled trial. *Pediatrics* **2010**, *126*, 526–533. [CrossRef] [PubMed]
65. Szajewska, H.; Gyrczuk, E.; Horvath, A. Lactobacillus reuteri DSM 17938 for the management of infantile colic in breastfed infants: A randomized, double-blind, placebo-controlled trial. *J. Pediatr.* **2013**, *162*, 257–262. [CrossRef] [PubMed]
66. Sung, V.; Hiscock, H.; Tang, M.L.; Mensah, F.K.; Nation, M.L.; Satzke, C.; Heine, R.G.; Stock, A.; Barr, R.G.; Wake, M. Treating infant colic with the probiotic Lactobacillus reuteri: Double blind, placebo controlled randomised trial. *BMJ* **2014**, *348*, g2107. [CrossRef] [PubMed]
67. Chau, K.; Lau, E.; Greenberg, S.; Jacobson, S.; Yazdani-Brojeni, P.; Verma, N.; Koren, G. Probiotics for infantile colic: A randomized, double-blind, placebo-controlled trial investigating Lactobacillus reuteri DSM 17938. *J. Pediatr.* **2015**, *166*, 74–78. [CrossRef] [PubMed]
68. Mi, G.L.; Zhao, L.; Qiao, D.D.; Kang, W.Q.; Tang, M.Q.; Xu, J.K. Effectiveness of Lactobacillus reuteri in infantile colic and colicky induced maternal depression: A prospective single blind randomized trial. *Antonie Van Leeuwenhoek* **2015**, *107*, 1547–1553. [CrossRef] [PubMed]
69. Sung, V.; D'Amico, F.; Cabana, M.D.; Chau, K.; Koren, G.; Savino, F.; Szajewska, H.; Deshpande, G.; Dupont, C.; Indrio, F.; et al. *Lactobacillus reuteri* to Treat Infant Colic: A Meta-analysis. *Pediatrics* **2018**, 141. [CrossRef]

70. Savino, F.; Garro, M.; Montanari, P.; Galliano, I.; Bergallo, M. Crying Time and RORγ/FOXP3 Expression in Lactobacillus reuteri DSM17938-Treated Infants with Colic: A Randomized Trial. *J. Pediatr.* **2018**, *192*, 171–177. [CrossRef] [PubMed]
71. Fatheree, N.Y.; Liu, Y.; Taylor, C.M.; Hoang, T.K.; Cai, C.; Rahbar, M.H.; Hessabi, M.; Ferris, M.; McMurtry, V.; Wong, C.; et al. Lactobacillus reuteri for Infants with Colic: A Double-Blind, Placebo-Controlled, Randomized Clinical Trial. *J. Pediatr.* **2017**, *191*, 170–178. [CrossRef] [PubMed]
72. Pärtty, A.; Lehtonen, L.; Kalliomäki, M.; Salminen, S.; Isolauri, E. Probiotic Lactobacillus rhamnosus GG therapy and microbiological programming in infantile colic: A randomized, controlled trial. *Pediatr. Res.* **2015**, *78*, 470–475. [CrossRef] [PubMed]
73. Baldassarre, M.E.; Di Mauro, A.; Tafuri, S.; Rizzo, V.; Gallone, M.S.; Mastromarino, P.; Capobianco, D.; Laghi, L.; Zhu, C.; Capozza, M.; et al. Effectiveness and Safety of a Probiotic-Mixture for the Treatment of Infantile Colic: A Double-Blind, Randomized, Placebo-Controlled Clinical Trial with Fecal Real-Time PCR and NMR-Based Metabolomics Analysis. *Nutrients* **2018**, 195. [CrossRef] [PubMed]
74. Dupont, C.; Rivero, M.; Grillon, C.; Belaroussi, N.; Kalindjian, A.; Marin, V. Alpha-lactalbumin-enriched and probiotic-supplemented infant formula in infants with colic: Growth and gastrointestinal tolerance. *Eur. J. Clin. Nutr.* **2010**, *64*, 765–767. [CrossRef] [PubMed]
75. Kianifar, H.; Ahanchian, H.; Grover, Z.; Jafari, S.; Noorbakhsh, Z.; Khakshour, A.; Sedaghat, M.; Kiani, M. Synbiotic in the management of infantile colic: A randomised controlled trial. *J. Paediatr. Child Health* **2014**, *50*, 801–805. [CrossRef] [PubMed]
76. Xinias, I.; Analitis, A.; Mavroudi, A.; Roilides, I.; Lykogeorgou, M.; Delivoria, V.; Milingos, V.; Mylonopoulou, M.; Vandenplas, Y. Innovative Dietary Intervention Answers to Baby Colic. *Pediatr. Gastroenterol. Hepatol. Nutr.* **2017**, *20*, 100–106. [CrossRef] [PubMed]
77. Indrio, F.; Di Mauro, A.; Riezzo, G.; Civardi, E.; Intini, C.; Corvaglia, L.; Ballardini, E.; Bisceglia, M.; Cinquetti, M.; Brazzoduro, E.; et al. Prophylactic use of a probiotic in the prevention of colic, regurgitation, and functional constipation: A randomized clinical trial. *JAMA Pediatr.* **2014**, *168*, 228–233. [CrossRef] [PubMed]
78. Pärtty, A.; Luoto, R.; Kalliomäki, M.; Salminen, S.; Isolauri, E. Effects of early prebiotic and probiotic supplementation on development of gut microbiota and fussing and crying in preterm infants: A randomized, double-blind, placebo-controlled trial. *J. Pediatr.* **2013**, *163*, 1272–1277. [CrossRef] [PubMed]

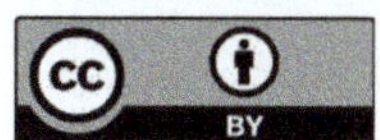

© 2018 by the authors. Licensee MDPI, Basel, Switzerland. This article is an open access article distributed under the terms and conditions of the Creative Commons Attribution (CC BY) license (http://creativecommons.org/licenses/by/4.0/).

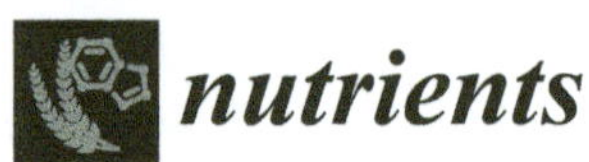

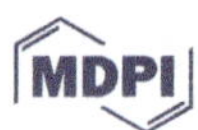

Article

Role of *Lactobacillus rhamnosus* (FloraActive™) 19070-2 and *Lactobacillus reuteri* (FloraActive™) 12246 in Infant Colic: A Randomized Dietary Study

Sergei Gerasimov [1,*], Jesper Gantzel [2], Nataliia Dementieva [3], Olha Schevchenko [3], Orisia Tsitsura [4], Nadiia Guta [5], Viktor Bobyk [5] and Vira Kaprus [6]

1 Department of Pediatrics #2, Lviv National Medical University, 69 Pekarska str., 79010 Lviv, Ukraine
2 BioCare Copenhagen A/S, Ole Maaløes Vej 3, 2200 Copenhagen, Denmark; jg@biocarecph.com
3 Dnipro State Children Hospital, 13 Kosmichna str., 49100 Dnipro, Ukraine; dementievana@ukr.net (N.D.); oshevchenko2202@ukr.net (O.S.)
4 Ivano-Frankivsk State Children Hospital, 132 Yevhena Konovaltsya str., 76014 Ivano-Frankivsk, Ukraine; vmatsalac@gmail.com
5 Lviv City Children Hospital, 4 Pylypa Orlyka str., 79059 Lviv, Ukraine; nadiia.guta@gmail.com (N.G.); vbobyk@yahoo.com (V.B.)
6 Lviv Community 4 Clinical Hospital, 3 Yaroslava Stetska str., 79007 Lviv, Ukraine; kaprus4mkl@gmail.com
* Correspondence: dr.gerasimov@gmail.com; Tel.: +38-067-937-5951

Received: 30 October 2018; Accepted: 10 December 2018; Published: 13 December 2018

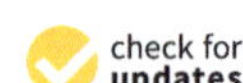

Abstract: Infant colic is a common condition of unknown pathogenesis that brings frustration to families seeking for effective management. Accumulating evidence suggests that some single strains of lactobacilli may play a positive dietary role in attenuation of colic in exclusively breastfed infants. The objective of this study was to evaluate a mixture of two *Lactobacillus* strains in decreasing infant cry and fuss in this population. Infants aged 4–12 weeks received *L. rhamnosus* 19070-2 and *L. reuteri* 12246 in a daily dose of 250 $\times$ 10^6 CFU, 3.33 mg of fructooligosaccharide, and 200 IU of vitamin D_3 (84 infants, probiotic group) or just vitamin D_3 (84 infants, control group) for 28 days. Cry and fuss time were measured with validated Baby's Day Diary on days 0 and 28. At baseline, mean (SD) duration of cry and fuss time was comparable in the probiotic and control groups: 305 (81) vs. 315 (90) min., respectively ($p = 0.450$). On day 28, mean cry and fuss time became statistically different: 142 (89) vs. 199 (72), respectively ($p < 0.05$). Mean change in cry and fuss time from day 0 through day 28 was −163 (99) minutes in the probiotic and −116 (94) minutes in the control group ($p = 0.019$). Our findings confirm that lactobacilli decrease cry and fuss time and provide a dietary support in exclusively breastfed infants with colic.

Keywords: infant; colic; lactobacilli

1. Introduction

Infant colic (IC) represents a temporary self-limited condition, which occurs in about one of five infants within the first months of life, and is characterized by inconsolable cry and fuss of unknown cause [1]. Wessel et al., who coined and brought the term into a wide medical use, defined IC as a stable symptomatic pattern with timing as a rule of three threes in an infant "who is otherwise healthy and well-fed, has paroxysms of irritability, fussy or cry, lasting for a total of three hours a day, occurring on more than three days in any one week for a period of three weeks" [2]. Despite its benign nature, IC serves a significant source for maternal anxiety, and depression [3], impaired family functioning [4], and the most common reason for seeking medical advice in this age group [1]. Infant colic had been linked to poor sleep and disorders in mental health in school age [5]. Due to universal prevalence, economic burden associated with IC is great for the healthcare system. In the UK, annual estimates for financial losses due to IC has been 65 million pounds [6]. At the same time, there is no consensus on the treatment of IC. Most of the current interventions have been found ineffective, unequivocal, or unsafe [7].

There is accumulating evidence that lactobacilli may play a role in IC. Earlier findings showed that infants with IC had more gas-forming *Clostridium difficile*, *Klebsiella pneumoniae*, and *Escherichia coli* in their intestines and lesser microbial diversity than their non-colic counterparts [8–10]. Probiotic bacteria can also theoretically influence sulfate reducing bacteria, methanogens and/or acetogens playing an important role in the functioning of the gut [11]. It was hypothesized that inoculation of antagonizing probiotic species into the gut of such infants could potentially decrease gas production, thereby alleviating abdominal distress. However, probiotic supplementation studies are not fully consistent, and their results ranged from significant and meaningful effects through the absence of efficacy [12–17]. Meta-analysis of personal data from randomized clinical trials showed that exclusively breastfed infants significantly benefited from probiotic supplementation, while this effect in the formula-fed infant was not evident [18].

The objective of our study was to explore the effect of *Lactobacillus rhamnosus* 19070-2 and *Lactobacillus reuteri* 12246 on the course of colic in the hypothetically susceptible population of exclusively breastfed infants.

The rationale for selecting a combination of *L. rhamnosus* 19070-2 and *L. reuteri* 12246 was based on its safety and clinical efficacy in a series of pediatric studies. Two randomized clinical studies concluded that the combination of the mentioned strains significantly reduced the duration of acute diarrhea [19,20], and results of two other studies reported a reduction in atopic dermatitis relapse rate together with a decrease of associated intestinal permeability, and reduction of gastrointestinal symptoms [21,22]. These studies, which involved 196 children aged six months to thirteen years, suggested that use of *L. rhamnosus* 19070-2 and *L. reuteri* 12246 for five days to six weeks was safe and effective.

2. Materials and Methods

This was a phase II randomized parallel group prospective controlled multi-center dietary study. The case of IC was defined as cry and/or fuss lasting > 3 h a day, occurring > 3 days for the last seven days [23]. Other inclusion criteria were as follows: Informed consent form signed by parents, gender males and females, age on enrollment 4–12 weeks; gestational age 37–42 weeks; birth weight 2500–4200 g, stated availability throughout the study period, stated availability of mobile phone or phone with answering machine. Excluded from the study were infants who received any amount of formula feeding, those who failed to thrive (weight gain less than 100 g per week as averaged from the birth weight to the weight at entry) and those with present intake of antibiotics, prebiotics or probiotics by infant or mother. Also excluded were mothers with current maternal smoking, known moderate or severe disease of any systems (neural, skeletal, muscular, cutaneous, gastrointestinal, respiratory, genital, urinary, immune), difficulty of parents to comprehend study requirements as judged by physician, suspected parental alcohol or drug addiction as judged by physician. There were no changes made to eligibility criteria or other methods after the study commencement.

The study was performed at six (6) clinical centers, where data was collected: Three centers—tertiary care state or city children hospitals (Dnipro State Children Hospital, Dnipro; Ivano-Frankivsk State Children Hospital, Ivano-Frankivsk; Lviv City Children Hospital; Lviv), two centers—out-patient community clinic or out-patient department at hospital (Chernihiv Pediatric Outpatient Clinic #1, Chernihiv; Pediatric Outpatient Clinic at Lviv Community 4 Clinical Hospital, Lviv); one center—University Medical Center (Lviv National Medical University, Lviv). All centers were in Ukraine. Methods of advertisement included social media, verbal information and brochure given during hospital, outpatient visits and regular newborn visits. During newborn visit families were also supplied with a leaflet with study announcement and normal immunization schedule.

Infants in the probiotic group were administered *L. rhamnosus* 19070-2 and *L. reuteri* 12246 in a dose of 125 × 10^6 CFU (both strains), 2.5 mcg (100 IU) of vitamin D_3, and 1.667 mg of fructooligosaccharides (FOS) in sunflower oil drops (0.25 mL). Subjects in the control group received 2.5 mcg (100 IU) of vitamin D_3 per dose. Both probiotic and control groups were given a dose of the test dietary supplement (TDS) two times daily: One dose (0.25 mL) during the first morning (from 06:00) breastfeeding, and one dose (0.25 mL) during one of the evening (18:00−24:00) breast feedings. As a result, the probiotic group received a daily dose of 250 × 10^6 CFU of lactobacilli (125 × 10^6 CFU each strain) with 5 mcg (200 IU) of vitamin D_3, and 3.33 mg of FOS, while the control group received only 5 mcg (200 IU) of vitamin D_3. The TDS was dripped behind the gums just before feeding. Compliance was assessed with phone calls (days 12, 26) and 28-Day Study Diary (28-DSD), where caregivers checked morning and evening TDS intakes. The 28-DSD was also designed to screen for mothers' diet (cow's milk, eggs, chocolate, nuts), exclusive breast-feeding status, and adverse events that might be linked to infant TDS intolerance (regurgitation, vomiting, constipation, diarrhea, skin rash). To evaluate background conditions that might interfere with the assessment of intolerance events, parents were questioned whether infant ever experienced the above disorders.

The primary outcome measure was changed in mean cry/fuss time (min/day) from day 0 through day 28. Cry was not specifically defined, while fuss was defined as "behavior that is not quite cry but not awake and content either" [24]. The secondary outcomes included: Time to treatment success, a day when more than or equal to 25% and 50% reduction in cry/fuss time from difference between baseline value and 180 min, a cutoff for definition of IC; recovery success (percent) at 7, 14, 21, 28 days, defined as reduction in duration of cry/fuss time less than 3 h per day (unmet Wessel criteria). For calculation of time to treatment success, data obtained on the days 6–7, 13–14, 20–21, and 27–28, was averaged and means were ascribed to days 7, 14, 21, and 28, respectively. Based on mean values, for every infant we found a day on which cry/fuss time decreased more than 25% or 50% as compared with baseline—180 min value. These days were averaged and mean weekly time to 25% or 50% improvement was calculated for active and control groups. Tertiary outcome measures included: Infant sleep duration (min/day) on days 0, 7, 14, 21, 28; change in maternal depression score from day 0 through 28. There were no changes made to outcomes after the trial commencement.

Cry, fuss, and sleep time were assessed with Baby's Day Diary (BDD), a validated tool for the observation of infant activity [24]. Briefly, the BDD had four, six-hour time-rulers printed on a single page, used to capture babies' behaviors on a 24-h basis. Instructions were given verbally by investigators and pre-printed on each BDD. Parents ticked the start and end time of successive periods of behavior on the time rulers, painted these periods with relevant schematic patterns against a scale showing five-minute increments of time. The BDD was completed nine times: On day 0 (before inclusion), and then on pairs of consecutive days 6–7, 13–14, 20–21, 27–28 after the commencement of TDS intake. To improve compliance with BDD recording, parents received two phone call reminders (days 12, 26), and two text messages (SMS) (days 5, 19). During phone calls parents were also asked about their impression of colic ("better", "worse", "no changes"). Maternal depression score was estimated with the Edinburgh Postnatal Depression Scale (EPDS) [25]. The scale was linguistically validated. [26]. Formal permissions to use these assessment tools were obtained from copyright holders.

To detect a difference in change of cry/fuss time of 40 min between the probiotic and control groups on day 28, with power of 80% and confidence of 0.05, 140 infants should be enrolled. At a dropout rate of 20%, the final sample size was 140 × 1.2 = 168. The rationale for the number of infants stemmed from the five published reports on the efficacy of probiotics in IC. It has been estimated weighted mean difference in change of cry and fuss time (40 min) between probiotic and control arms, and population variance (7456) [12–15,27]. There were no interim analyses and stopping guidelines in this study.

Random numbers were generated by the Random Allocation Software v. 1.0.0 [28]. Randomization was restricted to a 4-block system to secure an equal number of infants in the probiotic and control groups. Random allocation was implemented by sticking the labels with sequential random numbers and sequential selection of packs by the investigator. Random numbers were generated by the technician who did not participate in the distribution of packs among centers or data analysis. Investigators and families were blinded to which supplement was given. The supplements looked the same on appearance, smell and consistency and differed only by the randomization numbers on packs.

Absolute number and percent were used to describe baseline characteristics of boys/girls, proportion of caesarean delivery, family history of atopy, proton pump inhibitor use. Mean and standard deviation described age at study entry (weeks), birth weight (g), gestation (weeks), duration (days) of IC before randomization, total daily cry/fuss time (min/day), fuss time (min/day), cry time (min/day), infant sleep duration (min/day), maternal mental health (EPDS score). Difference between the groups in percent data was assessed in z-test, and between means—in a two-tailed *t*-test. Distribution of data was checked with Kolmogorov-Smirnov test. Recovery from IC was plotted using the Kaplan-Meier method, and the difference in recovery rates was assessed with Cox's F-test. If not otherwise specified, data in the text is present as mean (SD), and the difference between means is assessed in a two-tailed *t*-test. Tests were performed with Statistica 9 (StatSoft., Inc., Tulsa, OK, US).

The study received positive decisions of Ethical committees at clinical centers (Dnipro State Children Hospital, protocol #6.4 of 29 June 2016; Ivano-Frankivsk State Children Hospital protocol #12 of 6 May 2016; Lviv City Children Hospital protocol #3 of 22 June 2016; Chernihiv Pediatric Outpatient Clinic #1 protocol #11 of 8 September 2016; Pediatric Outpatient Clinic at Lviv Community 4 Clinical Hospital protocol #8 of 21 March 2017; Lviv National Medical University protocol #3 of 14 March 2016). Before enrollment, parents signed an informed consent form. The study protocol was registered by the protocol registration system at Clinicaltrial.gov NCT02839239.

3. Results

Screening and enrollment of infants occurred continuously from October 2016 to February 2018. Of 323 initially screened infants, 22 met exclusion criteria (formula feeding, present intake of probiotics, current maternal smoking, failure to thrive), and 129 declined to participate because of the investigational nature of the trial (Figure 1). During continuous evaluation of data, nine infants who finished the trial, were excluded from the analysis due to carelessly drawn BDDs, or failure to return BDD. One hundred seventy-two infants were randomized and evenly allocated into probiotic or control supplementation groups (86 infants/group). During the study, four infants were lost to follow-up with no further wish to participate. Four infants started formula feeding, three infants had carelessly recorded or absent BDD, one infant in the probiotic group started prebiotics, and one infant in the control group had poor compliance with intake of TDS These infants were excluded from the analysis and replaced with newly enrolled infants to secure pre-determined sample size. Finally, data from 168 infants were evaluable for study purposes.

3.1. Baseline Description of Study Participants

Probiotic and control groups were comparable on major demographic and medical data (Table 1).

A small percent of mothers and infants used probiotics and antibiotics in the past. No statistical difference was found between the groups, except for the duration of mother use of antibiotics and duration of infant use of probiotics, which were both longer in the control group. All probiotic and antibiotic treatments were stopped seven days before enrolment of the infant in the study. The most common past medical condition was hypoxic ischemic encephalopathy. In all cases, the diagnosis was made 1–3 days after delivery. The disease had mild severity and resolved by the time of enrollment. Functional jaundice was observed in approximately 5% (probiotic group) to 10% (control group) of newborns with no significant difference between the groups. Cephalo-hematoma was observed in one newborn in the probiotic and two newborns in the control group. At the time of inclusion, no finding of neurological consequences for the condition was found. Hemolytic disease, arthrogryposis, and lymphadenopathy were all documented in the probiotic group. Diaper dermatitis was observed in two infants in the probiotic group and one infant in the control group. None of the past medical conditions were moderate or severe, or was clinically active at time of enrollment, except for arthrogryposis that represents life-long congenital pathology of extremities.

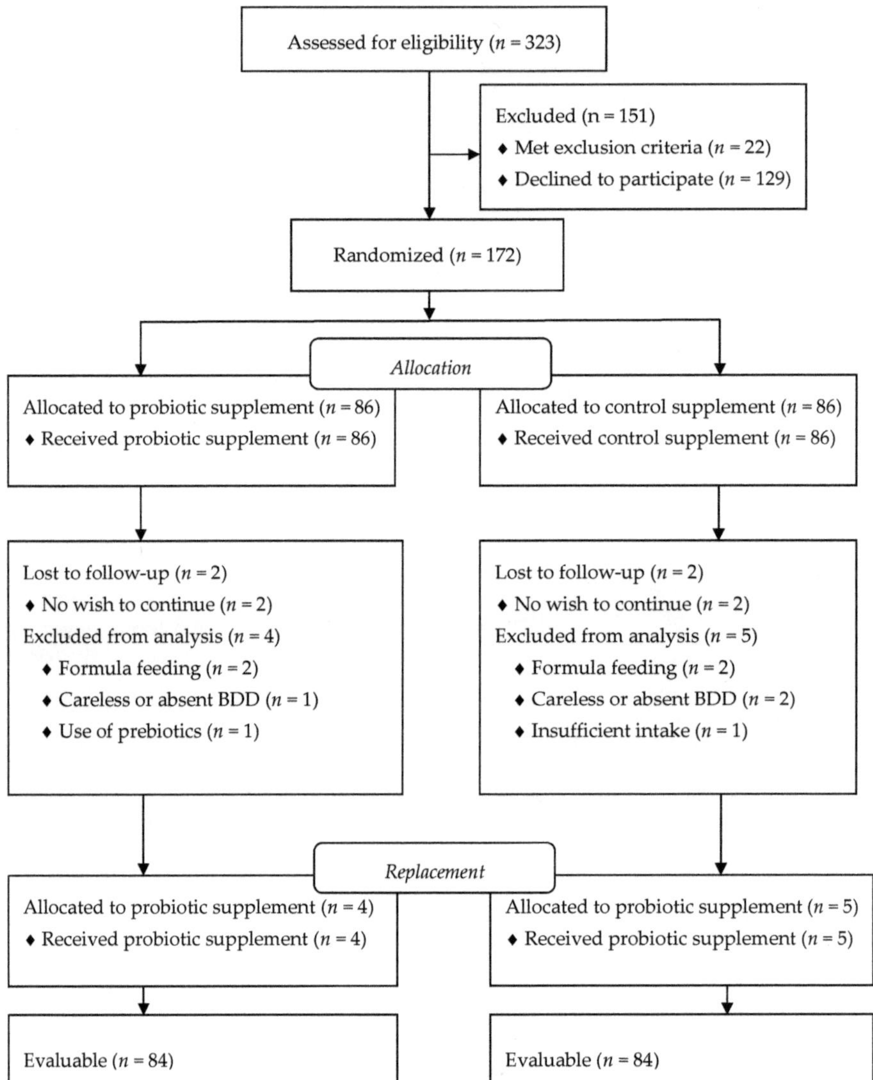

Figure 1. The Consolidated Standards of Reporting Trials flow diagram of the study participants. BDD: Baby's Day Diary.

Table 1. Baseline characteristics of study participants.

	Probiotic Group (n = 84)	Control Group (n = 84)	p-Value
Age, days, mean (SD)	44 (15)	45 (15)	0.666 [1]
Gender male, n (%)	40 (48)	44 (52)	0.605 [2]
Respiratory rate, mean (SD)	34 (3)	34 (3)	1.000
Heart rate, mean (SD)	132 (9)	132 (8)	1.000
Body weight, g, mean (SD)	4530 (637)	4581 (581)	0.588
Body length, cm, mean (SD)	55.9 (2.9)	56.6 (2.9)	0.119
Postnatal characteristics			
Weight at birth, g, mean (SD)	3427 (288)	3465 (278)	0.386
Length at birth, cm, mean (SD)	52.0 (2.0)	52.3 (1.9)	0.320
Head circumference, cm, mean (SD)	35.1 (1.7)	35.0 (1.5)	0.687
Gestation age, weeks, mean (SD)	39.4 (1.2)	39.5 (1.2)	0.589
Apgar score at 5 min., mean (SD)	8.3 (1.0)	8.2 (1.0)	0.518
Cesarean section, n (%)	7 (8.3)	9 (10.7)	0.597
Use of antibiotics and probiotics			
Use of antibiotic by mother, n (%)	7 (8.3)	8 (9.5)	0.785
Use of antibiotic by mother, days, mean (SD)	5.3 (2.1)	6.0 (1.1)	0.008
Use of probiotics by mother, n (%)	6 (7.1)	7 (8.3)	0.771
Use of probiotics by mother, days, mean (SD)	10.8 (5.4)	10.0 (6.2)	0.374
Use of antibiotics by infant, n (%)	3 (3.6)	2 (2.4)	0.649
Use of antibiotics by infant, days, mean (SD)	5.7 (1.5)	5.0 (9.4)	0.501
Use of probiotics by infant, n (%)	6 (7.1)	7 (8.3)	0.771
Use of probiotics by infant, days, mean (SD)	9 (3.3)	13 (9.3)	0.003
Hypoxic-ischemic encephalopathy, n (%)	11 (13.1)	16 (19.0)	0.299
Diagnoses			
Functional jaundice, n (%)	4 (4.8)	9 (10.7)	0.154
Umbilical hernia, n (%)	3 (3.6)	2 (2.4)	0.649
Cephalo-hematoma, n (%)	1 (1.2)	2 (2.4)	0.559
Hemolytic disease of a newborn, n (%)	1 (1.2)	0 (0.0)	0.315
Diaper dermatitis, n (%)	2 (2.4)	1 (1.2)	0.559
Arthrogryposis, n (%)	1 (1.2)	0 (0.0)	0.315
Lymphadenopathy, n (%)	1 (1.2)	0 (0.0)	0.315
Fever of unknown origin, n (%)	3 (3.6)	2 (2.4)	0.649

[1] Difference between the groups in the Student's t-test for means. [2] Difference between the groups in the z-test for proportions. SD, standard deviation; GIT, gastro-intestinal tract.

It was found that around half of the sample size had a history of regurgitation (Table 2).

Table 2. Any gastrointestinal events or skin rashes before study enrollment.

	Probiotic Group (n = 84)	Control Group (n = 84)	p-Value [1]
Regurgitation, n (%) [2]	46 (55)	53 (63)	0.293
Vomiting, n (%)	9 (11)	10 (12)	0.839
Constipation, n (%)	26 (31)	29 (35)	0.582
Diarrhea, n (%)	18 (21)	16 (19)	0.746
Rash, n (%)	9 (11)	10 (12)	0.839

[1] Difference between the groups in the z-test for proportions. [2] At least one episode of the listed events reported by parents was included in analysis.

More than one third of infants suffered from constipation, and fewer infants were observed to have a vomiting-like episode, diarrhea or skin rash. There was no significant difference in prevalence of these conditions between the groups before the study enrollment, and none of these conditions had criteria sufficient for diagnosis. They were commonly described as occasional events, not clinically meaningful, and did not influence the condition of the infant. In all cases these infants were included in the study, and per investigator judgment, an occasional and mild episode of these conditions could not serve a confounder.

One forth to one third of infants received treatments with claims for infant colic (Table 3).

Table 3. Prior treatment of colic.

	Probiotic Group (n = 84)	Control Group (n = 84)	p-Value [1]
Simethicone, n (%)	17 (20.2)	22 (26.2)	0.358
Dimethicone, n (%)	3 (3.6)	3 (3.6)	1.000
Lactase, n (%)	9 (10.7)	7 (8.3)	0.597
L. rhamnosus, n (%)	2 (2.4)	2 (2.4)	1.000
L. reuteri, n (%)	3 (3.6)	3 (3.6)	1.000
Fennel tea, n (%)	1 (1.2)	0 (0.0)	0.315
Homeopathic, n (%)	0 (0.0)	1 (1.2)	0.315
B. subtilis, n (%)	1 (1.2)	2 (2.4)	0.559
Prior treatment of colic, n (%)	26 (31.0)	31 (36.7)	0.436

[1] Difference between the groups in the z-test for proportions.

One fifth to one fourth of infants tried simethicone or dimethicone drops with no effects. Other treatments included probiotic dietary supplements, homeopathic drugs or fennel contained tea. All treatments were considered as ineffective by parents and finished at least seven days before entry in the study and were assumed not confounders for study outcomes.

3.2. Compliance

Generally, families complied well with the administration of the TDS and keeping the study diaries. During phone calls three families (3.6%) in the probiotic group reported one or more doses missed with a reference that this was due to forgetting and heavy daily routine. Two families (2.4%) in the control group reported doses missed for the same reasons. There was no statically significant difference in the number of infants who missed doses (p = 0.649). According to 28-DSD, of the total 4704 doses to be taken in one group (84 infants), only 11 doses (0.2%) were missed in the probiotic and 13 doses (0.3%)—in the control group (p = 0.331).

During phone calls, five families in the probiotic group and eight families in the control group reported significant troubles with recording in the BDD. In five cases in the probiotic group and four cases in the control group, the reason was difficulty in drawing graphical pictures. One family reported "difficulty to comprehend" on how to record in the BDD. Review and discussion of BDD in these families found consistent records.

3.3. Mother's Diet

All infants in the probiotic and control were breast fed during the entire study period. Cumulative groups daily intake by mother of foods that suspected to produce IC revealed no statistical difference between the groups (Table 4).

Table 4. Cumulative total-group days mother intake of foods suspicious to produce colic in breastfed infants.

	Probiotic Group (n = 84)	Control Group (n = 84)	p-Value [2]
Cow's milk, days, n (%)	973 (41.4) [1]	937 (39.8)	0.264
Eggs, days, n (%)	499 (21.2)	474 (20.2)	0.397
Chocolate, days, n (%)	260 (11.1)	267 (11.4)	0.745
Nuts, days, n (%)	232 (9.9)	234 (9.9)	1.000

[1] Data present as total days of intake of a specific food in the group (days of intake × number of mothers in the group) and percent days of all days of the study in the group (study duration (28) × size of the group (84) = 2352). [2] Difference between the groups in the z-test for proportions.

The most common food used in both groups was cow's milk that was consumed for approximately 40% of the study period. Approximately every 5th day mothers ate hen eggs, and approximately every 10th day chocolate and nuts.

3.4. Outcomes

There was no difference between the probiotic and control groups at baseline on the duration of fuss and cry (Figure 2).

After day 7, the probiotic group started demonstrating a faster reduction in cry and fuss time than the control group (upper boxes). Statistically significant results were found on days 14, 21, and 28 ($p < 0.05$). Mean change (SD) in cry/fuss time from day 0 through day 28 was −163 (99) minutes in the probiotic and −116 (94) minutes in the control group ($p = 0.019$). Success in controlling IC was more evident in the probiotic exposure group. Twenty-five percent reduction in cry/fuss times in the probiotic group was on day 8.2 (4.9) and day 9.6 (4.8) in the control group ($p = 0.063$). Fifty percent reduction in cry/fuss times in the probiotic group occurred after 8.9 (6.1) day and after 11.8 (7.4) day in the control group ($p = 0.006$).

Recovery from IC was illustrated in Kaplan-Meier analysis (Figure 3). Twenty-one infant (25%) in the probiotic group and 57 infants (68%) in the control group continued to have IC ($p < 0.001$). A significant difference between the groups was confirmed in Cox's F-test.

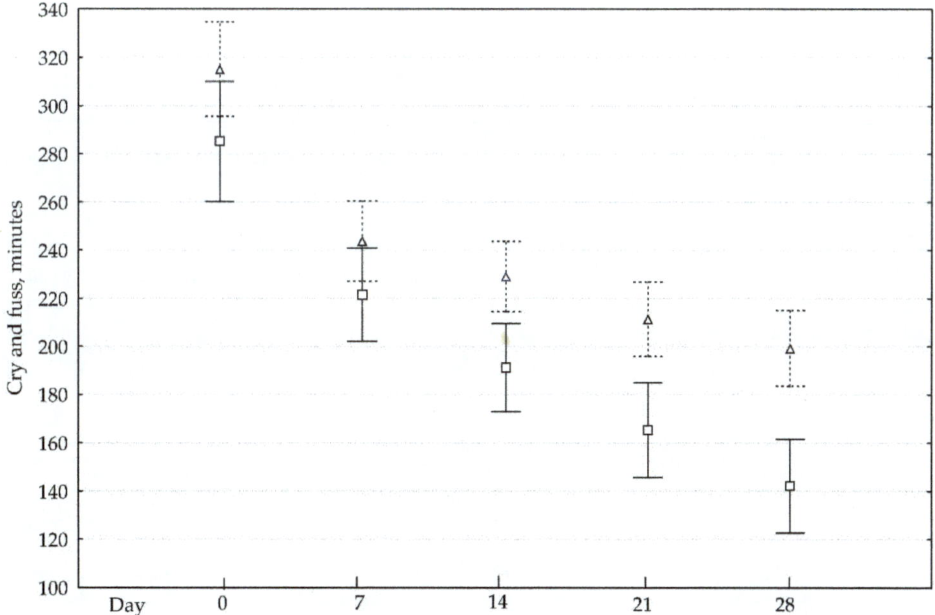

Figure 2. Cry and fuss time over study period. Data present as means (box mark – active; triangle mark - control group) and 2 standard errors (solid whiskers – active; dash whickers - control group).

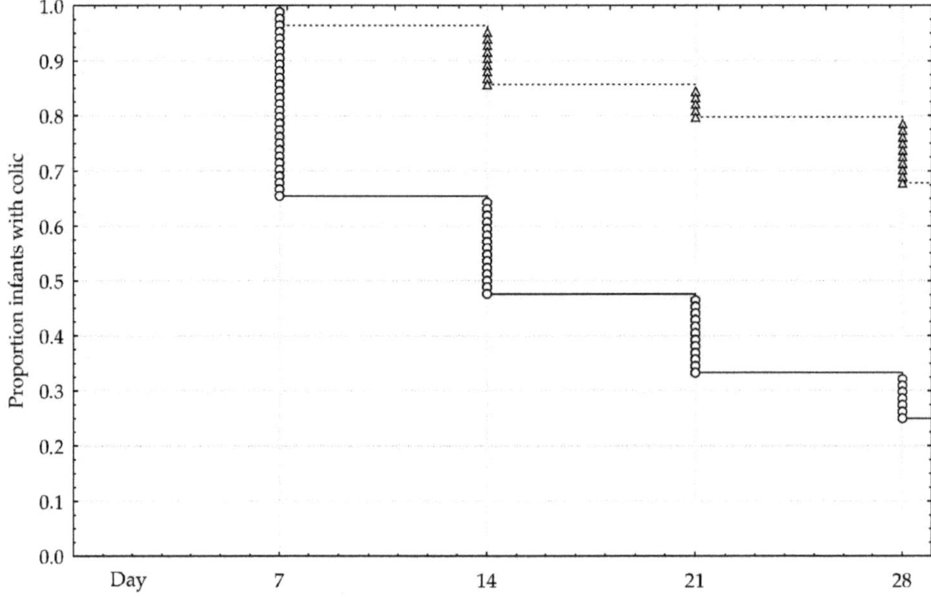

Figure 3. Recovery from colic. Solid line and round marks denote active group. Dash line and triangle marks denote control group.

Mean (SD) sleep duration did not change due to study intervention. On enrollment it was 770 (87) vs. 773 (112) minutes ($p = 0.847$); on day 28th—795 (104) vs. 805 (82) minutes ($p = 0.489$) in the probiotic and control group, respectively.

Both groups showed marginal changes in EPDS. On enrollment, EPDS was 6.2 (3.3) vs. 6.0 (2.5) ($p = 0.603$); on day 28th—5.1 (1.8) vs. 5.4 (2.8) ($p = 0.391$) in the probiotic and control group, respectively. Mean EPDS changed −1.0 (2.9) in the probiotic and −0.4 (2.9) in the control group ($p = 0.247$) over the duration of the study period.

On follow-up calls, parents in the probiotic group reported better course of IC than parents in the control group (Table 5).

Table 5. Parental impression of colic during the study.

	Probiotic Group (n = 84)	Control Group (n = 84)	p-Value [1]
Phone call 1			
Better, n (%)	58 (69.0)	39 (46.4)	0.035
Worse, n (%)	2 (2.4)	4 (4.8)	0.405
No changes, n (%)	24 (28.6)	41 (48.8)	0.008
Phone call 2			
Better, n (%)	78 (92.9)	66 (78.6)	0.008
Worse, n (%)	3 (3.6)	1 (1.2)	0.311
No changes, n (%)	3 (3.6)	17 (20.2)	0.001

Phone call 1 and 2 were made on 12 and 26 days of TDS intake. [1] Difference between the groups in the z-test for proportions.

Phone call 1 elicited a greater number of infants with "better" colic in the probiotic group and fewer infants with "no changes" colic on day 12th of the study. Two infants from the probiotic group and four infants from the control group had worsening colic, however, the difference was not statistically significant. After phone call 2, the number of infants with a better condition was still greater, as well as fewer cases without changes. Three infants from the probiotic group and one infant from the control group had worsening colic, and the difference was also not statistically significant.

3.5. Intolerance Events

As reported by investigators, both probiotic and control interventions were tolerated well (Table 6).

Table 6. Intolerance events.

	Probiotic Group (n = 84)	Control Group (n = 84)	p-Value [1]
Diarrhea, n (%)	1 (1.2)	3 (3.6)	0.311
Constipation, n (%)	0 (0.0)	1 (1.2)	0.315
Intense cry, n (%)	1 (1.2)	4 (4.8)	0.173
Regurgitation, n (%)	1 (1.2)	3 (3.6)	0.311
Intolerance events total, n (%)	3 (3.6)	11 (13.1)	0.027

[1] Difference between the groups in the z-test for proportions.

The most common intolerance in the control group was the intensification of cry, followed by diarrhea and regurgitation. In the probiotic group these events were evenly presented by one infant per event, except for constipation. Eleven total intolerance events were observed in the control group compared to three total events in the probiotic group ($p = 0.027$).

4. Discussion

Study participants were between the ages of 30 to 60 days with equal representation of male and female gender. The age at entry was comparable with previous studies and averaged the age when the manifestation of colic was the most severe [29]. Earlier age at entry might theoretically underestimate the role of any intervention as infant cry/fuss, as well as cry/fuss in colic normally intensifies from the 4th to the 6th week of life, remaining relatively stable for the next two weeks. If infant cry/colic includes congenital/inherited component, infants entering the study before two weeks or after eight weeks might not respond to probiotic treatment. This might explain why studies with less or greater mean/median age failed to show probiotic effect [13,16].

In this study we showed that the combination of *L. rhamnosus* 19070-2 and *L. reuteri* 12246 was effective in alleviation of colic in breast fed infants. Our results are consistent with the recent meta-analysis of four randomized trials that differentiated outcomes of probiotic intervention in infants with different types of feeding. Generally, breast-fed infants receiving probiotics had a mean change in cry and/or fuss time from day 0 to day 21 of −156.0 min compared to −101.9 min in the control group ($p < 0.05$) [18]. In our study, the mean change was −163 and −116 min, respectively ($p = 0.019$). Lack of standard deviation figures in the mentioned study did not allow for study comparisons however trends were similar. Difference between the probiotic and control groups was −47 min (−163 − 116 = −47 min) with −40 min difference was planned during calculation of the sample size. The real time difference outnumbered the planned one, and this secured statistical power of the data obtained.

In the meta-analysis data, the effect of lactobacilli assumed statistical significance from day 7, while in our research the difference was evident from day 14 [18]. This discrepancy at least partly can be explained by different approaches to collect primary data. In the referenced trials, only two used validated BDD on fixed days [13,15], while two others used non-standard scales with no indication on when these scales were used [12,17]. Even in the case of using a validated instrument, one may encounter a variability of data caused by the number of measurements. In a sample of 20 mothers, it was found that adequate monitoring of baby's activity required at least a 3-day period [30]. As per correlation coefficient, the reliability of measurement of cry increased 0.329, 0.546, 0.989 with the incremental number of days (1, 2, or 3, respectively) the activity was recorded [30]. In the latter trial, mothers kept diaries only once for three days, while multiple measurements were planned in our study. To improve compliance, we requested parents to fill in the BDD one day before enrollment, and, thereafter, on pairs of consecutive days 6, 7, 20, 21, 27, 28. The double-day approach was also used in the study by Sung et al. to reduce daily variability of cry and fuss time [18].

Treatment success, defined as a 50% reduction of colic manifestation, was statistically significant in the breast-fed infants that received lactobacilli [18]. We followed a different methodology for the assessment of treatment success: (1) We calculated a mean time (days) when 25% or 50% reduction in cry and fuss was achieved, while other researchers assessed percent of infants experienced 50% reduction of cry/fuss at the end of intervention period; (2) We calculated 25% or 50% relative reduction in presentation from baseline 180 min, which is a cut-off for the diagnosis. As a result, 50% relative reduction of cry and fuss time was observed almost three days earlier in the probiotic group. In Kaplan-Meier analysis we found significantly faster total recovery from colic in the probiotic group as well. As with previous studies, it was not possible to determine the precise time to treatment success, as measurements were made weekly and not daily.

The effect of lactobacilli was documented at a daily dose significantly lower than one advocated by some regulatory authorities for probiotics [31]. In our study, the daily dose was 0.25×10^8 CFU, while the minimum recommended number had been 1×10^9 viable cells per day [I]. The rationale for the higher dose of probiotic in this statement was largely based on the results of studies in adults that cannot be directly translated for young infants. In IC, other investigators reported the positive effects of probiotics at daily doses of 10^8 CFU [12,15,17,27]. Conversely, there had been a report that a dose as high as 10^9 CFU/day did not exert the effect in IC [16], suggesting a lack of consensus on the dose.

Sleep duration, as a tertiary outcome measure, did not change in the study and was within normal limits for age [32]. Three of the present probiotic intervention studies did not report sleep duration as an outcome measure [12,15,17]. One study found no changes during probiotic or control feedings [13]. This could be due to extreme biological importance and dominance of sleep over other infant activities. It might be for the same reason that the feeding duration was not changed significantly as well.

The role of breast-feeding modality on the positive effect of lactobacilli in infant colic is not understood. The situation is aggravated with the fact that breast-feeding itself did not affect the occurrence of colic [33,34] despite the fact it serves excellent nutrition medium for bifido- and lactobacilli [35,36]. The study performed by the Medical University of Vienna (Austria) also found a positive effect of probiotics on prevention of necrotizing colitis in the group of breast-fed infants [37]. Authors postulated that the effect can be explained by the presence of unique oligo-saccharides that promote optimal growth of lactobacilli, but direct studies comparing the potential of native human milk and herbal oligo-saccharides are not available. An alternative explanation of the lack of probiotic effect in formula fed infants may be due to a less "comfortable" physical and/or chemical environment of freeze-dried milk reconstituted in water for lactobacilli, however, direct data is also lacking.

The strength of our study was the randomized double blind controlled prospective parallel group design and the use of validated EPDS for measurement of maternal depression, and BDD for monitoring infant cry and fuss. The BDD tool was checked across sound records and found a reliable method for observation of infant cry and fuss [24]. Despite, there was not linguistic adaptation and validation of BDD, we believed that the translation of simple nouns, or combination of few words with clear meaning, could not significantly affect primary outcome measure. Linguistic validation of EPDS was available in the local language before the study started [26]. We retained almost all families primarily included in the trial, with phone calls and SMS notification messages. This gave an opportunity for evaluation and reassurance of the product storage, use of TDS, controlling for intolerance events, and timely filling the BDD.

The study limitation was the inclusion of infants that were treated with antibiotics or/and received probiotics before inclusion in the study. The number of such infants was small (5 and 13 cases in the probiotic and control group, respectively), and all these interventions were finished more than seven days before study enrollment. The effect of this was known neither in our study nor in the referenced literature. Any history of antibiotic or probiotic use served exclusion criteria in the Canadian study [15]. In two studies, infants, who were treated with antibiotics or probiotics on the week before study enrollment, were excluded [12,17], while in another one only current intake of probiotics and antibiotics was an exclusion criterion [13]. No data was available for infants who received these treatments before the week of enrollment in any study, except for the study of Australian group, which reported that 22 infants took any probiotic before entry to the study [13].

The weakness of the study was the use of not validated 28-day study diary. The diary contained questions about maternal diet and possible gastro-intestinal upset symptoms in the infant. It was not known how much this truly reflected real life events.

None of the infants received any treatments for colic during the study period. However, prior to the study more than 30% of infants received any type of treatment of colic that included simethicone or a similar drug, lactase, herbal medicine or homeopathic formulation. No consistent results were obtained for the efficacy of all the listed interventions except for fennel tea [7]. Only one randomized study successfully compared a herbal tea containing fennel with some other herbs with placebo. After one week of treatment, 57% of the infants in the active and 26% of the infants in the placebo group got rid of colic [38]. In our study, we had only one infant in the probiotic group who received a tea with fennel with no effect, and who stopped this treatment earlier than seven days before enrollment.

Another limitation was due to the inclusion of infants with hypoxic-ischemic encephalopathy, whose brain injure may obscure colic or otherwise interfere with cry and fuss patterns in infants. Particularly, these infants may present transient behavioral abnormalities, such as poor feeding, irritability, or excessive crying or sleepiness in an alternating pattern. However, we included only infants with a mild course of the pathology, which recovers within a few days without consequences. [39]. Potentially, infants with cephalohematoma could influence the study results, as it sometimes presents with behavioral changes, such as increased sleepiness, and increased crying [40]. However, we included infants, who were fully asymptomatic, and at the discretion of investigator did not have any symptoms linked to this condition before enrollment. The criterion for this was symptom free interval before colic commenced. Other background health conditions as being all mild or producing no constitutional symptoms could not confound the study results.

Notably, that in this study we assessed pre-existed functional conditions/episodes to avoid labelling them as intolerance events. Indeed, regurgitation was seen in 55% and 63% of all infants before enrollment the study, in the probiotic and control groups, respectively. According to previous estimates, the infant may have functional regurgitation in up to 67% that meet our data [41]. As per the Rome criteria prevalence of functional constipation was 12.1%, vomiting 1.7%, and diarrhea 2.4% vs. in our study rates for constipation 31%/35%, vomiting 11%/12%, and diarrhea 21%/19% in the probiotic/control groups, respectively. The difference in rates of these conditions could occur due to different definitions of the cases. We defined the conditions once only one episode was seen, while according to Rome criteria, these conditions should last more than four weeks and occur more frequently than one time for the past period [42]. These functional conditions were similar in rates at baseline. However, analysis of total symptom load showed fewer days with regurgitation, constipation, or rashes in the probiotic group. Indrio F. et al., demonstrated that infants with functional regurgitation benefited from the use of lactobacilli [43]. In the probiotic group infants had fewer episodes of regurgitation that correlated with an increase of the gastric emptying rate and reduction of median fasting antral area. Later the same researchers reported more frequent stools in infants with functional constipation [44]. There were no identifiable reports about the efficacy of probiotics in pediatric functional diarrhea. Studies in adults with irritable bowel syndrome and diarrhea showed a decrease in stool frequency, but it is not known if this finding can be extrapolated for infants [45,46].

The significance of our findings is difficult to assess, as the frequency of gastro-intestinal symptoms was not pre-screened. It remains unknown if this was due to probiotic effect, or pre-study features of infants in two groups.

Finally, our study design did not permit ascribing positive effect of *L. reuteri* 12246, *L. rhamnosus* 19070-2, and FOS mixture to its separate constituents or their combinations. Most of previous studies explored a role of *L. reuteri* [12,15,17,27], *L. rhamnosus* [16], and FOS separately [47]. While *L. reuteri*-based showed consistent beneficial effects in breastfed infants, the study with *L. rhamnosus* showed no effect in nonhomogeneous group of breast- and formula-fed infants. Our infants were all exclusively breastfed, so the role of *L. rhamnosus* is difficult to discuss. Reduction in the manifestation of IC in the study of infants fed with FOS fortified formula also prevents from extrapolation of beneficial results obtained [47]. In this study, we calculated that one-month old infants received approximately 576 mg of FOS per day, assuming concentration of FOS of 0.8 g/100 mL and the normal daily volume of formula, of 720 mL. In our study amount of FOS was 3.33 mg, more than 170 times less of that in the mentioned study. However, we cannot exclude that FOS played a role in the propagation of lactobacilli in an infant's intestines [48].

5. Conclusions

Our findings confirm that oral use of a mixture of *L. rhamnosus* 19070-2 and *L. reuteri* 12246 decreases cry and fuss time, and provides useful dietary support in exclusively breastfed infants with colic.

Author Contributions: Conceptualization, S.G. and J.G.; methodology, S.G. and J.G.; investigation, N.D., O.S., O.T., N.G., V.B., V.K.; formal analysis, data curation, original draft preparation, project administration, funding acquisition S.G.

Funding: This research was funded by BioCare CPH.

Acknowledgments: We thank Ronald Barr for permission to use Baby's Day Diary in this project, and Michael Tvede for his contribution to protocol development and manuscript review.

Conflicts of Interest: S.G. received funding for this research. Funder did not participate in the collection, analyses or interpretation of data, the writing of the manuscript and in the decision to publish the results.

References

1. Wake, M.; Morton-Allen, E.; Poulakis, Z.; Hiscock, H.; Gallagher, S.; Oberklaid, F. Prevalence, stability, and outcomes of cry-fuss and sleep problems in the first 2 years of life: Prospective community-based study. *Pediatrics* **2006**, *117*, 836–842. [CrossRef] [PubMed]
2. Wessel, M.A.; Cobb, J.C.; Jackson, E.B.; Harris, G.S.; Detwiler, A.C. Paroxysmal fussing in infancy, sometimes called "colic". *Pediatrics* **1954**, *14*, 421–434. [PubMed]
3. McMahon, C.; Barnett, B.; Kowalenko, N.; Tennant, C.; Don, N. Postnatal depression, anxiety and unsettled infant behaviour. *Aust. N. Z. J. Psychiatry* **2001**, *35*, 581–588. [CrossRef] [PubMed]
4. Smart, J.; Hiscock, H. Early infant cry and sleeping problems: A pilot study of impact on parental well-being and parent-endorsed strategies for management. *J. Paediatr. Child. Health* **2007**, *43*, 284–290. [CrossRef]
5. Brown, M.; Heine, R.G.; Jordan, B. Health and well-being in school-age children following persistent cry in infancy. *J. Paediatr. Child Health* **2009**, *45*, 254–262. [CrossRef] [PubMed]
6. Morris, S.; James-Roberts, I.S.; Sleep, J.; Gillham, P. Economic evaluation of strategies for managing cry and sleeping problems. *Arch. Dis. Child.* **2001**, *84*, 15–19. [CrossRef]
7. Hall, B.; Chesters, J.; Robinson, A. Infantile colic: A systematic review of medical and conventional therapies. *J. Paediatr. Child Health* **2012**, *48*, 128–137. [CrossRef]
8. Savino, F.; Cordisco, L.; Tarasco, V.; Calabrese, R.; Palumeri, E.; Matteuzzi, D. Molecular identification of coliform bacteria from colicky breastfed infants. *Acta Paediatr.* **2009**, *98*, 1582–1588. [CrossRef]
9. Rhoads, J.M.; Fatheree, N.Y.; Norori, J.; Liu, Y.; Lucke, J.F.; Tyson, J.E.; Ferris, M.J. Altered fecal microflora and increased fecal calprotectin in infants with colic. *J. Pediatr.* **2009**, *155*, 823–828. [CrossRef]
10. de Weerth, C.; Fuentes, S.; de Vos, W.M. Cry in infants: On the possible role of intestinal microbiota in the development of colic. *Gut Microbes* **2013**, *4*, 416–421. [CrossRef]
11. Nakamura, N.; Lin, H.C.; McSweeney, C.S.; Mackie, R.I.; Gaskins, H.R. Mechanisms of microbial hydrogen disposal in the human colon and implications for health and disease. *Annu. Rev. Food Sci. Technol.* **2010**, *1*, 363–395. [CrossRef] [PubMed]

12. Szajewska, H.; Gyrczuk, E.; Horvath, A. *Lactobacillus reuteri* DSM 17938 for the management of infantile colic in breastfed infants: A randomized, double-blind, placebo-controlled trial. *J. Pediatr.* **2013**, *162*, 257–262. [CrossRef] [PubMed]
13. Sung, V.; Hiscock, H.; Tang, M.L.; Mensah, F.K.; Nation, M.L.; Satzke, C.; Heine, R.G.; Stock, A.; Barr, R.G.; Wake, M. Treating infant colic with the probiotic *Lactobacillus reuteri*: Double blind, placebo controlled randomised trial. *BMJ* **2014**, *348*, g2107. [CrossRef] [PubMed]
14. Savino, F.; Ceratto, S.; Poggi, E.; Cartosio, M.E.; Montezemolo, L.C.; Giannattasio, A. Preventive effects of oral probiotic on infantile colic: A prospective, randomised, blinded, controlled trial using *Lactobacillus reuteri* DSM 17938. *Benef. Microbes* **2015**, *6*, 245–251. [CrossRef] [PubMed]
15. Chau, K.; Lau, E.; Greenberg, S.; Jacobson, S.; Yazdani-Brojeni, P.; Verma, N.; Koren, G. Probiotics for infantile colic: A randomized, double-blind, placebo-controlled trial investigating *Lactobacillus reuteri* DSM 17938. *J. Pediatr.* **2015**, *166*, 74–78. [CrossRef] [PubMed]
16. Pärtty, A.; Lehtonen, L.; Kalliomäki, M.; Salminen, S.; Isolauri, E. Probiotic *Lactobacillus rhamnosus* GG therapy and microbiological programming in infantile colic: A randomized, controlled trial. *Pediatr. Res.* **2015**, *78*, 470–475. [CrossRef] [PubMed]
17. Savino, F.; Cordisco, L.; Tarasco, V.; Palumeri, E.; Calabrese, R.; Oggero, R.; Roos, S.; Matteuzzi, D. *Lactobacillus reuteri* DSM 17938 in infantile colic: A randomized, double-blind, placebo-controlled trial. *Pediatrics* **2010**, *126*, e526–e533. [CrossRef]
18. Sung, V.; D'Amico, F.; Cabana, M.D.; Chau, K.; Koren, G.; Savino, F.; Szajewska, H.; Deshpande, G.; Dupont, C.; Indrio, F.; et al. *Lactobacillus reuteri* to treat infant colic: A meta-analysis. *Pediatrics* **2018**, *141*, e20171811. [CrossRef]
19. Rosenfeldt, V.; Michaelsen, K.F.; Jakobsen, M.; Larsen, C.N.; Møller, P.L.; Pedersen, P.; Tvede, M.; Weyrehter, H.; Valerius, N.H.; Paerregaard, A. Effect of probiotic *Lactobacillus* strains in young children hospitalized with acute diarrhea. *Pediatr. Infect. Dis. J.* **2002**, *21*, 411–416. [CrossRef]
20. Rosenfeldt, V.; Michaelsen, K.F.; Jakobsen, M.; Larsen, C.N.; Møller, P.L.; Tvede, M.; Weyrehter, H.; Valerius, N.H.; Paerregaard, A. Effect of probiotic *Lactobacillus* strains on acute diarrhea in a cohort of nonhospitalized children attending day-care centers. *Pediatr. Infect. Dis. J.* **2002**, *21*, 417–419. [CrossRef]
21. Rosenfeldt, V.; Benfeldt, E.; Nielsen, S.D.; Michaelsen, K.F.; Jeppesen, D.L.; Valerius, N.H.; Paerregaard, A. Effect of probiotic *Lactobacillus* strains in children with atopic dermatitis. *J. Allergy Clin. Immunol.* **2003**, *111*, 389–395. [CrossRef]
22. Rosenfeldt, V.; Benfeldt, E.; Valerius, N.H.; Paerregaard, A.; Michaelsen, K.F. Effect of probiotics on gastrointestinal symptoms and small intestinal permeability in children with atopic dermatitis. *J. Pediatr.* **2004**, *145*, 612–616. [CrossRef] [PubMed]
23. Reijneveld, S.A.; Brugman, E.; Hirasing, R.A. Excessive infant cry: The impact of varying definitions. *Pediatrics* **2001**, *108*, 893–897. [CrossRef] [PubMed]
24. Barr, R.G.; Kramer, M.S.; Leduc, D.G.; Boisjoly, C.; McVey-White, L.; Pless, I.B. Parental diary of infant cry and fuss behaviour. *Arch. Dis. Child.* **1988**, *63*, 380–387. [CrossRef] [PubMed]
25. Cox, J.L.; Holden, J.M.; Sagovsky, R. Detection of postnatal depression: Development of the 10-item Edinburgh Postnatal Depression Scale. *Br. J. Psychiatry* **1987**, *150*, 782–786. [CrossRef]
26. Pushkareva, T.N. Postpartum depression: Prevalence, clinic, dynamics. *Ment. Health* **2005**, *3*, 31–36.
27. Savino, F.; Pelle, E.; Palumeri, E.; Oggero, R.; Miniero, R. *Lactobacillus reuteri* (American Type Culture Collection Strain 55730) versus simethicone in the treatment of infantile colic: A prospective randomized study. *Pediatrics* **2007**, *119*, e124–e130. [CrossRef]
28. Random Allocation Software. Available online: https://random-allocation-software.software.informer.com/1.0/ (accessed on 18 March 2016).
29. Brazelton, T.B. Crying in infancy. *Pediatrics* **1962**, *29*, 579–588.
30. Thomas, K.A.; Burr, R.L. Accurate assessment of mother & infant sleep: How many diary days are required? *MCN Am. J. Matern. Child. Nurs.* **2009**, *34*, 256–260. [CrossRef]
31. Hill, C.; Guarner, F.; Reid, G.; Gibson, G.R.; Merenstein, D.J.; Pot, B.; Morelli, L.; Canani, R.B.; Flint, H.J.; Salminen, S.; et al. Expert consensus document. The International Scientific Association for Probiotics and Prebiotics consensus statement on the scope and appropriate use of the term probiotic. *Nat. Rev. Gastroenterol. Hepatol.* **2014**, *11*, 506–514. [CrossRef]

32. Galland, B.C.; Taylor, B.J.; Elder, D.E.; Herbison, P. Normal sleep patterns in infants and children: A systematic review of observational studies. *Sleep Med. Rev.* **2012**, *16*, 213–222. [CrossRef] [PubMed]
33. Lucassen, P.L.; Assendelft, W.J.; van Eijk, J.T.; Gubbels, J.W.; Douwes, A.C.; van Geldrop, W.J. Systematic review of the occurrence of infantile colic in the community. *Arch. Dis. Child.* **2001**, *84*, 398–403. [CrossRef] [PubMed]
34. Clifford, T.J.; Campbell, M.K.; Speechley, K.N.; Gorodzinsky, F. Infant colic: Empirical evidence of the absence of an association with source of early infant nutrition. *Arch. Pediatr. Adolesc. Med.* **2002**, *156*, 1123–1128. [CrossRef] [PubMed]
35. Rautava, S.; Luoto, R.; Salminen, S.; Isolauri, E. Microbial contact during pregnancy, intestinal colonization and human disease. *Nat. Rev. Gastroenterol. Hepatol.* **2012**, *9*, 565–576. [CrossRef] [PubMed]
36. Harmsen, H.J.; Wildeboer-Veloo, A.C.; Raangs, G.C.; Wagendorp, A.A.; Klijn, N.; Bindels, J.G.; Welling, G.W. Analysis of intestinal flora development in breast-fed and formula-fed infants by using molecular identification and detection methods. *J. Pediatr. Gastroenterol. Nutr.* **2000**, *30*, 61–67. [CrossRef]
37. Repa, A.; Thanhaeuser, M.; Endress, D.; Weber, M.; Kreiss, A.; Binder, C.; Berger, A.; Haiden, N. Probiotics (*Lactobacillus acidophilus* and *Bifidobacterium infantis*) prevent NEC in VLBW infants fed breast milk but not formula. *Pediatr. Res.* **2015**, *77*, 381–388. [CrossRef]
38. Weizman, Z.; Alkrinawi, S.; Goldfarb, D.; Bitran, C. Efficacy of herbal tea preparation in infantile colic. *J. Pediatr.* **1993**, *122*, 650–652. [CrossRef]
39. Hypoxic-Ischemic Encephalopathy. Available online: https://emedicine.medscape.com/article/973501-overview (accessed on 18 March 2016).
40. Cephalhematoma. Available online: https://www.ncbi.nlm.nih.gov/books/NBK470192/ (accessed on 18 March 2016).
41. Campanozzi, A.; Boccia, G.; Pensabene, L.; Panetta, F.; Marseglia, A.; Strisciuglio, P.; Barbera, C.; Magazzù, G.; Pettoello-Mantovani, M.; Staiano, A. Prevalence and natural history of gastroesophageal reflux: Pediatric prospective survey. *Pediatrics* **2009**, *123*, 779–783. [CrossRef]
42. Benninga, M.A.; Faure, C.; Hyman, P.E.; Roberts, J.I.; Schechter, N.L.; Nurko, S. Childhood functional gastrointestinal disorders: Neonate/toddler. *Gastroenterology* **2016**, *150*, 1443–1455. [CrossRef]
43. Indrio, F.; Riezzo, G.; Raimondi, F.; Bisceglia, M.; Filannino, A.; Cavallo, L.; Francavilla, R. *Lactobacillus reuteri* accelerates gastric emptying and improves regurgitation in infants. *Eur. J. Clin. Invest.* **2011**, *41*, 417–422. [CrossRef]
44. Indrio, F.; Di Mauro, A.; Riezzo, G.; Civardi, E.; Intini, C.; Covaglia, L.; Ballardini, E.; Bisceglia, M.; Cinquetti, M.; Brazzoduro, E.; et al. Prophylactic use of probiotic in the prevention of colic, regurgitation, and functional constipation: A randomized clinical trial. *JAMA Pediatr.* **2014**, *168*, 228–233. [CrossRef]
45. Andresen, V.; Layer, P.; Keller, J. Efficacy of freeze-dried Lactobacilli in functional diarrhea: A pilot study. *Dtsch. Med. Wochenschr.* **2012**, *137*, 1792–1796. [CrossRef] [PubMed]
46. Ki Cha, B.; Mun Jung, S.; Hwan Choi, C.; Song, I.D.; Woong Lee, H.; Joon Kim, H.; Hyuk, J.; Kyung Chang, S.; Kim, K.; Chung, W.S.; et al. The effect of a multispecies probiotic mixture on the symptoms and fecal microbiota in diarrhea-dominant irritable bowel syndrome: A randomized, double-blind, placebo-controlled trial. *J. Clin. Gastroenterol.* **2012**, *46*, 220–227. [CrossRef] [PubMed]
47. Vandenplas, Y.; Ludwig, T.; Bouritius, H.; Alliet, P.; Forde, D.; Peeters, S.; Huet, F.; Hourihane, J. Randomised controlled trial demonstrates that fermented infant formula with short-chain galacto-oligosaccharides and long-chain fructo-oligosaccharides reduces the incidence of infantile colic. *Acta Paediatr.* **2017**, *106*, 1150–1158. [CrossRef] [PubMed]
48. Kaplan, H.; Hutkins, R.W. Fermentation of fructooligosaccharides by lactic acid bacteria and bifidobacterial. *Appl. Environ. Microbiol.* **2000**, *66*, 2682–2684. [CrossRef] [PubMed]

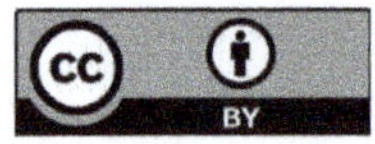

© 2018 by the authors. Licensee MDPI, Basel, Switzerland. This article is an open access article distributed under the terms and conditions of the Creative Commons Attribution (CC BY) license (http://creativecommons.org/licenses/by/4.0/).

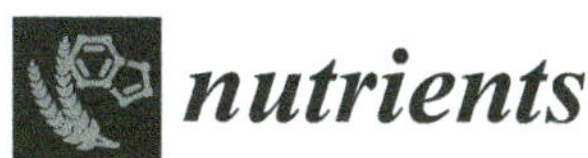

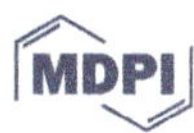

Letter

Letter to the Editor Re: Diaz M., et al. *Nutrients* 2018, *10*, 1481

Benjamín Martín Martínez * and Maria José López Liñán

Unidad de Gastroenterología y Nutrición Infantil, Hospital de Terrassa, 08227-Terrassa, Barcelona, Spain; mjlopez@cst.cat

* Correspondence: bmartingastro@hotmail.com

Received: 1 February 2019; Accepted: 19 February 2019; Published: 23 February 2019

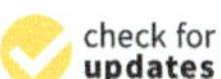

Keywords: fecal microbiota; protein hydrolyzed formulas; cow's milk protein; tolerance acquisition; non-IgE mediated allergy

---

Dear Editor,

We have read with interest the article published by Diaz et al. about the effects of extensively hydrolyzed cow's milk formulas (eHF) or vegetable formulas (soy and rice) on the microbiota in children with a non-IgE mediated (NIM) cow's milk protein allergy (CMPA) under a restrictive diet [1]. Although we believe it is a very interesting topic, we do not agree on some points and conclusions that are derived from this study, as explained below.

Guidelines and recommendations on the nutritional treatment of infants diagnosed with a mild to moderate cow's milk protein allergy (CMPA) advise the use of eHF formulas as the first option, whereas elemental formulas based on free amino acids are recommended in case of failure of the eHF formulas. Soy formulas (SF) are an option in CMPA infants older than six months, due to the presence of phytoestrogens.

In recent years, hydrolyzed rice protein formulas (HRFs) have been included in the protocols and guidelines as a first option in the treatment of CMPA, as rice is one of the less allergenic foods (<1%) and does not contain phytoestrogens [2,3]. Moreover, HRFs have a better palatability and are a good option in children who reject the eHF formulas or in vegetarian or vegan families, with efficacy and nutritional safety similar to eHF [4]. Therefore, according to the latest published recommendations on CMPA, HRFs are a first line option in infants with CMPA from the first day of life, at the same level of eHF, in those countries where HRFs are available.

The research topic in the study of Diaz et al. is interesting, but the number of infants both in the study group (n = 17), as well as in the control group of healthy children of same sex and age (n = 10), is too low. Moreover, if we look at the number of infants in each formula group, the number of cases studied is even lower: n = 12 in the eHF group, n = 2 in the SF group and n = 3 in the HRF group.

Since this is a cohort study, it is assumed that infants were not randomly assigned to each formula, and we think this is an important limitation for the interpretation of the results of the study, particularly with regard to causality between the type of formula ingested, the observed pattern of the microbiota and tolerance acquisition to cow's milk proteins. The authors neither explain what the criteria to allocate the infants to the eHF were, nor what the vegetable (soy or hydrolyzed rice) formula groups were.

Secondly, the authors do not provide enough information about the diet of the infants before their inclusion in the study. The study was carried out in infants with non IgE mediated CMPA with ages between 13 and 23 months, with a mean age of 17 months. Considering that diagnosis of NIM-CMPA is usually performed at ages below six months, the authors should provide information about the type of diet they received from diagnosis until the beginning of the study. We think this is a key factor because it can clearly influence the pattern of the microbiota in these infants, and this factor could explain, at least in part, the observed differences in the acquisition of tolerance between infants in the eHF, SF, and HRF groups; that is, none of the three infants who were fed with HRF acquired tolerance, whereas the infants fed eHF and SF acquired tolerance by the end of the study. Another important difference between controls and infants with NIM-CMPA is that the latter followed a diet free of dairy products for six months. Indeed, this can be a factor modifying the microbiota (e.g., fermented dairy products are an important source of lactobacillus at this age).

Another important missing piece of information in the article is related to the type of formula eHF used in the study. The authors do not provide information about the type of milk hydrolysate used in the eHF group (casein or whey proteins), and whether they were lactose free or with added lactose (with prebiotic effect of undigested lactose). All these factors may have a strong impact on the microbiota of the children.

The third point is related to the analysis of microbiota composition in the infants. Diaz et al. find that those infants who do not become tolerant in the study (those fed HRF) present less abundance of *Coriobacteriaceae* and *Bifidobacteriaceae* than those who become tolerant. However, they also mention that infants fed vegetal protein formulas, both rice and soy, have less *Coriobacteriaceae* than those fed eHF formulas. They do not provide any hypothesis to the fact that infants fed SF with lower *Coriobacteriacea* levels become tolerant (unfortunately, they do not provide details on the levels per feeding group). Also, the authors do not explain the fact that *Coriobacteriaceae* are also less abundant in healthy controls and vegetal formula in comparison with NIM-CMPA infants. Ultimately, the lack of data on diet composition in the different feeding groups, as well as the lack of longitudinal data on microbiota composition, makes it difficult to interpret or make conclusions about the microbiota results in this study.

Finally, the authors suggest in the discussion of the article that the use of vegetable formulas may impair the acquisition of tolerance due to the absence of exposure to immunomodulatory peptides. We believe that this conclusion cannot be drawn from the results of the study from Diaz et al., given the small number of infants in each study group, as well as the other confounding factors, mentioned in the previous paragraphs, that were not controlled in the present study and may have influenced the obtained results. The role of immunomodulatory peptides in the acquisition of tolerance was suggested in the study performed by Canani et al., which is a non-randomized study, with an eHF formula with LGG (*Lactobacillus Rhamnosus* GG) [5,6].

Contrary to the suggestion of the authors, several clinical trials in infants have found similar rates for the acquisition of tolerance between infants with CMPA fed extensively hydrolyzed cow's milk protein formulas and hydrolyzed rice formulas [7], besides being effective for the treatment of CMPA [7,8]. Moreover, a study published by Terracciano et al. in 2009 found that infants and children with CMPA who received hydrolyzed rice or a soy-based formula for the dietary management of their condition achieved tolerance earlier than their peers on an extensively hydrolyzed cow's milk formula. This fact led to the consideration that the elimination from the diet of any cow's milk protein residue may accelerate the induction of tolerance and would be adequate for the management of CMPA [9].

Conflicts of Interest: All the authors declare no conflict of interest.

References

1. Díaz, M.; Guadamuro, L.; Espinosa-Martos, I.; Mancabelli, L.; Jiménez, S.; Molinos-Norniella, C.; Pérez-Solis, D.; Milani, C.; Rodríguez, J.M.; Ventura, M.; et al. Microbiota and Derived Parameters in Fecal Samples of Infants with Non-IgE Cow's Milk Protein Allergy under a Restricted Diet. *Nutrients* **2018**, *10*, 1481. [CrossRef] [PubMed]
2. Koletzko, S.; Niggemann, B.; Arato, A.; Dias, J.A.; Heuschkel, R.; Husby, S.; Mearin, M.L.; Papadopoulou, A.; Ruemmele, F.M.; Staiano, A.; et al. Diagnostic approach and management of cow's-milk protein allergy in infants and children: ESPGHAN GI Committee practical guidelines. *J. Pediatr. Gastroenterol. Nutr.* **2012**, *55*, 221–229. [CrossRef] [PubMed]

3. Fiocchi, A.; Dahda, L.; Dupont, C.; Campoy, C.; Fierro, V.; Nieto, A. Cow's milk allergy: Towards an update of DRACMA guidelines. *World Allergy Organ. J.* **2016**, *9*, 35. [CrossRef] [PubMed]
4. Fiocchi, A.; Schunemann, H.; Ansotegui, I.; Assa'ad, A.; Bahna, S.; Canani, R.B.; Bozzola, M.; Dahdah, L.; Dupont, C.; Ebisawa, M.; et al. The global impact of the DRACMA guidelines cow's milk allergy clinical practice. *World Allergy Organ. J.* **2018**, *4*, 2. [CrossRef] [PubMed]
5. Berni Canani, R.; Nocerino, R.; Terrin, G.; Frediani, T.; Lucarelli, S.; Cosenza, L.; Passariello, A.; Leone, L.; Granata, V.; Di Costanzo, M.; et al. Formula selection for management of children with cow's milk allergy influences the rate of acquisition of tolerance: A prospective multicenter study. *J. Pediatr.* **2013**, *163*, 771–777. [CrossRef] [PubMed]
6. Martin, B. Fórmulas extensivamente hidrolizadas. Importancia del grado de hidrólisis. *Acta Pediatr. Esp.* **2018**, *76*, 115–122.
7. Reche, M.; Pascual, C.; Fiandor, A.; Polanco, I.; Rivero-Urgell, M.; Chifre, R.; Johnston, S.; Martín-Esteban, M. The effect of a partially hydrolysed formula based on rice protein in the treatment of infants with cow's milk protein allergy. *Pediatr. Allergy Immunol.* **2010**, *21*, 577–585. [CrossRef] [PubMed]
8. Vandenplas, Y.; De Greef, E.; Hauser, B. Paradice Study Group. Safety and tolerance of a new extensively hydrolyzed rice protein-based formula in the management of infants with cow's milk protein allergy. *Eur. J. Pediatr.* **2014**, *173*, 1209–1216. [CrossRef] [PubMed]
9. Terracciano, L.; Bouygue, G.R.; Sarratud, T.; Veglia, F.; Martelli, A.; Fiocchi, A. Impact of dietary régimen on the duration of cow's milk allergy: A random allocation study. *Clin. Exp. Allergy* **2010**, *40*, 637–642. [CrossRef] [PubMed]

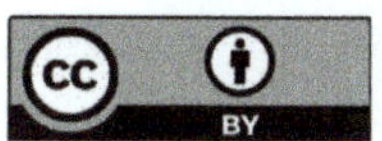

© 2019 by the authors. Licensee MDPI, Basel, Switzerland. This article is an open access article distributed under the terms and conditions of the Creative Commons Attribution (CC BY) license (http://creativecommons.org/licenses/by/4.0/).

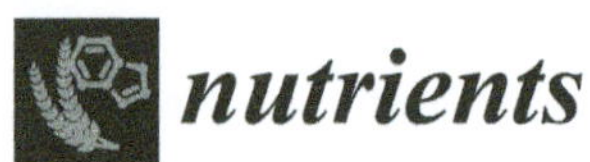

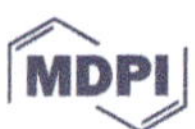

Reply

Reply: "Letter to the editor Re: Diaz M., et al. *Nutrients* 2018, *10*, 1481"

María Díaz [1], Lucía Guadamuro [1], Irene Espinosa-Martos [2], Leonardo Mancabelli [3], Santiago Jiménez [4], Cristina Molinos-Norniella [5], David Pérez-Solis [6], Christian Milani [3], Juan Miguel Rodríguez [2], Marco Ventura [3], Carlos Bousoño [4], Miguel Gueimonde [1], Abelardo Margolles [1], Juan José Díaz [4,*] and Susana Delgado [1,*]

1 Department of Microbiology and Biochemistry of Dairy Products, Instituto de Productos Lácteos de Asturias (IPLA)-Consejo Superior de Investigaciones Científicas (CSIC), 33300 Villaviciosa-Asturias, Spain; Maria.Diaz@quadram.ac.uk (M.D.); luciagg@ipla.csic.es (L.G.); mgueimonde@ipla.csic.es (M.G.); amargolles@ipla.csic.es (A.M.)

2 Department of Nutrition and Food Science, Universidad Complutense de Madrid (UCM), 28040 Madrid, Spain; irene.espinosa@probisearch.com (I.E.-M.); jmrodrig@vet.ucm.es (J.M.R.)

3 Laboratory of Probiogenomics, Department of Chemistry, Life Sciences and Environmental Sustainability, University of Parma, 43121 Parma, Italy; leonardo.mancabelli@genprobio.com (L.M.); christian.milani@unipr.it (C.M.); marco.ventura@unipr.it (M.V.)

4 Paediatric Gastroenterology and Nutrition Section, Hospital Universitario Central de Asturias (HUCA), 33011 Oviedo-Asturias, Spain; principevegeta@hotmail.com (S.J.); ringerbou@yahoo.es (C.B.)

5 Paediatrics, Hospital Universitario de Cabueñes, 33394 Gijón-Asturias, Spain; cristinamolinos@gmail.com

6 Paediatrics, Hospital Universitario San Agustín, 33401 Avilés-Asturias, Spain; doctorin@gmail.com

* Correspondence: juanjo.diazmartin@gmail.com (J.J.D.); sdelgado@ipla.csic.es (S.D.)

Received: 13 February 2019; Accepted: 19 February 2019; Published: 24 February 2019

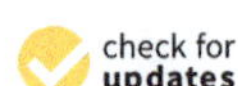

The objective of this letter of reply is to provide answers to the doubts and critical issues that Martín Martinez and López Liñan [1] raised in their letter to the editor with respect to the work published last year in *Nutrients* in the field of microbiota, diet and non-IgE cow's milk protein allergy (NIM-CMPA).

As authors of this publication, we understand and welcome the controversial issues that unavoidably surround any novel research results with implications for the dietary management of cow's milk protein allergy (CMPA).

First, we would like to point out that in the latest published recommendations on CMPA, the allergologic and nutritional safety of hydrolyzed rice protein formulas (HRF) according to DRACMA (Diagnosis and Rationale for Action against Cow's Milk Allergy) guidelines are clearly stated. However, according to this review it is advisable that debate is ongoing about the best substitute for infants with CMPA, and it concludes that "in the substitute choice, clinicians should be aware of recent studies that can modify the interpretation of the current recommendations" [2]. The letter to the editor of Martín Martinez and López Liñan argues in favor of the use of HRF, which is a reasonable position but which must be open to debate in the light of new data. As mentioned in our publication, "the data found in this pilot study need to be confirmed in a larger population" [3], thus, we cannot disagree with Martín Martinez and López Liñan that the main limitation of our study is the small number of patients included. Nonetheless, this limitation is already mentioned in our paper. Further research studies are of course needed and we remain open-minded, but a lack of consensus does not represent a lack of evidence.

With respect to the first questionable aspect of our study; as stated in the publication [3], our work is a prospective cohort study, so infants were not randomly assigned to each formula, however, we really do not think this constitutes a limitation of the study since it was an observational, not an interventional study. In this case, randomization was not intended in the study, which focused on the description of what was happening (microbiota and biochemical parameters of fecal samples) at the intestinal level in non-IgE mediated cow's milk protein allergy (NIM-CMPA) infants as compared with healthy controls, for the first time as far as we know. Infants with proven NIM-CMPA determined by positive standardized oral challenge (SOC) and negative IgE tests to cow´s milk proteins (CMP) were included in our study when they were on a cow´s milk elimination diet for at least 6 months. The substitution formula was decided by the attending physician, and therefore, the number of infants on each formula simply reflects the formula selection by pediatric gastroenterologists in Spain. In a recently published survey, extensively hydrolyzed whey or casein formulas were those of choice, followed by amino acid-based formulas, HRF and soy formulas [4]. Furthermore, formula selection was not the primary variable outcome of our study.

Secondly, Martín Martinez and López Liñan [1] mentioned that the authors did not provide enough information about the diet of the infants before inclusion, and because the studied infant ages ranges between 13 and 23 months, we should provide information about the type of diet that infants received from diagnosis until the beginning of the study. Probably we did not make these points clear enough in our manuscript. The age of the infants was recorded at the time of fecal sampling, after a period of at least 6 months using therapeutic hypoallergenic formulas as the main dietary food, and matching with the age of the control group (median 18 months versus 17 months in the NIM-CMPA group). That means that at the time of diagnosis, the NIM-CMPA infants were at least 6 months younger than at sampling. In their letter [1], Martín Martinez and López Liñan argue that "another important difference between controls and infants with NIM-CMPA is that the latter followed a diet free of dairy products for 6 months. Indeed, this can be a factor modifying the microbiota". We believe that their interpretation overlooks important points of our study. Control infants are healthy infants that consume milk and dairy without restriction, and of course, infants with NIM-CMPA are on a restricted diet for at least 6 months. Hence, we did not conclude that differences in microbiota are only due to the allergic condition of the infants, and of course, we think that a milk restricted diet is at least partially responsible for the observed differences.

It is also suggested that another missing piece of information in our study is related to the type of formula, which has a strong impact on microbiota. It is true that we have not provided detailed information on the type of hydrolyzed formula used in our study (trademarks) apart from extensively hydrolyzed formula (EHF), soy protein-based formulas, and HRF, and maybe this has contributed to some of the confusion. Nevertheless, significant differences in microbiota composition were found between those infants fed with vegetable protein-based formulas and those consuming EHF, but not among the last group. Additionally, regarding the argument focusing on lactose, it is important to underline that in infants with IgE mediated CMPA, formulas containing lactose are sometimes used. However, in NIM-CMPA cases, these formulas are usually avoided.

Surprisingly, another point that is criticized is the analysis of the microbiota. Our microbial sequences are deposited in a public database and openly available [3], allowing further analyses by other authors. We found that those infants who do not become tolerant in the study (fed HRF) present significant differences and less abundance of Coriobacteriaceae and Bifidobacteriaceae members than those who become tolerant. It is also noticeable in our study, that infants fed vegetal protein formulas, both rice and soy, have significantly less Coriobacteriaceae than those fed EHF formulas. The details on the levels are displayed on page 5: "Coriobacteriaceae were significantly diminished in NIM-CMPA infants consuming vegetable protein-based formulas (n = 5), both rice and soy, (mean of 0.64% of total assigned reads, range 0.02–2.38%) compared to those infants fed with EHF (mean of 4.45%, range 0.08–13.44%)", and in Table 1 (Coriobacteriaceae mean abundance in infants consuming HRF = 0.26%) [3]. A potential explanation for these observations is mentioned in the discussion section of our article in relation to cross-feeding mechanisms among lactate microbial users and butyrate producers, although it is true that the exact role of the Coriobacteriaceae in the infant gut microbiota is still unknown. Moreover, we do not have a clear response to the authors of this letter as to why these Coriobacteriaceae members are enriched in those infants fed with EHF, as compared also with healthy controls infants, although, a positive significant correlation was found between this family and butyrate levels [3]. In addition, a statistical association was detected between this important microbial metabolite and the excretion of the mediator TGF-β, implicated in tolerance, so there is a potential relationship among all these factors.

Regarding the comment on the use of vegetable formulas and the possible impairment of tolerance acquisition, Martín Martinez and López Liñan [1] indicate that "this conclusion cannot be drawn from the results of the study from Diaz et al". However, although these issues are discussed within the discussion section, our manuscript does not establish such a conclusion. Actually, our conclusions are that type of formula can determine microbiota composition, and that this, through the production of microbial metabolites and modulation of immune mediators, may influence tolerance acquisition. Of course, in the discussion we are allowed to comment on possible explanations for our results, based on current knowledge such as exposure to immunomodulatory peptides.

We hope this letter will help to clarify the points raised by Martín Martinez and López Liñan and appreciate the interest of these authors and the opportunity to engage in a dialogue around NIM-CMPA tolerance, diet and microbiota.

Author Contributions: The corresponding authors J.J.D. and S.D. wrote this reply in agreement with the rest of co-authors of the original publication.

Conflicts of Interest: All the authors declare no conflict of interest.

References

1. Benjamín, M.M.; Maria, J.L.L. Letter to the editor Re: Diaz M., et al. Nutrients 2018, 10, 1481. *Nutrients* **2019**, *11*, 468. [CrossRef]
2. Fiocchi, A.; Dahda, L.; Dupont, C.; Campoy, C.; Fierro, V.; Nieto, A. Cow's milk allergy: Towards an update of DRACMA guidelines. *World Allergy Organ. J.* **2016**, *9*, 35. [CrossRef] [PubMed]
3. Díaz, M.; Guadamuro, L.; Espinosa-Martos, I.; Mancabelli, L.; Jiménez, S.; Molinos-Norniella, C.; Pérez-Solis, D.; Milani, C.; Rodríguez, J.M.; et al. Microbiota and derived parameters in fecal samples of infants with non-IgE cow's milk protein allergy under a restricted diet. *Nutrients* **2018**, *10*, 1481. [CrossRef] [PubMed]
4. Pascual Pérez, A.I.; Méndez Sánchez, A.; Segarra Cantón, Ó.; Espin Jaime, B.; Jiménez Treviño, S.; Bousoño García, C.; Díaz Martín, J.J. Attitudes towards cow's milk protein allergy management by Spanish gastroenterologist. *An. Pediatr.* **2018**, *89*, 222–229. [CrossRef] [PubMed]

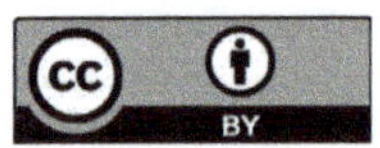

© 2019 by the authors. Licensee MDPI, Basel, Switzerland. This article is an open access article distributed under the terms and conditions of the Creative Commons Attribution (CC BY) license (http://creativecommons.org/licenses/by/4.0/).

MDPI
St. Alban-Anlage 66
4052 Basel
Switzerland
Tel. +41 61 683 77 34
Fax +41 61 302 89 18
www.mdpi.com

Nutrients Editorial Office
E-mail: nutrients@mdpi.com
www.mdpi.com/journal/nutrients

www.ingramcontent.com/pod-product-compliance
Lightning Source LLC
Chambersburg PA
CBHW051726210326
41597CB00032B/5622

* 9 7 8 3 0 3 8 9 7 9 5 0 0 *